The Esther M. Wilkins Story As Told by Her Friends

AN AUTHORIZED BIOGRAPHY

Pamela J. Bretschneider, BA, MEd, PhD
With Esther M. Wilkins, BS, RDH, DMD

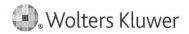

Wolters Kluwer

Philadelphia • Baltimore • New York • London
Buenos Aires • Hong Kong • Sydney • Tokyo

Acquisitions Editor: Jonathan Joyce
Editorial Coordinator: Alexis Pozonsky
Marketing Manager: Leah Thompson
Production Project Manager: Marian Bellus
Design Coordinator: Stephen Druding
Manufacturing Coordinator: Margie Orzech
Prepress Vendor: Absolute Service, Inc.

9 8 7 6 5 4 3 2 1

Printed in China

Library of Congress Cataloging-in-Publication Data

Names: Bretschneider, Pamela J., author.
Title: The Esther M. Wilkins story : as told by her friends : an authorized
   biography / Pamela J. Bretschneider ; with Esther M. Wilkins.
Description: Philadelphia : Wolters Kluwer, [2019] | Includes bibliographical
   references.
Identifiers: LCCN 2018013968 | ISBN 9781975106249
Subjects: | MESH: Wilkins, Esther M. | Dental Hygienists—history | Schools,
   Dental—history | History, 20th Century | History, 21st Century | United
   States | Biography
Classification: LCC RK43.W54 | NLM WZ 100 | DDC 617.6092 [B] —dc23 LC record available at
https://lccn.loc.gov/2018013968

DEDICATION

This book is dedicated to the many friends, colleagues, and students of Dr. Esther M. Wilkins, to those who are dedicated to the dental professions, and with special mention to the families of Dr. Pamela J. Bretschneider and Dr. Esther M. Wilkins who are remembered with much appreciation for their support in the writing of this biography.

TO THE READER: DR. PAMELA J. BRETSCHNEIDER

This book is a labor of love for both the process and subject of this biography. In 2008, I asked Dr. Wilkins why a biography about her had not yet been written. Her response was that she *didn't think anyone would be interested in reading it.* I thought differently, as did the plethora of friends who kindly and with tremendous respect for this icon of dental hygiene responded to our request for their stories of how Esther Wilkins had impacted their lives. As Lois Barber stated, "This is a woman whose story needs to be told and remembered."

Esther preferred her biography to be written by someone who was not a dental professional, so the many facets of her life could unfold. She was active throughout the process, and I was delighted to incorporate her revisions and suggestions, which often came in the form of what she called *little pearls* to be added to her life story.

One of the goals of a biographer in retelling the life of a person is to let the individual drive the story. In an effort to highlight Esther's voice and distinguish it from the innumerable voices of family, students, colleagues, and friends, Esther's own words as the speaker or writer appear in *italics* without the use of quotation marks. She preferred to write several stories herself to assure I would *get it down right,* and she carefully selected introductory quotes or phrases at the beginning of each chapter, all of which had meaning for her.

Esther truly enjoyed reflecting on her life not because of her many accomplishments, but because of the people she met. She wrote early in the biography process: *I don't believe I ever thanked you for undertaking this bio thing. When I see the interesting letters, with their fabulous memory-inducing thoughts, I am so appreciative of what you are doing. Of course, no wonder my eyes get a little damp occasionally, especially reading what my friends wrote. It's that big head swelling up and squeezing the juice out.* She never truly realized what a precious jewel she was to the world not only for her contributions to dentistry and dental hygiene but also for the relationships, both personal and professional, she cultivated along the way.

TO THE READER: DR. ESTHER M. WILKINS

It was important to me that my biography was written by the people who know me best, my friends. Developing social connections with colleagues, friends, and family members profoundly impacts personal happiness, health, and longevity. These connections can provide sound advice when treating a difficult case, validation when your confidence is shaken, help when needed, and perspective.

The connections I have made are some of my greatest treasures. I remain close to my family, traveling to my hometown of Tyngsborough, Massachusetts, each year when I get to visit with my cousins and one of my grade school and high school classmates. A few of my Simmons College and Tufts Dental School classmates are still able to make reunions. The relationships I have developed with colleagues in dentistry and dental hygiene over the past 80 years are some of the most valued of all. The contributions to my textbook, my students, university colleagues, and the many dental hygienists round the world, have all added greatly to my life.

Foreword

Whenever I talk about my Aunt, Dr. Esther Wilkins, to someone new, I always start out by saying that she made major contributions to public health in the United States. Then I amend that to the world. I think she would be happy with this expansion beyond oral health, as her focus was really the overall health of the individual.

If you consider the progression of her career, her consistent push for fluoridation, the continual expansion of chapters in her textbook, and her never ending examination of the literature, you can see her commitment. Her journal subscriptions and the books she read were not limited to dentistry and dental hygiene.

And of course, her vigorous insistence on strengthening the education of both dental hygienists and dentists to integrate the practice of both for better patient care had her traveling the globe, lecturing and learning constantly.

She was tough on her students. In fact she was tough on anyone who worked with her, including faculty, administrators, and contributors to her book. She had high standards and expected everyone to live up to those standards.

It is hard for most of us to imagine living with that kind of drive and high expectations of oneself. She pushed herself most of all.

As a child, in fact through most of my adult life, I rarely saw my Aunt. My mother, her sister, kept us apprised of her whereabouts and activities. When I did see her she wanted to make sure I was working hard at school or my career. She was a strong example to me of a successful woman, a feminist leader.

Her leadership will have a lasting impact on the fields of dental hygiene and dentistry, particularly periodontics. This book tells the story of her legacy.

Betsy Tyrol, October 2017

Acknowledgments

The author is very grateful for the detailed review, edits, suggestions, photographs and content provided for this biography by many special people: Christina Clarke Bell, Linda Boyd, Lana Crawford (our cheerleader), Tina Daniels, Dr. Timothy Hempton, Susan Jenkins, Jonathan Joyce, Dr. Paul Levi, Janet Clarke Lorman, Louise Lorman, Barbara Connell Magoon, Anna Pattison, Dr. Robert Rudy, Betsy Tyrol, and Charlotte Wyche; with special thanks to my son, Matthew Bretschneider, my wordsmith; and, of course, the inspiration of Dr. Esther Wilkins.

Of significant note are the contributions of Esther's niece, Betsy Tyrol, who reviewed every chapter of this biography before submission. I am truly thankful to Betsy for her keen eye, helpfulness, wisdom, and friendship through the 9 years of writing this biography. Thanks to Charlotte Wyche for her meticulous review of the chapter on *CPDH*. I thank our mutual friend, Tina Daniels, for her encouragement, shared tears of remembrance, and special spiritual connection with Esther.

I also acknowledge with thanks the expertise of the following people: Pauline Anderson (MCPHS) for developing the Family Tree; Andy Bretschneider, Kathie Gonzales, Craig Pasco, and Charlotte Wyche for proofreading; Sarah Anne Burns, Lillian Corricelli-Gauthier, and Matthew Bretschneider for Estherisms; Maggie Kuch for CPDH content and contributors; faculty and staff of MCPHS and TUSDM for photos; my editorial coordinator from Wolters Kluwer Health, Alexis Pozonsky; and the board of directors of the MetroWest Humane Society in Ashland, Massachusetts, for assuming my responsibilities as a board of directors member during the last year as this book was completed. I am also appreciative of the archivists of Simmons College, The University of Washington, and Tufts University School of Dental Medicine for their assistance.

Special thanks and all my love to my husband, Andy, whose patience and helpfulness throughout the writing of this book was vital to its completion, just as it was during my doctoral dissertation writing. Thanks to my mother, Pauline Redding, my children, Kimberly Cahill and Matthew Bretschneider, and my granddaughter, Sarah Anne Burns, for their insight throughout the process. I will also be forever grateful to Fr. James Woods, S.J., who believed in me during my years as a student and employee at Boston College and who encouraged me to excel.

This work would not have been possible without family members, friends, and colleagues of Esther who contributed their photos and stories, especially those of Esther's early years. Through their words, the impact of Esther's life can be realized. Thank you all very much.

TABLE OF CONTENTS

Table of Contents

CHAPTER 1

Early Life and Family

I'm amazed at what's happened in my lifetime!

On a June evening in Albuquerque in 2008, the matriarch of dental hygiene was poised to deliver yet another speech at the American Dental Hygiene convention. Sitting nearby was a second highly anticipated speaker, and while "America's sweetheart" was more widely recognized, she was no more visible, no more exalted than Esther in this environment. Debbie Reynolds's appearance at the convention was also recurring, and although Esther was not willing to reveal her actual age at the time, she was not going to be outdone as the senior speaker at the convention. The exact date of Esther's birth was kept a secret from the dental hygiene world and was discussed with great speculation. Esther's long-time friend, Caren Barnes, "summoned the courage to ask her and she avoided the question as if I didn't even ask it. But isn't she really ageless to us all?" In a 2009 *Dimensions of Dental Hygiene* article, Esther clarified her rationale for finally acknowledging her real age:

> We know that oral health along with general physical health is directly related to quality of life. At 93, I am often asked how old I am. When the question is worded "How old are you, really?" it seems to imply that whatever I answer can't be the truth. Sometimes I answer "What is your guess?" or "Unpublished number." In 2008, I shared the stage with the beautiful, charming, and famous Debbie Reynolds. She said she was 75. Not to be outdone, I said I was older—76
>
> (WILKINS, 2010, P. 20).

Esther was in fact 92 years old at the time. "Every moment adds up to a life," were some parting words from Reynolds in her last year (Rice, 2016, n.p.). And just as she would soon follow another icon in leaving us, so it was for Esther that a life of such achievement could not be summed up with a number. She could not resist an opportunity to share her enthusiastic and wry sense of humor with those closest to her: *After several public celebrations of my 90th birthday, I decided the whole world seemed to know my age so I could stop being coy.*

World War I was already underway when Edith Rose Packard Wilkins and Ernest Warren Wilkins welcomed Esther Mae Wilkins into the world on December 9, 1916, in Chelmsford, Massachusetts. Esther's middle name was for her great aunt Mae Bonney, whom Esther described as

> my mother's favorite aunt. She had a son [Clinton] about the same age as my mother, and they lived in Auburn, Maine. Clinton had plans to go across the river to Bates and Aunt Mae invited my mother to live with them and go to college, too. My grandmother had passed away when her little sister was born, so her father [Fred] was looking out for the two little girls. Mostly I guess they were "farmed out" to Aunts around Hebron. Anyway, when

1

mother finished at Hebron Academy, ready to go to college, my grandfather put his foot down and said she couldn't. She had to learn a way to support herself!

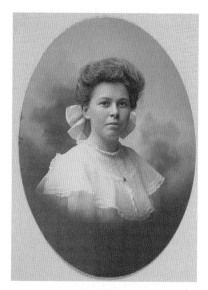
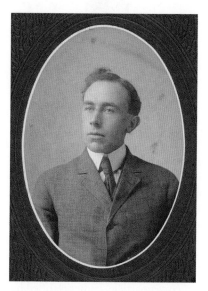

FIGURE 1.1: Edith Rose Packard Wilkins, Esther's mother.

FIGURE 1.2: Ernest Warren Wilkins, Esther's father.

At the start of her life in 1916, Woodrow Wilson was president of the United States, the price of bread was 7 cents a loaf, milk delivered to your door was 18 cents a half gallon, gas was 16 cents a gallon, and it cost only 2 cents to mail a first-class letter. There were no nylon toothbrushes, band aids, dial telephones, TV, SAT tests, penicillin, or fluoridated water.

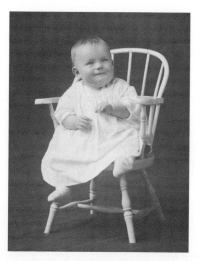

FIGURE 1.3: Esther Mae Wilkins's baby picture.

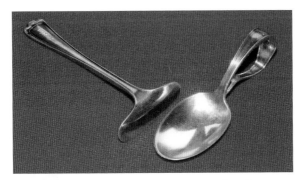

FIGURE 1.4: Esther Mae Wilkins's spoon and pusher.

❧ TOWN OF TYNGSBOROUGH ❧

Shortly after her birth, the family moved to Tyngsborough, which Esther called her hometown. Esther recalled,

> *We moved to Tyngsboro. My older sister, Ruth Ellen, was 2 years old at that time.*

In a story written for her 90th birthday, Chris Camire (2006), writer for the *Lowell Sun*, said that Esther's "expertise has taken her across the globe, but the woman known as the 'grandmother of dental hygiene' has her roots in Tyngsboro" (p. 1).

Now a residential community with a number of technology-based companies, at the time, Tyngsborough had been known as a small, rural community, settled in 1661. It is named after Col. Jonathan Tyng. Tyngsborough was incorporated in 1809 with a population of 870 inhabitants. Tyngsborough celebrated its 200th birthday in 2009. It had been known for "its ferries, quarries, and box companies" (Merrimack Valley Economic Development Council, 2009). The 18-mile stretch of land is divided by the Merrimac River and borders the towns of Dunstable, Groton, and Dracut as well as the city of Lowell and the State of New Hampshire. Its green-painted, single-arched iron bridge built in 1931 replaced the original bridge made of wooden blanks.

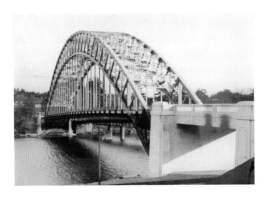

FIGURE 1.5: Tyngsborough bridge, circa 1931.

Tyngsborough's rich history includes Native American presence, as evidenced by the arrowheads and tomahawks found in the area as well as ties to the Lowell and Nashua railway line. This branch of the Boston and Maine (B&M) Railroad opened in 1838 and would later provide Esther her means of daily transportation to the Ruggles/Huntington stop, where she would transfer to a streetcar taking her to Simmons College.

⚜ ESTHER'S EARLY LIFE ⚜

When asked to name her favorite pastime, Esther would always say with a big, reminiscent smile: *dancing, of course.* Her mother, Edith, loved to dance and instilled this love in Esther at an early age. She taught her daughter to learn without the music as they had no records, and they glided on the kitchen floor humming the music as they waltzed. In springtime, they would decorate the front of their home with geraniums, carried in pots from the living room where they had been sheltered during the winter. When asked to expound on her childhood memories, Esther fixated on these two moments—on dancing in the kitchen and bringing out the geraniums—the images she seemed to hold forever in her mind.

While her marriage was somewhat troubled, Edith's relationship to both her children was strong and her impact on her daughters was profound. For Ruth and Esther, independence and strength were foremost in the qualities she imparted. As young women, they were not going to be dependent on a man, and there was no question, ever, that they would go to college and have careers of their own. This solidarity between Edith and her two girls is one they would find in future relationships and especially with one another.

The sisters were inseparable growing up and, as Ruth was 2 years older, she had the honor of being Esther's *original mentor. She was probably motherly when we were little.* As a preeminent educator and self-proclaimed perpetual student, Esther attributed most of her innate skill in this area to Ruth, who was a lifelong source of lessons, advice, and support. As Lynda McKeown (2017) reflected,

> Esther apparently learned from her older sister, Ruth, the importance of education and the potential power of acquired knowledge" (p. 57).

Esther and Ruth found serenity in simple childhood pursuits and gave one another confidence in knowing they had a companion. Esther remembered one such afternoon with stark clarity:

> *There was a sloping front lawn to the highway with a very large rock where Ruth and I would sit to watch the trolley car and what few automobiles passed by. A major train track was farther in the distance across a large field as it followed the Merrimack River north to New Hampshire. We could count the box cars and listen to the train whistle as it went through the village.*

While the family moved in Tyngsborough several times during her youth, the stability she found in her sister and mother remained constant. And although her father was more distant to her growing up, she possessed a well-rounded sense of family, and with each move it became more solidified.

> *After moving again as my father changed employment, the home I remember most in the preschool years [1920–1921] was known as the "Sinclair" farm. My mother and my*

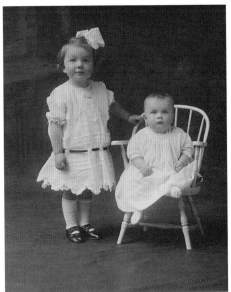

FIGURE 1.6: Esther and Ruth in chairs, 1917.

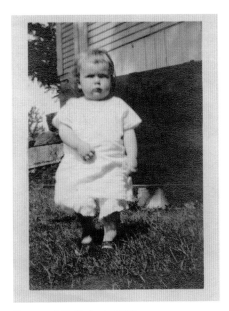

FIGURE 1.7: Esther, 1918.

grandfather, Fred Packard, had a huge vegetable garden and sold vegetables at a roadside stand. Sometimes a customer would wait while my grandfather went to pick fresh corn.

Through the summer, many a supper was composed of 10 to 12 vegetables without meat, and with fresh melon for dessert. Of course, we had the bent cucumbers, spotted tomatoes, and other produce unsuitable for sale at the stand, but it was delicious and fresh.

When I was a small child, sometimes my father would get home from work and go to the village for errands in his little Ford car. Often he would let me "drive." I would sit between his legs and hold onto the wheel, feet straight out. As we went along he would toot the horn to friends and wave, and they waved and laughed. We were probably moving at 15 to 20 miles per hour.

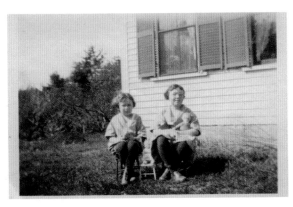

FIGURE 1.8: Esther and Ruth, 1922.

5

The Wilkins family lived on Kendall Road while the girls attended grade school. Many believe that *Clinical Practice of the Dental Hygienist* (*CPDH*) was Esther's first book, but in actuality, she wrote (and illustrated) her first book in 1924, when she was 8 years old. Her short story, *Thanksgiving*, consisted of three handwritten pages in cursive, bound in twine with two pilgrim caricatures on the cover. The second book was small—2 inches by 2 inches—bound by two paperclips and entitled *The Knight*. The third book bound by a single staple was coauthored by Ruth and entitled *Poems and Pictures*. The front page listed Esther Wilkins as "president" and Ruth E. Wilkins as "secretary." The two sisters worked tirelessly as a team, writing, illustrating, and using cutout color pictures from magazines.

My mother had two daughters, Esther [me] and Ruth. Her younger sister, Grace, also had two daughters, Dorothy and Carol Baker. Ruthie and Dorothy were within a month of being the same age, whereas Carol was one year younger and tall for her age, and I was two years younger and short. Auntie, as their mother Grace was called by nearly everyone [even by her son-in-law after Carl and Dorothy were married] brought the girls to visit us when they were little, but it is when we were somewhere in the 10 to 12 age range, that I remember a few special connections. They lived in Revere, while we were in Tyngsboro. During a few of those years, Ruthie initiated a family "publication" called the "Hayseeds and the Seaweeds" all made by hand, providing news and other items of the "country hayseeds" and the "ocean-side seaweeds." Dorothy offered the news from their side.

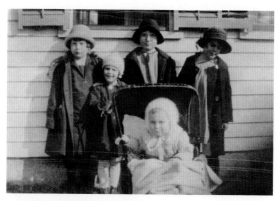

Figure 1.9: Esther and cousins (Esther is far left).

Big news for a few summers came from our summer visits when Dorothy and Ruthie would be in Tyngsboro, while I visited Carol in Revere. The second week Carol and I would be in Tyngsboro while Dorothy and Ruthie were in Revere. Every morning Carol and I would get ready to go to the beach for the day. Auntie would make us sandwiches to take, often baloney sandwiches which I had never had at home. I can still remember enjoying the aroma and the taste of those delicious baloney sandwiches, and associate them to my first visits to a salt water beach.

Some days we walked up the beach and across the street to watch the high roller coasters and other amusements. The roller coasters were very scary, going so fast and so steep. Later once when all of us were at the Beach entertainment section, watching various contests, riding dodgems, and enjoying popcorn and junk food, they convinced me to ride the low built roller coaster. It was two tracks side by side that ran as though racing. I don't recall any seatbelts but I held on tight. I'm still not convinced there's any real thrill while riding roller coasters.

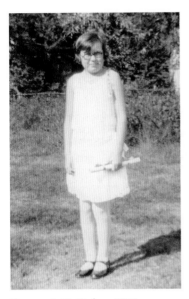

FIGURE 1.10: Esther, 1925.

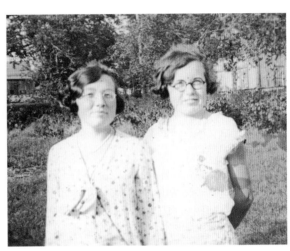

FIGURE 1.11: Ruth and Esther, 1927.

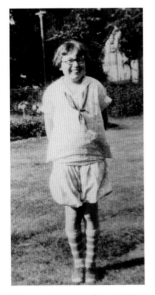

FIGURE 1.12: Esther, 1928.

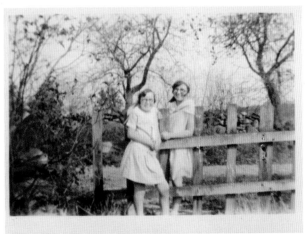

FIGURE 1.13: Esther and Ruth, 1929.

The *Magpie* was a *modest* monthly journal written by 14-year-old Esther M. Wilkins (president), 16-year-old Ruth E. Wilkins (editor), and their cousins, Dorothy and Carol Baker (secretary and treasurer, respectively).

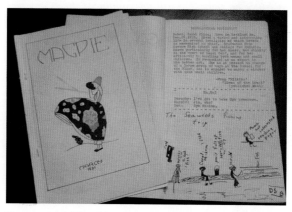

Figure 1.14: The *Magpie*.

The first issue of the *Magpie* was dated September 1930, and the final issue was dated March of 1932. Esther kept a copy of every issue, all of which were typed on a standard typewriter, illustrated by hand and bound with staples, measuring 8 ½ × 5 ½ inches. The issues were filled with editorials, poetry, plays, jokes, songs, crossword puzzles, stories, summaries of school activities (such as high school activities, town plays, church activities, and girl scouts), and "society notes." Hand-drawn illustrations corresponded to holidays the girls spent together, and a "biographical dictionary" outlined made-up accomplishments of the writers of the journal.

Esther seemed to be in charge, encouraging writers to get their material in on time for the next month's publication. For those *CPDH* chapter contributors, the following might sound familiar to the instructions Esther gave during chapter development and editing, including ALL CAPS and underline for emphasis.

> *Each member is requested to complete one <u>whole</u> page. IMPORTANT**—I haven't got time, aw quit it! Seems as though you could make time somehow. Material MUST be in by June 28, so get it in before then. BE ORIGINAL IF POSSIBLE!* (*Magpie*, April 1931).

Roles changed with the 1931 June edition, as Ruth became editor-in-chief, Esther's title changed to business manager and publishing editor, Carol became art editor, and Dorothy became society editor. A table of contents was also added to the publication, the treasury of which totaled $1.70, and their motto remained Bigger and Better!

Esther's passion for writing continued as she completed a full-length play entitled *The Spirit of Music by E. M. Wilkins,* and she began her lifelong love of writing poetry. Her early work included a poem entitled "The Flower Talk."

All the Tyngsborough children went to the Winslow Grammar School, and often, the students from an entire grade took up a single classroom. In several cases, multiple grades were grouped together. Barbara Magoon, Esther's best friend, recalled that their principal, Ms. Grace Henderson, whom they referred to as Miss Henny Penny (from the children's story, *Chicken Little*), "was the one who applied the Rat-ton [ruler]!"

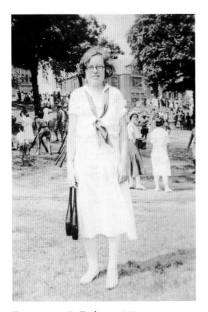

FIGURE 1.15: Esther, 1930.

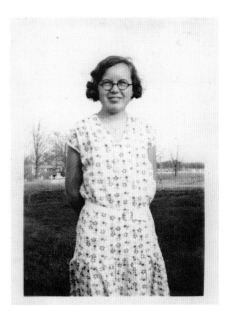

FIGURE 1.16: Esther, 1931.

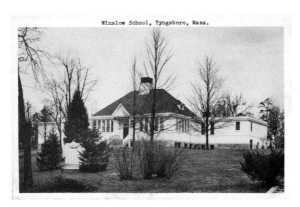

FIGURE 1.17: Winslow School, Tyngsborough.

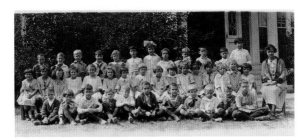

FIGURE 1.18: Winslow School, 1921 class photo (Esther is row 2, ninth from the left).

As Ruth began high school, Esther grew more independent. Her grades were steadily *A*'s and *B*'s; however, she was more inclined to earning *A*'s in creative subjects, such as music and drawing, but only *B*'s in arithmetic and hygiene!

When Ruthie first started school, she rode on the trolley—and I would be out on the rock to watch for her when she came home. Of course she brought home all the childhood diseases, so I was well-immunized by the time I went to school. I missed very few school days all the way through school. We still lived at the Sinclair Farm until I was in the 3rd or 4th grade, and then we moved to our next home on Kendall Road where we lived all through high school.

For each room and teacher I have brief memories. In the second grade the teacher was young and attractive and wore very pretty clothes. Sometimes when she had a dress made of silky material, I would put my hand on the edge of my desk as she went by so I could feel the lovely softness of her skirt as it swished by. The third-grade teacher, Miss Wylie, was older. About the only memory of that room was one day when we had all just returned from lunch. A little boy came in and held his pants down. I turned and pointed my finger at him, saying rather loud "oooooh" in an up and down tone, just as Miss Wylie walked into the room. She made me stand outside in the hall. I was so humiliated and fearful that my sister or someone else I knew would see me. Fortunately, she only left me out there a few minutes, but was truly scary thinking that she might tell my mother.

What happened in the 4th grade really changed my whole life. Apparently the earlier teachers had realized that I couldn't see very well. In both the 2nd and 3rd grades I had a front seat, which I thought was because I was short. They may have told my mother about my sight. I recall that one time my mother, Ruthie, and I went to see a program at the church where a speaker showed some old time moving pictures. At one point there were little small dark figures moving over the large white background. My mother asked me what they were. I guessed, saying "bugs crawling?" and she said, "no, they were people skiing down a snow covered hill." That led to getting my eyes tested for glasses. I will never forget that first day at school wearing the glasses.

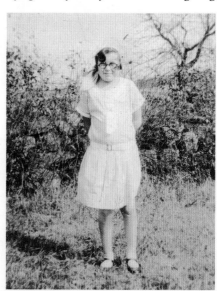

FIGURE 1.19: Esther, 1925, with glasses.

Everyone was looking at me! I was in a different world. My school work must have improved considerably, because during the 5th and 6th grades, Miss Norris decided that Barbara Connell and I could do the two grades in one year. From then, and the next year when we went into the room with the 7th–8th graders, we were isolates, and never really belonged to any class.

Each summer during her grade school years, aged 8 to 12 years, her family drove in *a very slow Ford* to Hebron, Maine, located west of Augusta, to visit her aunts and cousins. Esther truly enjoyed these excursions to visit *country people* with their farms and horses. *We always visited Aunt Mae. She let us cut paper dolls from her old fashion magazines.*

Despite living through the Great Depression, *Esther's lifelong friend,* Barbara Connell Magoon, described her joy in graduating from grade school with Esther:

❝ The big day came. Tuesday evening, June 19, 1929, at 8 o'clock. We all had speaking parts in the graduation program: Spirits of Song: Esther Wilkins, Mae Stevens, Nellie Pierce, and Phyllis Currier. Mother Nature: Barbara Connell."

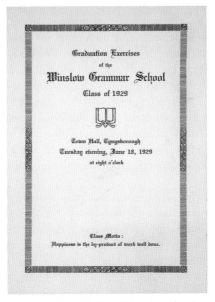

FIGURE 1.20: Winslow School graduation program, 1929.

❝ We then went on to Lowell High School. During the first year the trolleys stopped running so we were bussed. We were graduated in with a class of nearly 800 students."

Barbara exceeded the call of duty in her response to our request for artifacts and pictures she might still have of her friendship years with Esther. "I hope you realize that you are asking us to remember the days of our youth when we are not sure how many calories we had for breakfast today! Esther and I played together and my Mom gave Esther her first Hydrox Cookie," a fact Esther remembered later in life. They both rode by trolley to the Winslow Grammar School, "flew up" from Brownie Scouts to Girls Scouts, and together took piano lessons from Mrs. Winifred Symonds, who lived on Farwell Road in a charming house almost consumed by a sea of lilacs. There was a friendly competitive spirit between the girls, as Barbara recalls Esther's piano playing abilities far exceeded her own. "Esther did well and could play 'Nola,' while I was struggling with 'I Love Coffee, I Love Tea.'"

Esther's height at 45 inches tall was well below her peers in first grade and earned her the nickname (now outdated) of "Pygmy." Betsy said her "mother's nickname was Tink, short for Tinkerbell, even shorter than Esther when they reached full height." Barbara maintained that no one can remember who came up with that nickname, but she was in fact, taller than Esther. She shared all her wonderful photographs, including those of her and Esther performing in a school play. She evidently knew Esther quite well, as she added that rather than return these mementos to her, "give them to Esther," as "I'm sure she has a chair for it!" Barbara was referring to Esther's filing system, notorious among her friends, in which each piece of furniture in her home was covered with papers, boxes, and files, which temporarily had to be removed for guest seating.

Her roots in Tyngsborough remained important to Esther throughout her life. It was a country town with a culture of connectedness. *The Village Improvement Association Annual,* published every year by the Tyngsborough Village Improvement Association, dated February 1941 (one of the many artifacts Esther kept from her childhood) brought the news: School District Updates, Improvement Association Report, The Village Players (local theater production), The Industrial Club, the Tyngsborough Grange No. 222, Historical Society, Mother's Club, Girl Scouts, Ladies' Alliance, The Playground, Bird Notes, Marriages, Deaths, Changes in Residences, Junior Red Cross, outings, an Honor Roll during World War II, as well as advertisements for the local stores, bowling alleys, and A Teacher of Pianoforte.

Although she traveled the country and was busy working on her book or teaching, beginning in 2000, Esther returned to Tyngsborough on Memorial Day to visit the graves of her parents and her husband, Jim, at Sherburne Cemetery in Tyngsborough. Several of her Wilkins cousins still lived in town, so Esther made a special visit with the "girls" each year, including Janet and Louise Lorman and Christina Bell, who passed away in 2015 (see "The Family Tree"). Frances Clarke, whom Esther visited until she passed away, said that when the family reunited for the annual picnic, there could be over 90 people there, counting babies and everyone. Esther's cousins remained extremely important to each other. They were the daughters of her Aunt Ethel Clarke (her father's sister), who was very close to Esther.

She was a sweet lady, always smiling and cheerful, though she was busy with 8 children, house, and taking care of her elderly mom, my grandmother, who lived to 99 yrs., 11 months. Esther later elaborated, *When pressed with the question of genetics, I love to share about my paternal grandmother. She was a frail old lady, but my memories are clear of her busily sewing—by hand primarily—to help her many grandchildren get ready for back to school.*

As for my other grandparents, my maternal grandmother died in childbirth in the late 1800s. Her husband, my grandfather, lived into his late 80s in spite of the daily evening pipe that filled the kitchen with smoke while he read the newspaper after supper.

This warmth was reciprocated on both sides of the family as related by Esther's first cousin, Christina Clarke Bell.

❝ Since I've known Esther, she's never forgotten where she's come from. I'll always admire her bubbly personality and warm smile. I'm proud to know her and happy for all of her successes!"

In 2012, Christina recalled, "up until 2 years ago, Esther would drive herself to and from Tyngsboro by herself 45 miles each way." Esther frequently reminded everyone that although they were over 80 years old, they still referred to one another as "girls." One of the "girls," Janet Clarke Lorman, who practiced as a dental hygienist for 42 years, related a particular visit from Esther: "Esther came to Tyngsboro in May to put flowers on her parents' and husband Jim's grave and to spend time with us, my sister, Louise, and my sister, Christina, and Esther's friend Barbara Magoon."

The "girls" shared endless conversations about their childhood adventures, as evidenced by additional recollections from Christina Clarke Bell: "Esther and I [were] both family and lifelong friends. We [were] both natives of Tyngsboro and grew up within a mile of each other. Esther belonged to and was very active in the Evangelical Church in town, where she taught Sunday school as a teenager. Esther's mother, Edith Packard Wilkins, directed plays, which were presented once a year in the Tyngsboro Town Hall. Esther was intelligent enough to complete grammar school in 7 years and upon graduation attended Lowell High School for four years. At the time, Tyngsboro did not have its own high school."

❧ HIGH SCHOOL YEARS ❧

Esther graduated from Lowell High School in 1933 in one of the largest classes during that decade. On the subject of these formative years she recalled:

All the high school aged students in towns surrounding Lowell, Massachusetts, commuted into Lowell High School. My class had 789 graduates, which was one of the largest during that decade. We were dependent on first the trolley and later a bus with one schedule choice. Since we lived over a mile from the trolley stop, it meant an early morning walk for Ruthie and me.

My sister was two years ahead, so paved the way for me. She was my original mentor all the way from preschool to college. My mother was determined that we would both get to college, so our high school college preparatory program was very important. Most courses required at least an hour of homework. The dining room table was devoted to our evenings with Ruth on one end and I on the other. In those early days, our house was not wired for electricity, so we studied using kerosene lamps.

Ruth had taken Latin I and II during her Freshman and Sophomore years, so was now taking French I, which she had advised me to do because she thought it would be easier than the Latin I to start. She was taking the same course I was taking with a different teacher.

When I came up to the first few weeks about ready to flunk French, she became my tutor, and each evening she would drill me in an earlier lesson and the lesson for the next day, until I managed to pass that first test with a C! As Esther related many years later, *the intricacies of foreign language didn't make sense to me at all, so she took it upon herself to make sure I wouldn't flunk* (Esther, as cited in Ray, 1996, p. 8).

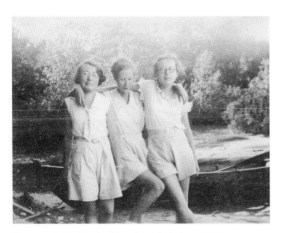

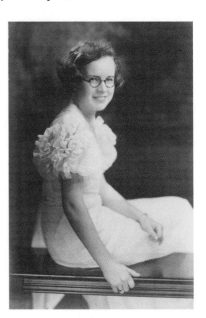

FIGURE 1.21: Ruth, friend, and Esther, 1933.

FIGURE 1.22: Esther's graduation photo.

Ruth was Esther's *personal hero*, and Ruth was devoted to her. Their closeness and teamwork is perhaps best revealed in Esther's recounting a simple Saturday morning:

At the risk of sounding like living Abe Lincoln style, studying by the fireplace with a candle, we had kerosene lamps. Saturday morning while our mother was at her secretarial position [everybody with full time jobs worked Saturday morning] Ruth and I cleaned house, changed the beds, and it was Ruth's special assignment to clean, wash, and fill the kerosene lamps and wash the lampshades, because she was bigger and more sensible. My responsibility was cleaning the bathroom. Part of those Saturday mornings we would play the piano, sing, read poetry out loud or do other "fun" things. Ruth had been inspired to love poetry by her high school English teacher [Miss Stickney] who took a special interest in her prize "A" student. Ruth's inspiration rubbed off on me as she would read poems out loud. Then, of course, when the clock began to near the time when Mama would be arriving home, we would scramble to finish our work. Mama would get home and be upset if everything wasn't clean and straightened out.

There was a framed motto which hung in the family's New England home: *The beauty of the house is order.*

In high school, Esther belonged to the Grange. Founded in 1867, the Grange is "a non-profit, non-partisan, fraternal organization that advocates for rural America and agriculture . . . with a strong history in grassroots activism, family values and community service" (National Grange, 2011, p. 1). Grange halls existed as community centers, much like the Masons, in which residents gathered for educational programs, events, dances, potlucks, meetings, and rallies. It was here Esther found another venue to enjoy her love for dancing.

❧ THE FAMILY TREE ❧

Esther had a remarkably good time developing her family tree.

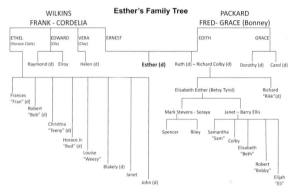

FIGURE 1.23: Esther's family tree.

Esther admired her mother, Edith Rose Packard Wilkins, who was born in Auburn, Maine, on July 6, 1889.

> *When I was 4 years old my mother's mother died after her little sister, Grace, was born. Their father was Fred Packard, my grandfather. The little girls, according to information my sister, Ruth, gave me later, were passed around among their several aunts who lived in the area of Hebron and Buckfield, Maine. Eventually they went to the Hebron Academy, which was high school. My mother [Edith] wanted to go to college. Aunt Mae and Uncle Sherm Bonney offered for her to live with them in Auburn, Maine, and go to Bates College [across the river in Lewiston] with their son, Clinton, who was about the same age as Edith.*

Edith's father, however, *put his foot down* and insisted that she would go where she could learn something more practical in order to earn a living. Women attending college in those days wasn't considered practical. The family moved to Massachusetts, and Edith attended business school and became a highly skilled secretary and office manager. Esther recalled that her mother *was a crackerjack secretary* who worked for the president of a blanket company in Lowell. *As a result of her own experience, she spent her life as a mother seeing to it that HER daughters went to college, as she had been cheated out of college herself.* Esther recalled that, although she never knew the details, as a young woman, Edith worked in the area of Chelsea, Massachusetts. During this time, she met Esther's father, Ernest Wilkins. They were married in 1910 and moved to Chelmsford where Ruth was born in 1914.

Later when Ruth and I were in school our mother went back for a brush-up program and was employed in the office of a big blanket mill in Lowell. When we were in high school we usually rode in with her [to Lowell High School], but came back on the bus after school in the afternoon.

Mama always worked very hard. She had a 5 ½ day workweek, and then kept her family and home responsibilities always ahead.

After a busy Saturday of cooking and doing housework, Ruth, Esther, and Edith, drove into town to the library. Ruth was an avid reader from the early days, and Esther developed this passion as well. Esther wanted assurance that the family going to the library was important to include in her biography: *You know how much I love libraries!* While many people cannot remember what they read last week, Esther recalled that 90 years ago, her favorite book was *Dotty Dolly's Tea Party* (Wheeler & Wheeler, 1914).

Most Saturdays there was a pot of beans baking all day in the oven, sometimes brown bread. My mother baked bread, made doughnuts, and did other cooking Sunday morning while she sent us off to Sunday school. She was the treasurer for the Sunday school, so it was our responsibility to bring home the collection, a small bag, mostly pennies with a few nickels. On special Sundays when we had a "piece" to speak, or sang a duet, she would always attend, and sometimes my father also went. For a few years we sang a duet on Girl Scout Sunday wearing our uniforms.

Although she was known for writing a highly scientific book on the practice of dental hygiene, Esther was a gifted storyteller as well. The family's first cat was Timmy Tiptoes, a black and white tomcat with white paws, who spent his nights out and slept in all day. *Sleeping all day wouldn't keep the mice at bay. He lived well into his teens. Not long after Timmy Tiptoes, Chippy arrived when Grampa Wilkins died. Tippy was Maltese, grey with a pointed face, and he squeaked to be let out. He took a liking to a spot on top of the piano, which was warm from the radiator next to it.* Chippy lived to be 19 years old. Esther affectionately remembered her childhood pets as part of the family.

Because a childhood friend broke his back skiing, Esther's mother decided she was not a fan of sports for the "girls." Other than skating as a young child, Esther didn't participate in sports, but the sisters had sleds and skates, and according to Esther, *skating was fun. Skates strapped right onto your boots back then.* In the warmer months, they swam at Willowdale. Ruthie and Esta (as it was pronounced) had dolls and other toys, *but the favorite was paper dolls cut from fashion magazines and furniture from Sears or other catalogs. We would spread them out over the dining room table and then begged our Mama to plan eating dinner in the kitchen. Sometimes they covered the dining room carpet.*

Esther was quite proud of her roots and her family, especially her mother, whose rule was you did not buy anything until you saved enough money to purchase it. Esther said that her mother saved until she had enough money to wire the cottage with electricity and opted to buy a washing machine instead of a dryer. In those days, having electricity depended on where you lived. As long-time friend, Barbara Magoon, related, "Esther and

I never outgrew being frugal—a lesson from the Great Depression." That frugality continued to be a lifestyle for Esther throughout her life, and in response to my question of why she doesn't spend more money on herself, she replied that if she *doesn't need something there is no need to buy it.*

When Esther was in high school, her mother drove her and her sister *on an adventure* to Washington, DC. While attending the American Dental Hygienists' Association (ADHA) convention in DC in 2009, Esther related this family trip with great detail and fondness. While atop a two-decker bus, with great precision and moving from stop to stop in Washington, she explained that neither Esther nor Ruth had ever been to the nation's capital. Esther's mother wanted the girls to learn about history and education. They were given passes to the House of Representatives from Edith Nourse Rogers, who was their district representative to Congress at the time, having taken over the office when her husband died. She often came to the village of Tyngsborough to talk, and Esther both respected and liked her; *everyone did.*

This adventure was one among many such memorable experiences for Edith and her two girls. As the Brown Owl, their Girl Scout troop leader, Edith cherished her time with her daughters. Edith had long hair, which Esther enjoyed combing and brushing for her occasionally. When Esther was away at Girl Scout camp, her mother came to visit and arrived with a "bob" haircut; Esther was crushed, but she *never told anyone.*

Edith passed away in January of 1946, at 57 years old, while Esther was a first-year dental student at Tufts. It was midwinter exam week, so she had to make up a few exams when she got back from the funeral. The service was held at the church on a frigid day and the ground was frozen. Many years later when friend and neighbor, Laura Weinrebe, moved from her apartment located in Esther's building in Boston, she gave her flower boxes to Esther to place on her own balcony. The geraniums reminded Esther of her mother, who took her geraniums in each fall and put them back out in spring. Esther grinned with pride and affection every time she spoke about her mother, what she taught her, and the value system she practiced.

Esther's father, Ernest Warren Wilkins, was born in 1879 in Ludlow, Vermont, the oldest of four children, Ernest, Vera, Edward, and Ethel, who had eight children, some of whom Esther referred to as "the girls" (see "The Family Tree"). Ernest worked at Chelsea Clock Company when he met Edith. Having little money, they had a small wedding. Ernest read a lot but didn't graduate from high school, which was not unusual for the time. *He was born and grew up in Tyngsboro, was a general workman for several years, drove the truck for a lumber company, and for several years worked on a chicken farm. He rode a bike to work, and he was never without employment, even all through the Depression.*

After Edith died, Ernest lived in a tiny cottage and did odd jobs on the grounds of an estate. He was active in coaching Little League teams in Tyngsborough, which Esther says was his *little haven.* Ernest was an honorary coach for the Tyngsboro Tigers of the Interstate Little League in the mid-1950s (Collins, 2009). Ernest took the whole team to the game in his little Ford, often taking them for ice cream or swimming after the game. Over the years, the folks in Tyngsborough called him *Uncle Toot.* Ernest was also a sports enthusiast and, as Esther recalled, *an extreme Red Sox fan.* He played baseball on a town team and took her and Ruth to games. Although they didn't have a radio back then, when they went to cousin Dorothy's house in Revere, they listened to the Red Sox games on the radio.

Esther's family was extremely important to her. Esther conveyed that she and her father were not letter writers, so had little correspondence, and he wasn't able to visit her when Esther was at the University of Washington. In 1953, when she visited for the first time since leaving Tyngsborough, she and Ernest made a day of it and called it a *date*. Her father met her at the train and they spent the afternoon together, including going out to lunch at the Green Ridge Turkey Farm in Nashua, New Hampshire. They talked about the family in Tyngsborough and the baseball team he coached, travelling around to relatives, and visiting *Grammie Wilkins at Aunt Ethel's*.

At the time of Ernest's passing in 1957, he was the park commissioner for Tyngsborough. Esther seemed pleased to note that the current Little League team, in uniform, attended his funeral. It was not the team he coached, but it was important nonetheless. *It was a testimonial to the connection he had with the league.* Ernest's own mother went to his funeral, carried by her grandsons, and she herself died the following year at 99 years, 11 months. *She died quietly away 1 month before her 100th birthday. She was a frail little old lady, but my memories are clear of her busily sewing—by hand primarily—to help her many grandchildren get ready for back-to-school.*

Esther had two sisters, Ruth and Doris Elizabeth, born in 1918, but Doris passed away as an infant. This may partly account for the closeness between the two sisters. Just mentioning Ruth's name to Esther would elicit a wide smile; she was a dear friend and an integral part of her life. *She studied for teaching nursery school and kindergarten* and subsequently *taught in a nursery school in Nashua, New Hampshire.* Ruth's daughter, Betsy, remained very close to her aunt as well and toward the end of Esther's life became her primary caregiver.

❧ THE COLLEGE SEARCH ❦

Esther's college search process was an unusual one.

My sister graduated and went to Boston University. About the middle of my senior year in high school, she started asking what I was going to do and which college I would choose. I had no idea, so she would go over the options. Did I want to teach school? Be a nurse? And after much discussion I thought maybe I could be a nurse. So my mother decided I would go to the best, which she thought had to be the Children's Hospital in Boston. We made the appointment, and she drove me to Longwood Avenue and parked across the street to wait for me. I met Miss Goostray, the Head of Nursing, in her office. In a crisp nurse's uniform and cap, she was very pleasant and I was impressed. She looked over my transcript, and asked questions, then said, "But, Esther, you are not old enough. You wouldn't be able to take the State Board when you graduated." She went on to advise that I enroll at Simmons in their nursing degree program. "Then if you still want this program we will be happy to accept you."
That disappointment led to my application at Simmons.

During their college years, both sisters helped their mother at the New England Telephone and Telegraph switchboard, where Edith was the office manager. The office for the branch was located in their white house overlooking the center of town. *The switchboard was in the front window and it required 24/7 duty. The police car often parked in view of the switchboard, and if someone wanted to know if the chief was there, they would call the switchboard. That's small-town stuff.* Mama slept in the room next to the switchboard to take care of any calls during the night, until her day shift relief came at 8:00. If the bell rang in the middle of the night, she would get up, connect it, and go back to sleep—*she did get to sleep through the night sometimes.*

Edith hired Barbara Connell to be the "day girl," and when Esther arrived home from college, she would take over while her mother made dinner, doing her homework while on the switchboard.

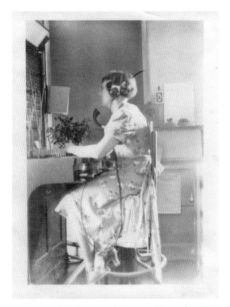

FIGURE 1.24: Esther at the switchboard, 1937.

Barbara related that "Mrs. Wilkins took over the agency in Tyngsboro for N. E. T & T. She asked me to work for her, as I had no money to go back to school (Massachusetts School of Art). The agent had to live in the first-floor apartment and the switchboard was in the right front corner room. I worked days, Esther and Ruth evenings, and Mrs. Wilkins all night. The job paid the agent $100 per month and she had to pay me out of that. I got 20 cents per hour for 5 ½ days per week ($8.80 per week, no benefits!) I gave 41 ½ years to Ma Bell. The summer of 1936 Esther worked at an Inn in Manchester-by-the-Sea next to Coast Guard Station #22. One day in July her mother and I visited her and took her bike to her."

Barbara remained a close and devoted friend to Esther and the family. She shared a page from her "autograph book" from Friday the 13th, 1930, which according to Barbara were the "in thing" at the time. Esther had written:

What! Write in your booklet?
For poets to spy?
And critics to laugh at?
No, not I!

❧ RUTH, RICHARD, AND FAMILY ❧

Esther related her sister, Ruth's, meeting of her future husband.

Ruth had dated a Boston University classmate, Richard G. Colby, who was in the same year of undergraduate college of liberal arts as Ruth was at Boston University, although they did not date when they were in college together. Then he went on to Boston University School of Theology. After he graduated in 1939, his first church was in southern New Hampshire. I remember they saw each other during that time. I remember him telling me about one time she visited him there because he told me about the dinner he made and mentioned vitamins and healthy things, such as tomato ketchup.

Ruth married Richard Colby on June 14, 1941, in the chapel at Boston University School of Theology, located then on Beacon Hill.

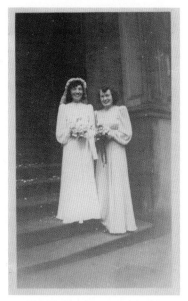

FIGURE 1.25: Esther as maid of honor, Ruth's wedding day 1941.

Esther was maid of honor, and she fondly described how she wore a yellow dress in the same pattern as her sister's white dress. It was not a large wedding, rather a small gathering of primarily their classmates and family members. Both Ruth's father and the groom, Richard, had white pants and dark jackets. In describing the ceremony, Esther does not remember where the dinner was afterward, *but it was not far away—in fact it seems as though we walked there.*

The couple lived in the parsonage in Sanbornville and had two children. Richard Jr. (Rikki) was born in Wolfeboro on June 19, 1943, and their second child, Elisabeth Esther (Betsy), was born on August 19, 1946, in Haverhill Massachusetts, while her father was overseas in Japan. As this was wartime in America, Richard Sr. (The Reverend Colby) enlisted as a chaplain in the Army in 1944, late in the war, and was originally stationed on Long Island. Although Ruth went along, Betsy related that "she came back to stay in Haverhill, Massachusetts, with his parents when he was sent overseas in the Army occupation of Japan." When The Reverend Colby was discharged in November, the family moved to Wellfleet, where he was put in charge of two churches, one in Wellfleet and another in neighboring Eastham. The community was very welcoming, and Betsy recalled, "The churches got together and bought them a new Pontiac, since their old car was not reliable and he had to give two services each Sunday."

For most of Betsy's childhood, Esther was in Seattle, but she remembers a particular anecdote told to her by her parents when they were living in Wellfleet (1946–1951); Esther was still in Massachusetts then. "On Christmas Eve, the milkman asked me if I knew who was coming to visit that night. I told him Auntie Esther, of course!"

The family moved to East Greenwich, Rhode Island, in 1951, where, as Betsy related,

    ❝ Ruth was very involved as a minister's wife—as Sunday School Superintendent, in the Women's Society for Christian Service, and in Church Women United. While they were in East Greenwich, they spent a lot of energy developing plans for a new church hall and Sunday School building and renovations for the church. In 1958 we moved to Brockton where my mother went to work in 1961 as a social worker for the Town of Stoughton. She bought a Rambler named Rosie [for Rosie the Riveter], like the women who went to work in World War II."

Rikki and Betsy graduated from high school in Brockton. The family moved to Warwick, Rhode Island, in 1967. Rikki went on to attend American University; he became an organist and held a teaching position outside Washington, DC. Betsy attended DePauw University in Greencastle, Indiana, and was later married at her father's church in Warwick. "Ruth continued working as a social worker in the projects in Providence. She really loved her work," recalled Betsy. Ruth and Richard moved to Osterville on Cape Cod in 1971. Betsy's own two children (Esther's niece and nephew) were born during this time. "Mark was born at White Sands Missile Range in New Mexico, and Janet in New Jersey." It is also at this time, as Betsy recalls, that her mother was first diagnosed and treated for ovarian cancer.

The family moved again, to Lynn, Massachusetts, in 1976 and then retired in 1978 to North Kingston, Rhode Island. Betsy said, "At that point they returned to the E. Greenwich church where they still had a lot of friends. Ruth has a Sunday School room dedicated to her, and the large meeting hall is dedicated to Dick." According to Betsy, they traveled a great deal in Canada and Europe. Ruth died in 1982, Rikki in 1986, and Dick in 1990, one day before their first great grandchild was born.

❧ TYNGSBOROUGH VISITS 2010 ❧

A drive up to meet the "girls" during a 2010 Memorial Day trip to Tyngsborough confirmed Esther's descriptions of the countryside and uniqueness of the terrain, the river, and historical bridge. The buildings, many of which are preserved original structures, include the Winslow School (although it is currently abandoned) and the homes in which Esther lived during her childhood. I met Esther and Betsy at cousin Weezie's home right outside the center of town, followed by a trip to the local library.

Our visit continued as Betsy followed Esther's directions as she guided us through a tour of her home town, beginning with a first stop for *a spring spruce up of the gravesites* of her husband and parents, a plot located on a small hill. As the three of us walked back to the car, we passed a few gravesites, and with her keen memory, Esther told in detail their stories and roles in the town in years past.

Our stops included a visit to the bridge over the Merrimac River as well as the home in which Esther lived in grade school. We visited the Windsor School, the large rock where Esther and her sister watched the trolleys, the church, and the train tracks. With precision, Esther related each element of her hometown and its significance to her and her family, truly enjoying her tour through her childhood.

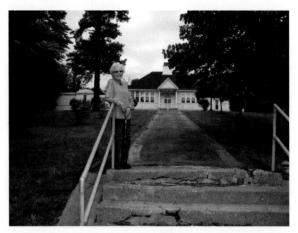

FIGURE 1.26: Esther in front of Winslow School, 2010.

There was much laughter as the "girls" looked at old pictures, remembering family, friends, and adventures. A few adjustments were made to the family tree as a result of their discussions as well as the topic of dental hygiene. Cousin Janet related her own dental hygiene career, traveling from school to school in the area, treating the children. She is proud that Esther Wilkins is the reason she enjoyed a profession so important to her.

The opportunity presented itself for an extensive discussion by the master herself on the topic of tooth sealants for children. With her usual expertise, we all learned a few new things on the topic. After she had spoken for about 10 minutes, Esther said that she would then collect a fee from everyone, as she was usually paid to provide this type of information. Everyone got quite a giggle from that one. A group picture captured the day when the "girls" got together in 2010.

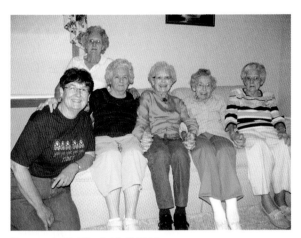

FIGURE 1.27: The "girls," 2010.

Early in the process of developing this biography and learning more about Esther's life, it became evident she had a keen mind and an astonishing sense of recall. How she could remember her early life with such detail was quite remarkable.

CHAPTER 2

Simmons

In September of 1934, Esther M. Wilkins began her college career at Simmons College, located on the Fenway in Boston, Massachusetts.

The history of early years of the college is well documented in the book, *Delayed by Fire: Being the Early History of Simmons College*, written in 1945 by Kenneth L. Mark, who was professor of chemistry and director of the School of General Science at Simmons. The book is a definitive guide to the heritage of John Simmons (his family can be traced back to the ship *Fortune* which came to America in 1621) as well as the character of John Simmons and the vision he had for a college for women. When a copy of the book was located in 2012, Esther spent quite a bit of time reading it.

Esther remembered Dr. Mark's gentlemanly manner when taking his Basic Chemistry class from 1934 to 1935. It was not her favorite subject, but *I liked it better than organic chemistry, for sure!* During the first days of class, Professor Mark himself uncrated the chemistry bottles as well as equipped the labs. Mark was one of the first professors at Simmons (since 1903) and had access, as evidenced by his extensive detail, to the founding documents,

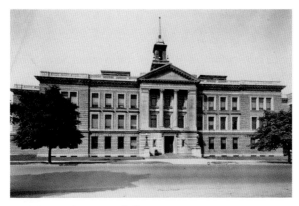

Figure 2.1: Simmons College, 1930s.

first speeches, and curriculum. Simmons's vision was for an institution for women for the purpose of "branches of art, science, and industry best calculated to enable the scholars to acquire an independent livelihood" (Mark, 1945, p. 25) (see Appendix D for historical information on the founding of Simmons College, which can be accessed via the online e-book).

All the higher educational institutions Esther attended as a student were within the City of Boston, two within ¼ mile of each other. Esther attended Simmons during its "growth years" (Goodwin & Wood, 2008), which were from 1920 to 1939. The College expanded its fundraising efforts in these years of growth, which Simmons archivists, Claire Goodwin and Jason Wood, described as a coordinated effort "from students selling pencils on street corners," to "alumnae selling used merchandise from the Simmons Salvage Shop," and "sandwiches and soda from a lunch wagon in Post Office Square" (p. 3).

Esther entered Simmons as a first-year nursing student on September 17, 1934. The first president, Lefavour, had retired in 1933, and a new president had taken office, Bancroft Beatley (1933–1955), who had been on the faculty of the Harvard Graduate School of Education. Jane Louise Mesick was dean. According to the Simmons College Bulletin (Simmons College, 1935), tuition was $250 per year, paid in two installments (which remained the same during Esther's 4 years). This was a hefty sum in those days, as Esther recalled quite vividly, especially for a student coming from a rural and not wealthy family. The cost of laboratory classes was between $1 and $9. The Simmons school day began at 8:45 AM and ended at 4:00 PM.

As Esther many years later reviewed the information from the Simmons College Bulletin, she eagerly recalled Professor Hilliard who taught Public Health, Catherine Witton (Biology), Dr. Richardson (Biology), Dr. Granara (Chemistry), Judith Matlack (English), and Dr. Hinton (Biology).

Esther changed majors from nursing to general science beginning in her sophomore year at Simmons, which was a program "leading to the degree of BS designed for students who wish to become teachers of biology, chemistry, physiology, or math, assistants in chemistry or biology to persons engaged in medicine or other scientific research" (Simmons College, 1935).

I did my first year in the nursing curriculum. By the end of the year I had decided to change majors, but since I was still unclear as to what career I wanted to enter, I was advised to stay with the "general science" curriculum. It was a very heavy program, and with the commute to Tyngsboro daily, it was difficult to be more than an "average" student, but I did work very hard.

The 64-credit-hour curriculum in 1934 for the General Science major encompassed the following courses:

1934–1935	1935–1936	1936–1937	1937–1938
Biology	Chemistry 4	Chemistry 5	Biology 7: Prevention
Chemistry I	Mathematics I	Biology 4	Biology 8: Public Health Lab
English I	Physics I	Physics 2: Principles	Public Health Science
History I	Fine Arts 3	Physics 5: X-ray Tech	Biology: Hospital Lab
Methods	Philosophy I	Government 2	Economics I
Biology 100		Psychology I	Hygiene

The grading system was A through F, with no minus or plus grades. A numerical weight had been added in 1926. Esther described the courses as *rigorous*. She excelled in Biology, Chemistry, English, and Physics, although Fine Arts, Economics, and Physics 5: X-ray proved not to be her strengths.

One of her Simmons classmates, Doris C. Spiegel, who entered the nursing program with Esther in 1934, commented that Esther was "brilliant and ambitious and she loved to dance." They walked down Huntington Avenue together, Doris to walk home to the South End and Esther to take the bus to North Station for her 5:14 PM train back to Tyngsborough. Sometimes, according to Doris, they would stop for a delicious jelly donut. "We would walk to save the carfare! That's a long walk from Simmons to North Station!" Doris recalled fondly that, although Esther transferred to the School of Science and their paths diverged, they kept in touch for many years. "We shared a love for Boston and science!"

Another nursing classmate, Roberta R. Strong, also kept in touch with Esther for nearly 74 years, although she had stayed in nursing and Esther transferred to general science. "We remained friends all these years, as Esther traveled worldwide." Esther also became friends with Roberta's sister, Betty, who was a coast guard wife when Esther was teaching at the University of Washington.

It certainly was a challenging pursuit of higher education for Esther. She remembered,

My train to Boston for Simmons had but one stop down at Tyngsboro in the morning and one stop back in the evening. There were three of us regular commuters. The conductor watched as the train started to slow up to be sure I wasn't running down the road to the station. I never could miss with such a fine helper.

It was a 50-cent ride home to Tyngsborough from Simmons. Decades later, she recalled these long trips as though they were yesterday, vividly enacting the call of the conductor *Lowell-Tyngsboro-Nashua Train*, delightfully singing the stops as she described them.

The 5:14 from North Station was the one stop each day back. So I would hurry to walk home and get on the switchboard so Mama could go to the kitchen and get our dinner.

We usually ate it in the office near the switchboard. Getting much homework done was difficult during those busy evenings after the long days at college and commuting.

Although the General Science program was extremely challenging, Esther enjoyed the experience and found her preparation useful for her many years in the professions of dental hygiene and dentistry. *I enjoyed the friends I made and Simmons opened the doors to graduate school for me.* Although she changed majors, Esther remained lifelong friends with several students who continued in the Nursing major.

Esther was a commuting student, which presented its own challenges for students. Although there was an absence policy, Esther didn't realize it existed; her attitude was: *I went every possible day; I can't waste all that money! And although I had colds, I wasn't really "sick." I know I missed about a week at the time of the 1936 big flood [flood was over the roads and railroad tracks that ran along the river]. Some of the snowstorms were pretty bad so there must have been a snow day or two!* There was a lunchroom available for nonresident students in the east wing of the main building. Esther remembered the Wasserman Lab and Bacteriology lab quite vividly.

Catherine McCarthy Murphy fondly recalled her days with Esther at Simmons:

" I first met Esther at Simmons. We were both commuters. In those days at least half of the students commuted. Money was scarce. We spent our days in the College on the Fens both classes and free time. We'd be in classrooms; in labs; in the library on the third floor; in the study hall, a large room with long tables on the first floor on the end of the building toward the Gardner Museum, a wonderful place to visit when time allowed; in the lounge where we could study or socialize or attend an occasional afternoon tea or club meeting. We all watched our pennies and our weight. The lunchroom was in the basement. We usually brought our lunches to save money. On a good day we might take our lunches out to the Backyard, a lovely area which is no longer there, due to new buildings. Also, in the basement there was a smoking room for commuters. Sometimes we'd stop in to see friends, even though we didn't smoke."

" Then, time to go home. Off we would go over to Ruggles Station to catch the Huntington Avenue trolley. Sometimes it was a leisurely walk; other times a wild dash if we happened to see or hear a trolley approaching. If we missed it, it might be a long wait for the next and it might make the difference between catching our trains; mine from Back Bay; Esther's from North Station. The trolley was a dime and we could get a discount on the Boston portion of the train until we were 21 by having a paper signed each month by Simmons College."

" On one of our first days at Simmons we all went to the large auditorium on the second floor for an orientation meeting. I wondered whether Esther would remember what the students were told at this meeting: Look to your left, look to your right, by mid-term, many of these people will no longer be here! What an upsetting greeting! But as the year progressed we realized that we were staying at Simmons. We relaxed and happily enjoyed many of the interesting programs that were presented each week in the auditorium."

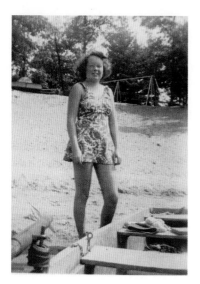

FIGURE 2.2: Esther at Simmons, 1935.

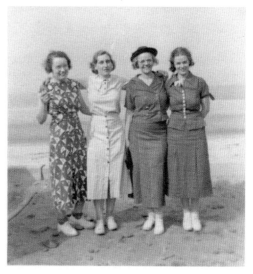

FIGURE 2.3: Simmons outing, 1936. Esther, Madeline, Mary, and Laura.

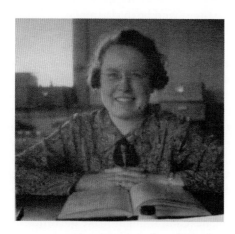

FIGURE 2.4: Esther at Simmons, 1937.

The Class of 1938 mascot was the penguin; class colors were red and white. In warm weather, the students had gym class in the open playing field area behind the main building, where now a new building, built in 2008, stands. Esther said it had a fence around it and they had to wear uniforms, which classmate Catherine McCarthy Murphy said looked like:

    ❝ baby's rompers, blue sleeveless jumpers with elastic around the legs. With them we wore short sleeved white blouses, yellow sweatshirts, white socks, and sneakers. In the gym on the first floor we would do exercises. The one I remember best is lying on the floor, putting our head and shoulders on the floor, and pulling in our tummy until our back touched the floor. The teacher told us that if we continued to do that exercise, we would have much better posture by Christmas."

Esther was not extremely active in nonacademic activities because she was a commuting student who needed to get home on the last train back to Tyngsborough. As a first-year nursing student, Esther belonged to the Anne Strong Club, whose purpose was "the promotion of friendships among the Nursing School students outside of their classrooms, and also the formation of a bond between the students at Simmons and those affiliated with various hospitals" (Simmons College, 1938, p. 131). As a General Science major, during her last 3 years, Esther belonged to the Ellen Richards Club, which "demonstrates to the girls how their laboratory work and scientific courses will be of use to them in later life by engaging men and women well informed in the various fields of science, in Chemistry, Biology, and Physics, to speak at their frequent teas" (Simmons College, 1938, p. 132).

Esther saw the Boston Pops (Boston Symphony Orchestra) multiple times. She and her friends had their favorite spots in the second balcony for the 25 cents it costs for those sections on special Friday rehearsal afternoons. She went to Boston Red Sox games for 5 cents a game on Ladies day Friday afternoons *for good seats*, and she went to the Gardner Museum to see the flowers: *It was free back then!* The Gardner is next door to Simmons and is on the Fenway, on the corner of Worthington Street (now named *Palace Road*).

In the three summers between academic years, Esther worked as a waitress at Straitsmouth Inn in Rockport, Massachusetts, an old inn out on the point, which provided money for her tuition, Betsy (Esther's niece), related

> " When Esther was waitressing in the summers, the place was a typical hotel back then in that it served three meals a day to the guests. She and the other girls shared quarters and worked all three meals with time off in between. They spent time sunning themselves on the rocks at the beach. She once spilled strawberries all over a male customer. She said they didn't have her back the next summer because of it!"

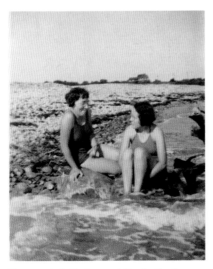

FIGURE 2.5: Esther and Ruth, Rockport, Massachusetts, near where she worked.

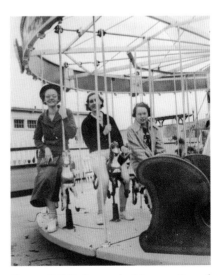

FIGURE 2.6: Esther on the Merry-go-Round at Nantasket Beach, Massachusetts, 1937.

29

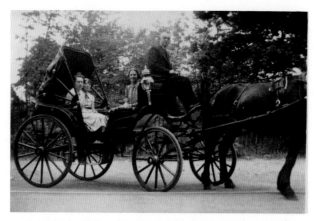

FIGURE 2.7: Esther and Ruth in Carriage on Mt. Royal, 1937.

Although Esther attended the senior prom in 1938, she was *not sure with whom*! She bought her dress in Filene's Basement in Boston for $5. Evidencing Esther's typical recall for detail, she remembered that it was a dress that had a white top connected to a black full skirt. In a yet another effort to save every penny possible, Esther kept that dress to wear to a Tufts party event decades later.

It was in her senior year the opportunity was presented to Esther to live with associate professor of English, Miss Myra Coffin Holbrook, who began teaching at Simmons in 1905.

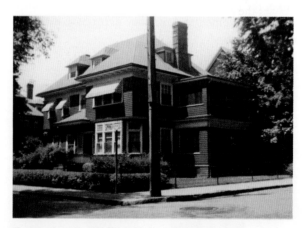

FIGURE 2.8: Dr. Holbrook's home where Esther worked while attending Simmons.

Esther slept in the front parlor room in exchange for *preparing her breakfast, polishing silver, and other small jobs*. Esther's studies were intense in her final year in the science program, which required hours of studying. This arrangement provided time for Esther to study at the library at Simmons, as well as Massachusetts College of Pharmacy (MCP) (to which she walked from Simmons, passing Boston Latin School, the first public school in the United States), and Harvard University. It was a long walk up the stairs to the top floor of Professor Holbrook's home. Esther called her *an interesting woman*, and she *learned a lot from her* (although Esther admitted she didn't like polishing silver). The 1938 Simmons yearbook, the *Microcosm*, was dedicated to Miss Holbrook. As was the custom, students asked professors and students to sign their yearbooks as graduation time neared. Ms. Holbrook's inscription to Esther read, "In memory of a year with a very pleasant and helpful housemate: Myra Coffin Holbrook."

Because she had no dinner privileges at Simmons, Esther often ate her evening meal at Sparr's Drug, which was, until 2008, on the corner of Longwood Avenue and Huntington Avenue, near MCP (later named Massachusetts College of Pharmacy and Health Sciences [MCPHS]), where the Esther M. Wilkins Clinic is now located, just a short walk from Simmons. Sparr's had a counter and a few tables, and Esther could have a meatloaf dinner with mashed potatoes for 35 cents. On several occasions later in her life, when visiting MCPHS, Esther fondly recalled her time at Simmons and Sparr's.

Included in the *Microcosm* were senior class pictures, group pictures of all the classes, club information, and sayings that were included for each graduating student. Everyone who knew Esther well realized that she would never part with her copy of her Simmons yearbook from 1938. She knew exactly where it was located in her apartment, despite the array of journals, boxes of articles, and piled up proofs.

Baccalaureate Service was on Sunday, June 12, 1938, at the auditorium, Riverway, in which seniors dressed in graduation gowns, followed by a reception by President Beatley for alumnae, seniors, and friends in South Hall. The Commencement of 1938, Simmons College, took place at Symphony Hall on Monday, June 13, 1939, at 11 AM, followed by a luncheon for seniors at the refectory.

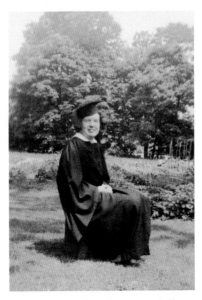

FIGURE 2.9: Esther, Simmons College graduation, 1938.

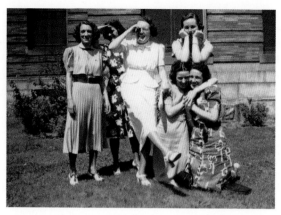

FIGURE 2.10: Esther and Simmons classmates, 1938.

The science preparation was excellent at Simmons, as Esther had

all the pre-requisite science classes I would later need for application to dental school. I didn't have to repeat any of the pre-requisites that others did, even though I was a little rusty. Chemistry was the toughest course for her, *but my classmates helped me!*

Classmate Catherine McCarthy Murphy related,

❝ Then came senior year. After we received our caps and gowns we wore them to classes! Everyone was looking for work and in 1938 jobs were scarce. Esther continued her education at Forsyth and I at BU. Esther, my other Simmons friends, and I were BIG TREND SETTERS. At that time most people and particularly women did not go to college. But we did!"

Esther was close friends with two alumni, Barbara Jasper Bales and Doris Larson Spiegel, with whom she corresponded for over 75 years. One summer, Esther and Barbara Jasper, who majored in English at Simmons, took a room for a week and biked on Nantucket, and another summer, they took their bikes on a train north to New Hampshire. *I had my father's antique bike and it was safe to sleep on the beach back then. We had stuff on our bikes to sleep on.* During one of their beach adventures on the North Shore, after sleeping on the beach, Esther took her glasses off. Then she broke the glasses and according to Esther, *had to bike home blind!*

Esther's career began at Simmons College, which she considered her roots. She spoke fondly of her experience as an undergraduate and of Simmons' influence on her accomplishments since graduation in 1938. Esther recalled with pride that *it all started at Simmons* and made special note of Dr. Hilliard, who inspired her on the subject of dental hygiene. Esther recalled approaching Dr. Hilliard to *find out more about how dental hygienists were educated.* This discussion launched the beginnings of her career.

When asked about her experiences at Simmons that she valued the most, she replied, *The friends I made and the doors to graduate school that Simmons opened.* She remained active in the alumni association, served as a class officer for 5 years, and in 1963 became the organization's 50th anniversary president. She had her 70th reunion in 2008, and six classmates were able to attend. Esther was the honoree at the Simmons Biology Symposium in 2011 and was the class agent for the Class of 1938 until 2013.

Esther enjoyed the long relationships she had with classmates, and she never failed to recognize the inspiration Simmons has had for her to achieve such significant results. She remembered her professors and the details of the curriculum, the values instilled by the College, and especially the emphasis placed on the potential greatness of its students.

During my senior year I began to realize that I didn't like the options I would have for using my sciences after commencement. The graduates of that major did a variety of types of hospital, research, or other clinical laboratory work; they could teach science in schools; and a few went on to obtain higher degrees. Esther later commented, *By my senior year I didn't know if I liked the available options, but I knew Simmons girls always were prepared to make a living.*

We only had one credit of elective courses each semester. For the spring semester elective of my senior year, I chose a once-a-week lecture program called "public health." The professor, Prof. Hilliard, was a public health official in a town outside Boston and gave us an overall picture of what public health included. One period he spent describing personnel, including sanitation engineers, public health physicians, nurses, dentists, and mentioned dental hygienists briefly. He described them in relation to dentists, even as registered nurses were related to medical doctors. After class I went up and asked him where dental hygienists went to school. He looked at me as though I were from Mars!! Then he asked if I didn't know where the Forsyth Dental Infirmary was located, just around the Fenway a short distance from Simmons College.

At lunch time that day, a nice spring day in March, I decided to walk around and find the Forsyth building. When I got there, a beautiful marble building, the big front doors were open wide to let in the nice spring air. I went in and asked at the reception switchboard if I could see someone about the program for dental hygienists. The lady said, "Oh there's no one here. They are all on spring break. Come back next week."

The next week, Esther *went into the large, bright clinic, with little children's chairs. I saw the teachers' caps with purple bands and all the students had white dresses, shoes, and hose. I was smitten! When I tell that story, I often end by saying, what if I hadn't gone back the next week, and made that second walk around the Fenway?*

In an interview with Julie Flaherty from Tufts many years later, Esther described how she had *never met a dental hygienist before, but something about it appealed to me.* Those who submitted stories to this biography wondered what the profession of dental hygiene would have been like without Esther Wilkins. As Mary Dole, very close friend of Esther Wilkins, wrote:

❝ What if Esther hadn't thought of dental hygiene as an interesting second career? Just think about what that walk to 140 The Fenway did for her, for us, and for dental hygiene and dentistry."

CHAPTER 3

Forsyth Training School for Dental Hygienists

Forsyth was built "for the children of Boston."

Forsyth School for Dental Hygienists began as the Training School for Dental Hygienists in September of 1916 (the year Esther was born), with the enrollment of "a small group of women who became dental hygienists, specializing in prevention, prophylaxis, and student education" (Millstein, 2002, p. 13). It was almost 2 years after the 1914 opening and dedication of the Forsyth Dental Infirmary for Children in Boston.

The cornerstone of the Forsyth Infirmary for Children, the first institution of its kind in the world, was placed on June 4, 1912. It is built with Vermont white/gray marble, with fountains, pathways, and landscaped grounds and was located near Fenway Park and the Museum of Fine Arts. In 1914, the infirmary was "dedicated to the children" (Brown, 1952, p. 10).

"The object of this is to care for children with defective teeth, adenoids and diseased tonsils, so that when they reach the age of sixteen years they shall be in good physical condition" (Taylor, 1922, p. 203). Esther stated, *local dentists volunteered time for providing care for the children. Eventually, Forsyth became a renowned clinic where intern-dentists from dental schools all over the world were trained in pediatric dentistry and orthodontics.* The poor or moderately circumstanced children of Boston now had an opportunity for proper dental care and education. "The new clinic was charged with providing complete oral therapy for children, with an emphasis on prevention of dental cavities (Forsyth Institute, 2014b, p. 1).

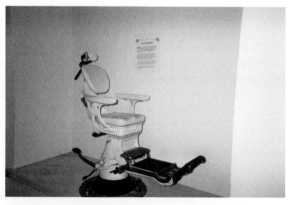

FIGURE 3.1: Children's chair.

Director of the infirmary and chief of dental staff during Esther's Forsyth year was Percy R. Howe. Brown (1952) called Howe "some kind of unusual person, with unusual background and training" (p. 33) and with an ever-inquisitive mind in refining studies of microorganisms associated with dental caries, in opening new avenues of study by questioning and researching and reading, by spreading his knowledge and influence around the globe, and by collaborative efforts in thinking and understanding. Esther was destined to do the same.

‪ FORSYTH TRAINING SCHOOL FOR ‪ DENTAL HYGIENISTS

The Forsyth brothers, founders of the Forsyth Institute, had sought quality dental care and established the Training School for Dental Hygienists in 1916 (later renamed the Forsyth-Tufts Training School for Dental Hygienists in 1919) (see Appendix E, accessed via the online e-book). This occurred after Massachusetts legalized the practice of dental hygiene in 1915. The first director was Dr. Harold DeWitt Cross. The first graduating class was in September 1917, with 13 hygienists receiving diplomas. The first meeting of the Forsyth Training School for Dental Hygienists was held on January 15, 1918, at the Forsyth Infirmary for Children (Forsyth, 1918, p. 285)

As the second oldest and the longest continuously operated dental hygiene program in the United States, Forsyth has served as a national model for other programs. According to Northeastern University Libraries (2004), "from 1917 to 1950, a one-year course (certificate) was offered to students. In 1947, the Council on Dental Education of the American Dental Association established a two-year minimum requirement for dental hygiene education that included academic courses" (p. 2).

In 1948, the school entered into an affiliation with Tufts University whereby through the College of Special Programs, Tufts University faculty taught courses in the 2-year degree programs at Forsyth, as students were bussed to the Medford campus. They were later affiliated with Northeastern University in 1964 where students could choose a 2-year or 4-year program. In 2002, the Forsyth program was acquired by Massachusetts College of Pharmacy and Health Sciences University (MCPHS), located a short distance from the building on the Fenway. It is now identified as Forsyth School of Dental Hygiene at MCPHS, where several different degree options in dental hygiene are now offered. According to MCPHS President Charles F. Monahan, Jr., the addition of the dental hygiene program expanded "the college's range of health science degree programs. The agreement brings together two historic institutions" (MCPHS, 2002, p. 14) (see Chapter 11, accessed via the online e-book).

The Forsyth building was sold by the Forsyth Institute in 2007 to the Museum of Fine Arts in Boston. Dr. Dominick P. DePaola, president and CEO of the Forsyth Institute, said, "It is fitting that this Boston landmark will be sold to another organization with longstanding ties to the Fenway. The Museum of Fine Arts shares Forsyth's historic commitment to the City of Boston and we are happy that this building will continue to serve as a resource for the community" (Forsyth, 2007, p. 1). Now located at 245 First

Street in Cambridge, "Forsyth is the world's leading independent research organization dedicated to improving oral health, and reducing interrelated systemic diseases and conditions" (Forsyth, 2014c, p. 1).

Esther as a Student at Forsyth

Forsyth Training School for Dental Hygienists had been educating dental hygienists for practice for over 22 years when Esther Mae Wilkins, bachelor's degree in general science in hand, enrolled in the school's 1-year (11-month) dental hygiene program on September 19, 1938. From that day forward, the profession of dental hygiene changed forever, especially by students who would follow in her footsteps.

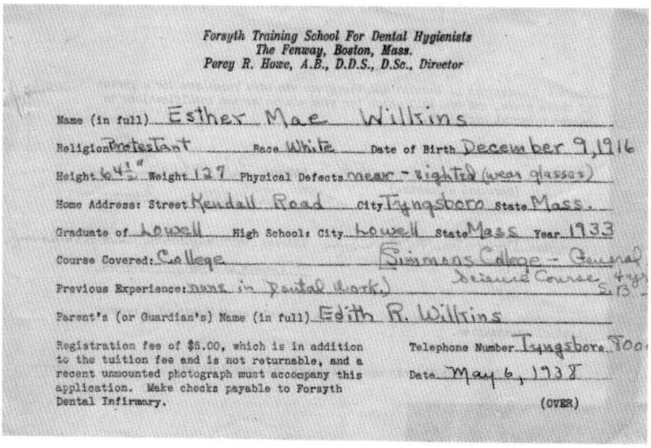

Forsyth Training School For Dental Hygienists
The Fenway, Boston, Mass.
Percy R. Howe, A.B., D.D.S., D.Sc., Director

Name (in full) Esther Mae Wilkins
Religion Protestant Race White Date of Birth December 9, 1916
Height 64½" Weight 127 Physical Defects near-sighted (wear glasses)
Home Address: Street Kendall Road City Tyngsboro State Mass.
Graduate of Lowell High School: City Lowell State Mass Year 1933
Course Covered: College Simmons College - General Science Course, 4 yrs S.B.
Previous Experience: none in Dental work.)
Parent's (or Guardian's) Name (in full) Edith R. Wilkins

Registration fee of $6.00, which is in addition to the tuition fee and is not returnable, and a recent unmounted photograph must accompany this application. Make checks payable to Forsyth Dental Infirmary.

Telephone Number Tyngsboro 100
Date May 6, 1938
(OVER)

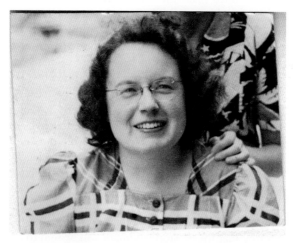

Figure 3.2: Esther's application to the Forsyth Training School for Dental Hygienists.

Figure 3.3: Esther, 1939.

Esther attended on a full tuition scholarship. In July 1938, students received notices of acceptance and in August became, according to the class history, the "proud owners of our probation uniforms" (Forsyth Training School for Dental Hygienists, 1939, p. 31). Two days after the first class, there was a hurricane: September 21, 1938. According to the National Weather Service (n.d.), it was "one of the most destructive and powerful storms ever to strike Southern New England" (p. 1). Winds clocked at 100 mph, boats were torn from moorings, the Constitution was tossed against the dock, rainfall caused significant flooding, Boston Common and the Public Garden suffered lost trees, and 685 people lost their lives. Many students could not get to class, and when they did arrive back to class, *there was a row of poplars, lying flat, like a row of dominoes, at least 6.*

One of the first classmates Esther met at Forsyth was Barbara L. Wilson, who related,

“ On my first day of class (September 19, 1938) at Forsyth, students were assigned seats in the lecture hall alphabetically. That was my good fortune, as Wilkins and Wilson sat side by side for the year. It was the beginning of a long friendship with Esther Wilkins. At that time Esther had her degree from Simmons and I was a young, shy, quiet person. I was in awe of her! But soon she became my mentor and I followed her directions and took on her interest in education.”

Barbara also recalled how Esther would climb over her every morning and "usually landed on my clean, white shoes!" Esther said that at that point in her life, *Barbara lived in the country and didn't know much about life.*

When Barbara later began as professor and department chair at the University of Rhode Island, she told her students that Esther Wilkins was her classmate at Forsyth, and they "would be overcome! Of course, we used her book and invited her to be a lecturer. It pleased them to talk with her." Barbara believed her success working in the dental field "was entirely due to the influence and association I had with Esther and our belief in education."

The grading system ranged from 0 to 100 for each course. The 11-month curriculum at Forsyth in 1939–1940 included the following courses:

Aseptic Technology	Dental Anatomy	Pathology
Anatomy	Anesthesiology	Bacteriology
Otology	Orthodontics	Oral Surgery and Pathology
Chemistry	Prosthetics	Pharmacology
Physical Chemistry	Histology	X-ray
Nutrition	Physiology	Common Diseases
First Aid		

On the first day back to Forsyth after the holiday break, January 9, 1939, Esther and her classmates received their caps, "a badge of honor which seemed to be the answer to all our ambitions" (Forsyth Training School for Dental Hygienists, 1939, p. 31).

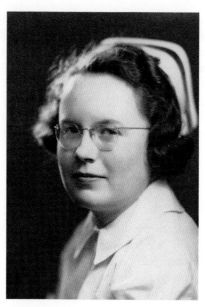

FIGURE 3.4: Esther in cap.

In the spring, Science and Literature was the early class. The school's director was Alice Leggat, RDH, a 1927 graduate, who was well liked and considered an understanding and skilled administrator who had "the difficult and seemingly unaccomplishable task of cor-relating the factual knowledge for a group of future Dental Hygienists" (Forsyth Training School for Dental Hygienists, 1939, p. 5). She left the year Esther graduated, and the year-book was dedicated to her. Esther held Director Howe in extremely high regard, *though the students didn't see him much.* The assistant supervisor was Forsyth graduate, Ethel E. Young, a close friend and confidante of Esther's and class advisor. She was one of 37 lecturers and instructors at Forsyth the year Esther attended. The day was full, with classes from 9 AM to noon and from 1:00 to 4:00 PM, with an occasional half day on Saturday. The students worked in the clinic with children when not attending classes. Beverly Whitford reminded that in those days at Forsyth, as in hers in the late 1950s, "dental hygienists were not allowed to scale below the gum line. We were indeed providing a 'dental manicure.'"

Esther recalled her days at Forsyth:

The children were called by groups to the clinic upstairs. They passed through the turnstile and deposited a nickel (later a dime) before going into the big beautiful high-ceilinged clinic where child-sized dental chairs lined the area adjacent each of the tall windows. A notable feature of the clinic was the multi-faucet sinks in the middle of the clinic where the dental hygiene students scrubbed their hands. Each faucet was turned on by a knee-activated device, clearly a forerunner of the modern infection control system. (From Esther's *Reminiscences Forsyth*)

During her year at Forsyth, Esther lived on the corner of 416 Marlborough Street in Boston in a small room, which she rented in exchange for tending the switchboard.

There were professional offices in the main part of the building, where upon completing classes and arriving home, Esther would take messages that came in after hours from patients. On her rare evenings off, she occasionally went to the movies at the Uptown Theatre, which showed the news in addition to two major movies; you could stay as long as you wanted. While most of her free time consisted of studying rigorously, she was still able to maintain some social life with her classmates.

The Class of 1939 attended the 75th Dental Convention held at the Hotel Statler (now Park Plaza) in Boston, where they registered in full uniform. "Crisply starched caps and uniforms certainly added an air of hospitality, meriting a fine reputation for Forsyth" (*The Forsythian*, 1938, p. 31).

The Class of 1939 also had the privilege of being the first class of the Forsyth Training School for Dental Hygienists to become junior members of the American Dental Hygienists' Association (ADHA). The members of this class took the state boards in June and graduated on July 28, 1939. Little did Esther realize the later impact that the ADHA would have on her life and she on the Association for over 75 years.

Forsyth's first yearbook, the *Forsythian*, was published in 1920. Esther ("Wilkie") was editor of the yearbook for 1938–1939, with Hilda Mandell as assistant editor.

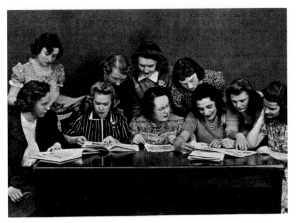

FIGURE 3.5: *Forsythian* Yearbook Staff 1939. Esther is front row center.

Keeping with the tradition of the day, classmates signed the yearbooks of their classmates. Esther's yearbook as one might expect contained some particularly standout quotes. One entry written by Etta Murgida read "Esther—the girl who always made it, no matter how late she came in!" and from Hilda Mandell "Wilkie, dear, you are the only girl of the class whose motto will ever be: veni vidi vici" (I came, I saw, I conquered). Esther would indeed persist, especially when it came to making her mark on the profession of dental hygiene.

Janet Clarke Lorman, Esther's first cousin and one of the "girls" from Tyngsborough, recalled, "When Esther graduated from Forsyth [in] '39, I was only 7 ½ years old. My mother loved Esther, and Esther was my mother's most favorite niece. As I was growing up my mother kept telling me I was going to be a dental hygienist. I didn't know what a dental hygienist was, and I didn't know how to spell it."

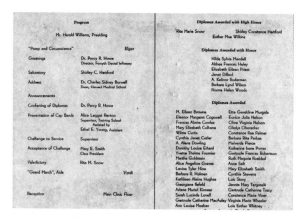

FIGURE 3.6: Forsyth graduation program, 1939.

Esther's friend Rita Marie Snow had straight *A*'s and was honored as valedictory (now referred to as valedictorian), and Shirley Hartford served as salutatory (now called salutatorian). The 26th graduating class from Forsyth Training School for Dental Hygienists held commencement exercises on July 28, 1939. Greetings were provided by Dr. Percy R. Howe, director, Forsyth Dental Infirmary, who also conferred diplomas. The commencement speaker was Dr. Charles Sidney Burwell, dean, Harvard Medical School. The program also included presentation of cap bands by Alice Leggat Renton RDH, supervisor, Training School, assisted by Ethel E. Young, followed by challenge to service by supervisor and acceptance of challenge in behalf of the graduating class by Mary E. Smith, president of the class. After walking in the "grand march" to Verdi's Aida, the graduates convened for a reception in the main clinic floor.

Esther graduated from Forsyth in 1939. She was very happy with her achievement and those of her classmates. Esther's grades resulted in her achieving high honors at the completion of the 11-month certificate program, with an average of 92.8, third in the class. Out of the 19 courses, she earned a perfect grade (100) in 6 of them: Physical Chemistry, Prosthetics, Physiology, Bacteriology, Pharmacology, and X-ray. Esther remembers *not doing that well in first aid!* It wasn't until she was in her 90s that Esther learned the grades she earned at Forsyth.

On July 12, 1939, Esther received notification:

❝ It is my duty to inform you that you have successfully passed your examination as a dental hygienist. This means that you may now practice dental hygiene in the State of Massachusetts, subject to such rules and regulations as may be adopted by the Board of Dental Examiners."

Classmate, Rita Snow, said that after graduation they went their separate ways, but she still kept in touch with Esther, including meetings, conventions, and continuing education courses "because Esther expected me to be there!" Rita knew Esther for over 70 years and remembered, "At the time we attended Forsyth, we had courses of various lengths throughout the year. When we would finish one subject, for example, anatomy, we would have the final exam for that. After each final, Esther and I would 'celebrate' by having English muffins and tea. I don't remember the name of the restaurant where we did all this, but I am betting Esther will remember." Just before Rita passed away in 2009, Esther spoke of her:

We do keep in touch and see one another when we can. I am honored to be her friend.

One particularly memorable story as told by Caren Barnes described a later-in-life meeting with one of Esther's faculty members from the 1938–1939 academic year.

" One of the first people whom I had met in Birmingham when I began to teach at U. Alabama was Louise W. Hord, RDH, who had retired to Birmingham after serving on the faculty of the Forsyth School of Dental Hygienists for over 40 years. [Louise had worked with Dr. Alfred Fones and had also taught Esther Wilkins in dental hygiene school]. When Esther came to Birmingham to present a continuing education program course, our dental hygiene faculty took Esther and Louise to dinner. What an historic moment this was for us. Of course, our wheels were turning—just how old were these two? The time we spent with them was surreal. There were these two pioneers of our profession interacting as though they were in their twenties and not a day had passed since they last saw each other. It was a special moment in time!"

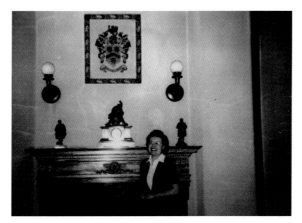

FIGURE 3.7: Esther in front of Founders Room, Forsyth Institute, 1945.

Esther's had a lifelong connection and commitment to Forsyth. She supported the institution through donations and served as adjunct clinical professor from 1973 to 1995 and staff dentist (supervising clinical dentist, 12 day each week). She made presentations to the students at the clinic on the topic of anesthesia. When Esther was a student, dental hygienists could not administer anesthesia to patients.

As she continued to present lectures and attend events at Forsyth (now Forsyth School of Dental Hygiene at MCPHS), she grew even more fond of the bond she had with dental hygiene students who were about to enter the profession. She stayed connected with many of her classmates from Forsyth and looked forward to many reunions over the years as an active alumnus, alumni officer, and often spearhead of the events.

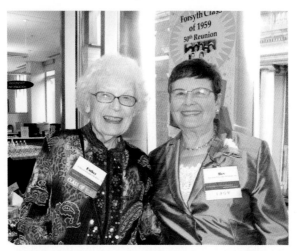

FIGURE 3.8: Forsyth reunion, 2009, Esther and Beverly Whitford.

CHAPTER 4

The Early Professional Years: Manchester-by-the-Sea

But the same tides flow;
And the same stars glow;
And the waves sing the same wild glee.
Just the same the seabirds' screech,
And the shining singing beach
Takes the kisses of the same old sea.

(From "The Same Tides Flow," called the Manchester Hymn by
N. B. Sargent, 1895, as cited in Lamson, 1895, p. 382;
Town of Manchester-by-the-Sea, 2017).

After Esther graduated from Forsyth, she began her professional dental hygiene career in the small town of Manchester-by-the-Sea, Massachusetts, a beautiful coastal community 25 miles north of Boston on Cape Ann, 18.2 square miles (9.2 land, 9.0 water), rich in history, originally a small fishing village.

Manchester-by-the-Sea became a popular location for society (from Boston; Washington, DC; New York City; and others) for summer residencies where they built summer estate cottages. Unique tourist attractions include Eaglehead rock composite, Singing Beach, Smith's Point, and Coolidge Reservation, a nature preserve.

Louise Hord, the director of the Forsyth School, had set up different interviews for Esther. When she interviewed with Dr. Frank Willis, a general practitioner and dentist in Manchester, Esther said she wasn't even sure how to answer the question of what she thought she would be doing in the position, although she knew she wanted to work with an independent practitioner. She briefly considered enlisting into the navy as World War II had broken out; however, she was not accepted due to her nearsighted vision, resulting in wearing glasses. She said the services were *fussy back then on whom they took*. Later in the war when there was a shortage, they relaxed their policies, but Esther had already invested in her commitment to working with Dr. Willis's practice. Dr. Willis had interviewed several dental hygienists before offering her the position. *He must have liked me more than the others.* Ultimately, she accepted the position *due to the location and its beauty.*

Esther began practicing in Dr. Willis's office as a full-time dental hygienist on November 13, 1939. She practiced there until 1945, living at 6 Lincoln Street, which faced the ocean across the street.

A dental hygienist had already been in practice with him for over 16 years when I started with Dr. Frank Willis in Manchester-by-the-Sea, Massachusetts, soon after my Forsyth graduation. The faithful group of patients were well-settled into their 3 or 6-months' maintenance programs. They had retained their teeth with many amalgam and gold restorations along with the careful scaling by the dental hygienist. Patients were all in really good shape—Dr. Willis didn't have an extraction to do once in a blue moon [sic]*—practically none on those regular patients who came on plan. The early practice specified no instrumentation under 2 millimeters below the gum-line, but of course we had been taught to take off all the calculus and really 'clean' and polish the teeth.*

Just think of the many millions of teeth those old-time classic dental hygiene practitioners saved.

Dr. Willis graduated from Tufts Dental School in 1912. He had been in the service during World War I, and when he arrived home from Europe in the early 20s, he *hunted around for a town* to set up his practice. Esther recalled, *fascinating to think so far back!*

Dr. Willis was in general private practice and provided dental services all year round. Four mornings per week during the school year, Esther and Dr. Willis walked to the local public middle school, which had a two-chair dental clinic in the attic, and treated the children in Grades 1 to 8 with a preventive orientation. Esther remembered *doing a lot of walking and climbing during those years.*

Dr. Willis had one dental chair for his dental practice, and Esther had one in the next room. She scheduled the adult patients every hour on the hour. Sometimes her responsibilities included answering the telephone, and since there were few rules back then for infection control, Esther doesn't recall whether she washed her hands before doing so. "Instruments were sterilized using boiling water, which seems funny to us now" (Esther, as cited in Gladstone & Garcia, 2007, p. 14). One of Esther's patients was Dr. Willis's son, Sonny. When he was a child, Dr. Willis had a difficult time getting him to go to the dental hygienist. Esther remembered when Henry was a teenager, he sometimes came to her right off the beach, *barefoot and in swim trunks.* When she passed a patient when walking to the grocery store, she did not mind at all when they asked, "Esther, what time is my appointment on Monday?"

As Julie Flaherty (2012) related as she discussed with Esther her long career that as much as she liked Manchester, she wasn't drawn to private practice.

Not that I didn't have idealism about how it should be. Dr. Willis gave me a wide background on how you can have a little practice in a little town and do a lot for a lot of people (p. 28).

Dr. Willis held a special place for Esther in her heart. She learned a great deal from working with him, especially with regard to the personal relationships he cultivated with his patients. Many of Esther's patients came for a checkup every 6 months, and some as frequently as every 4 months. *I was brought up right from Forsyth on what good regular attention should and could do.*

The memories she had of those days held *warm feelings for her,* and she said her patients were very proud to have their mouths healthy. Dr. Willis adhered to a philosophy that Esther considered to be well before its time. He had a small community practice and treated all the children, and he was *conscientious, honest, devoted, sincere, and hard-working.* Esther recalled with pride that

All the kids who lived in that town all their lives went on to high school from our clinic with all their own teeth. We just about never extracted anything except for the kids who moved in when they were older. I grew up in dentistry with a beautiful concept of preventative dental care—and how it can really be done. Dr. Willis planted the seed for me, and I have eternally been for preventive dentistry.

During her first year in Manchester, Esther rented a room, and the following year she shared an apartment with the school nurse, where they occupied the first floor of a big white house and each had their own rooms. They were both independent people and went their own ways after the year.

Also in that first year in Manchester, Esther met her first official and serious boyfriend. His name was Robert Colburn, and he was originally from Chelmsford, which is near Esther's hometown. Although Esther did not expand on her relationship with Robert, she said he *did bags for guests* at the Inn.

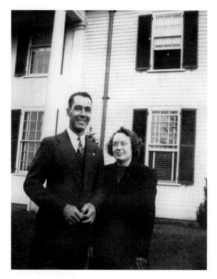

FIGURE 4.1: Esther and Robert Colburn, 1939.

In a letter dated 1983, Mae Saco, who worked in the bank in Manchester when Esther practiced dental hygiene with Dr. Willis, said,

❝ We have been friends for quite a while. How nice you still get *The Cricket*; it keeps you in touch with the town doings."

Esther decided to take a trip all by herself to New York City to attend the World's Fair of 1939–1940. The New York City subway cost was a nickel, and the Fair itself cost 75 cents to enter. Esther stayed in a hotel right in Times Square, and she remembered that trip in all its detail for the rest of her life: the hotel, the Futurama exhibit, and the adventure of travelling alone as a young woman.

Esther described her 6 years as a practicing dental hygienist in Manchester as *enjoyable*, although World War II was taking place.

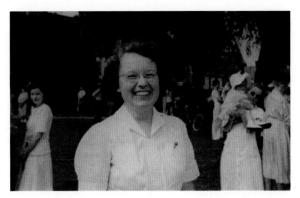

FIGURE 4.2: Civil Defense Parade, 1942.

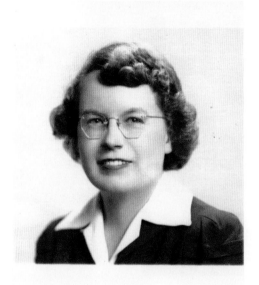

FIGURE 4.3: Professional photo, 1942.

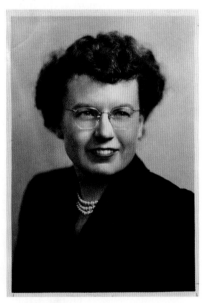

FIGURE 4.4: Professional photo, 1943.

Several lifelong relationships were made in Manchester-by-the-Sea, and Esther remained connected with them throughout her life. Esther met one of her closest friends, Deb Younger, whom she met at the local bank where she worked. Esther met another close friend, Trudy Sinnett, through Massachusetts Dental Hygienists' Association (MDHA), who became a strong advocate and supporter of Esther's career.

Together, Esther, Deb, and Trudy called themselves "The Three Musketeers" and spent endless hours with one another biking, beaching (including Esther's favorite, Singing Beach), and enjoying all that Manchester had to offer. Esther fondly remembered her *days off* and the parties on Singing Beach. Deb's bank director *took the bank people out boating* and Esther came along. Going to the beach as often as she could, she later shared, *see the freckles on my arm? That's from all the time I spent on the beach during my Manchester years.*

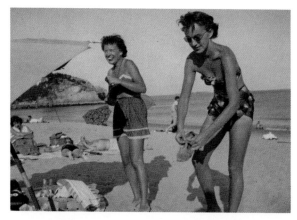

FIGURE 4.5: Two of the musketeers, 1942.

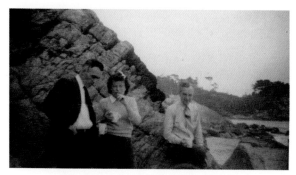

FIGURE 4.6: Esther on Singing Beach with friends, 1940s.

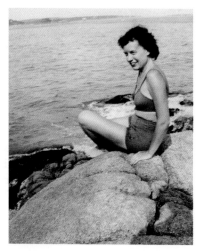

FIGURE 4.7: Esther on Singing Beach rock, 1942.

During Esther's tenure in Dr. Willis's dental office, she remained active in dental hygiene organizations, including MDHA.

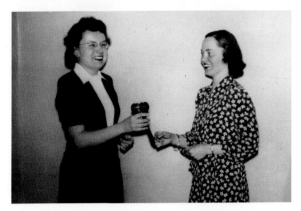

FIGURE 4.8: Esther's installation as president of Massachusetts Dental Hygiene Association, 1944.

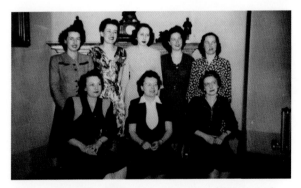

FIGURE 4.9: Officers. Massachusetts Dental Hygienists' Association, President of Massachusetts Dental Hygienists' Association, 1944.

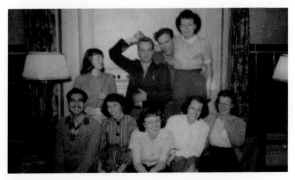

FIGURE 4.10: Esther with friends, Spring 1945.

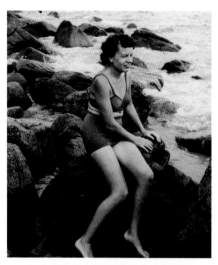

Figure 4.11: Esther, Manchester-by-the-Sea, 1945.

One summer during her Manchester days, Esther and Simmons friend Barbara Jasper took a room for a week on Nantucket and *spent their time biking for the most part.* During another summer, they took their bikes on a train north to New Hampshire.

In later years, after Esther and Trudy had left Manchester to attend school in Boston, Deb visited her two friends frequently. One of the most memorable adventures they had was to the Opera House in Boston to see

> *Swan Lake, sitting way up high where they could hardly hear the music and the people on stage appeared as though they were an inch tall. The dancers were like tiny toys way down there on the stage.*

The Three Musketeers went to the theater together as well, where they sat in the second balcony due to Esther's budget. They saw *My Fair Lady, Oklahoma,* and *other famous openings.* Trudy and Esther had a strong influence on one another, and while Trudy referred to Esther as her mentor, Esther contended it was Trudy who was in fact her own mentor. Debbie and Esther were equally involved and were glued to one another when back in Manchester for summer and holiday vacations. Their adventures took place many years ago, but they made such a strong impression that Esther remembered them fondly:

> *What a memory it was for me!*

The old Opera House in Boston was torn down during Esther's 12 years in Seattle. *I surely missed it when I got back!* Deb eventually left the Manchester bank and commuted daily to Boston. She joined the staff as office manager in Dr. J. Murray Gavel's dentist office, where Trudy was the dental hygienist. Sadly, both friends passed away several years ago, but their memories remained quite vivid for Esther as the surviving musketeer until her own passing in 2016.

When asked her reason for no longer practicing dental hygiene and leaving Manchester-by-the-Sea, Esther claimed, *I guess I just wanted something more.* In an interview with Esther in 1999, Wolff wrote, "One summer, a college girlfriend who had become a physician visited and urged Wilkins to go to dental school. *It sounded like a good idea*" (p. 17). Esther had practiced as a dental hygienist full-time for 6 years; her thirst for knowledge and passion for the industry, as well as her friends and colleagues, urged her to take another step forward. Later in her career, 1977, at a presentation she made at the Northeastern Vermont Regional Hospital, she reflected on the rationale for her decision:

> *I was a dental hygienist first you know. I became a dentist because at that time in the field you were more limited than you are now. I wanted to do more. So I became a dentist. The field of dental hygiene is more complete now* (Esther Wilkins, as cited in Gowan, 1977, p. 1).

When Esther decided to advance her education and move forward in her professional life by attending dental school, she had the burden of informing Dr. Willis she had to move on from his practice. *He practically blew the roof off.* She continued to practice part-time with Dr. Willis during her 4 years at dental school, summers, and vacations, staying with friends in Manchester. Dr. Willis needed her to stay in that capacity for the support she provided and the extent to which his patients loved her. Esther's view was *he was helping me, you see. He was allowing me to have my position with him to earn money for dental school.* After Esther graduated from Tufts, "he hired a dental hygienist within a matter of weeks (Flaherty, 2012, p. 3). It was then she realized he didn't have trouble hiring a dental hygienist after all; he just wanted Esther to continue. Jean Clooney (Forsyth, '49) replaced Esther in Dr. Willis's office.

They say you never can go back, but in Esther's case, you can indeed. A visit back to Manchester-by-the-Sea in 2008 brought back fond memories for Esther, of the town, the people, Singing Beach, and her first practice as a dental hygienist.

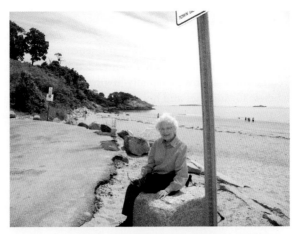

FIGURE 4.12: Esther returns to Singing Beach, 2008.

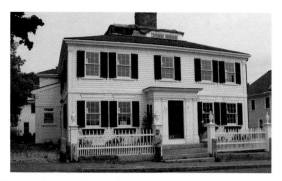

FIGURE 4.13: Esther in front of where she lived from 1939 to 1945, in Manchester-by-the-Sea, 2008.

Dr. Willis's daughter, Anne Willis, still lived in the family home, the detached rear building of which housed Dr. Willis's dental practice.

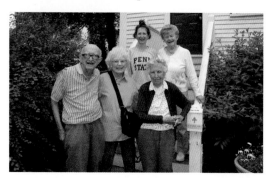

FIGURE 4.14: Dr. Willis's Family, Dr. Willis's Office, 2008.

Although many years had passed, Esther, Anne, and Anne's brother, Sonny, reminisced about those days during Dr. Willis's professional practice when they spent so much time together. After a conversation with Anne in January of 2009, Esther recalled, *we talked for about ¾ of an hour!!! Fun—about old friends.* Esther kept in contact with Anne Willis until she passed away in 2011. It was important for Esther that she return to Manchester to attend Anne's funeral, and she was greeted like a member of the family.

In almost every article that Esther wrote about her life and in almost every interview she gave, she praised Dr. Willis and her positive experience in her first professional position in Manchester-by-the-Sea. According to Ann-Marie DePalma (2002), "Esther wish[ed] that all new dental hygiene graduates could experience practicing with a sincere, honest, and devoted dentist like Dr. Willis, and know what a 'real' dental practice can mean to a community" (p. 1). Dr. Willis was not only Esther's first employer but also her professional hero. As she related to Tonya Smith Ray in 1996,

The clinic was his passion, and preventive dentistry was his concept of practice in an age when extractions were commonplace. He taught me that honest, practical, preventive dentistry is possible (Wilkins, as cited in Ray, 1996, p. 1).

51

CHAPTER 5
Tufts Dental School, 1945–1949

"Thru these portals pass the best dentists in the world."
(*Explorer*, Tufts College Dental School Yearbook, 1949)

TUFTS COLLEGE DENTAL SCHOOL

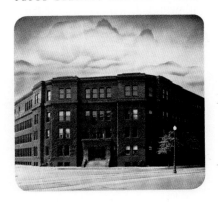

Thru these portals pass
the best dentists in the world

FIGURE 5.1: Tufts Dental College.

When Esther informed her mother she was going back to school, her response was "Oh no, not again!" Esther enjoyed relating this moment and reenacted her mother receiving the news. Her mother, of course, was immediately ready to offer support, which continued until her passing in January of 1946, the week before Esther's end-of-semester examinations at Tufts Dental School.

At the time Esther began pursuing her dental degree in 1945, "the first electronic computer that did not need a roomful of space to operate had just been manufactured" (Bailey, 1999, p. 16). Only 2% of dentists practicing in the United States were women, but Esther said this did not daunt her in the slightest. *I was motivated by my passion for learning. It drove me even further to complete post-graduate specialty training in periodontics.* She remembered her days of dental training with a surgeon's precision, unaware that she would be later called a "pioneer of dental medicine" (Bailey, 1999, p. 16).

My story about being a student at Tufts of Dentistry really starts with my interviews for entrance. I had made an appointment, and at the school I had a brief tour and talked with other professors before my appointment with Dean Basil Bibby. We had already been acquainted during the last few years because of my activities in the Massachusetts Dental Hygienists' Association. Dr. Bibby was very receptive to the application and asked "How do you expect to pay for this?" To this question, I replied that I have some savings and can work as a licensed dental hygienist. I went on to say to him that I knew he had employed a dental hygienist in some of his fluoride research studies and I hoped I might do something like that. He replied that was a possibility. Then he went on to say that he thought it would be better to apply not that fall, because there had been no women applicants for this next beginning class, but there is one woman definitely getting ready for Fall 1945. I decided that would be good and would give me another year to save more money.

I also had planned and made an appointment for an interview at the Harvard Dental School. I met with a very fine professor who politely listened to me as I answered the usual type questions about why I wanted to go to dental school. It was a nice visit which ended when he said very politely there was only one real problem, which was that Harvard had never had a female dental student. He didn't say there never would be, but there was a hidden implication. Fast forward about 70 years to the present when both Tufts and Harvard have over 50 percent of their dental classes who are women.

In 1868, Boston Dental College was established for the purpose of the "advancement of dental art and instruction in it for means of lectures and clinical exercises" (Bacon, 1916, p. 294). In 1899, it "became an incorporate part of Tufts College under a special act of legislature and was then called the Tufts College Dental School" (American Academy of the History of Dentistry, 1970, p. 14). A new curriculum was developed, and the degree awarded "was the Doctor of Dental Medicine (D.M.D,) rather than the Doctorate of Dental Surgery (D.D.S)" (American Academy of the History of Dentistry, 1970, p. 18). In doing

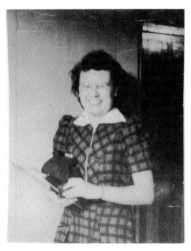

FIGURE 5.2: Esther as freshman, Tufts Dental School, 1945.

so, it "placed American dentistry at the head throughout the world" (Bacon, 1916, p. 295). The dental school on Huntington Avenue was built and opened in 1901 and renamed in 1955 to Tufts University School of Dental Medicine (TUSDM), its current name. (For a complete history of TUSDM, see American Academy of the History of Dentistry, 1970).

Esther began as a dental student at the "old" Tufts College Dental School in 1945 when tuition cost $600 per semester and when the institution was located at the corner of Huntington Avenue and Forsyth Street in Boston.

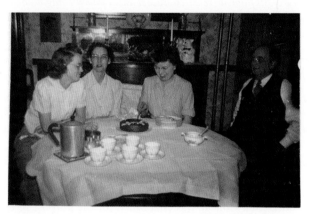

Figure 5.3: Esther celebrating her birthday with friends, December 9, 1945.

That first year I had found a room a few blocks from the dental school. It was a very densely rented place with many single students all using the same bath, but cheap. Come December it turned out to be poorly heated. One Sunday morning I was waiting for Trudy who came into the room, took one look, and said "you aren't staying here." She went to the closet to start grabbing my clothes out to pack to leave. I lived with her the rest of the first year, and was driven to school from Roslindale when she and her father went to work in Boston. The Sinnetts treated me as one of the family. Trudy's kid sister, Edith, sometimes loaned me something to wear, and for Christmas they gave me a skirt with matching bolero jacket and skirt to help keep me in style when an occasion arose.

The second and third years I lived at Norfolk House near Dudley Square. It was a real old community center where there were child and adult afternoon and early evening classes. About 20 students from a wide variety of colleges in Boston lived there. We paid a fee for a cook who made an evening meal.

Our work responsibilities depended on our individual abilities. The art students had art classes. Several students who could be home by the time public schools were out were playground supervisors. Others of us had office watch duties. It was a short walk to Tufts Dental School and so a real big help to me.

Dr. Willis had not been able to find a dental hygienist to replace the full-time position, and I was able to continue to practice there on all vacations and the long holiday weekends. During the summer following my first dental school year, he had taken on an associate dentist, so I had only part-time work at his practice. I also obtained a 6-week fill-in position in Hartford, Connecticut, at a psychiatric hospital. The full-time dental hygienist, Fumiko Saito, was able to have her first real vacation since she graduated from the Forsyth School and was going home to California to see her family.

When I arrived the day before she left, she was busily sewing new clothes to take. For one thing, she had made a beautiful fully-lined black and white checked coat. She was a very talented lady and loved art and music. It turned out to be an enlightening educational experience to practice dental hygiene with carefully guarded patients. We counted the instruments after each appointment. It also led to a lifetime friendship with Fumi Saito who entered my life again when I moved to Seattle, Washington.

❧ THE DENTAL SCHOOL EXPERIENCE ❧

The Class of 1949 started with 49 students, 3 of whom were women. We were a miscellaneous group of veterans, some of whom had been officers, and one who had been a prisoner of war. Others were young people, fresh out of two years of college. Admission required only 2 years at that time.

Starting in October a group of 24 students from Norway joined us. During the occupation of Norway many colleges were closed, and there was a shortage of professional people in the country. Nearly 50 students came to the USA for dentistry, one-half to Tufts and the others to Northwestern in Chicago. They were very studious and with their language difficulties, they had to work hard. One of the men had taught English in Norway, yet we had difficulty understanding his spoken English. They loved our ice cream, a treat that was hard to get and very expensive in Norway.

During the two years that Dr. Bibby was our Dean, I was privileged to participate in his early research testing the use of fluoride for dental caries prevention in children. There were studies in which lead fluoride solution was being compared to sodium fluoride with children in Medford schools.

Another study was with the children at the Perkins School for the Blind in Watertown, where they had a sodium fluoride tablet to chew on a daily basis. Each child came to the small, one-chaired dental clinic for my dental hygiene care. A dentist was there one day every week. He oriented me and told me to keep everything exactly where he did, because the children knew the clinic very well and would enter and go directly to sit in the dental chair when they arrived.

❧ CLASSES AT TUFTS ❧

It was a busy, heavy schedule Monday through Friday and some semesters Saturday morning. Lectures were daily at 8:00 and 4:00 and laboratory classes in the first and most of second year the rest of the time. I hadn't been to school with all that studying for nearly seven years, so some subjects were especially difficult. When I was suffering chemistry that first year, my dear classmate Ruth Lapen (who was young and fresh out of college with her BS degree), was afraid I might flunk out and leave her, so she took it upon herself to tutor me during our lunch hour. She quizzed me over and over and saved me from my fears of that low grade.

There were some of our teachers who were excellent, and I could enjoy learning more about dentistry after my several years practicing dental hygiene. Most of our morning lectures were in a room on the top floor of the old school, so with no elevator we climbed the creaky wooden stairs. One morning we waited nearly 15 minutes, but our professor did not arrive. We groaned and unhappily stomped our way back down. Near the foot of the stairs on the first floor we met Dr. Joseph Volker, who said "Well you are a sad looking group—what happened?" When we told him the professor didn't show up, he said, 'Come on back up, and I'll give you your 4 o'clock lecture now so you can get to go home early.' So back up we climbed. He took nothing with him, such as notes, slides, or other materials, and gave a beautiful lecture with references from the literature. How could he remember all that, I thought, and I later checked some of them in the library to make sure, but they were perfect. He was a remarkable teacher. Over the first 2 years, he taught several of our courses, including preventive dentistry.

*Another of our outstanding professors was Dr. Irving Glickman, who became internationally famous in periodontology. He was **not** noted for being humorous, but on St. Patrick's Day, he appeared for lecture wearing a brilliant green necktie. He walked to the center, put his books down, placed his hands firmly on each side of the bench top, looked up at us with a very serious glare, and announced: 'When in Rome, do as the Romans do.' The class howled with delight.*

There was a group of 3 or 4 very smart and studious men who were in serious competition at the top of the class. One of the examinations in Dr. Volker's preventive dentistry class (which was a favorite subject of mine), was a bluebook essay type, as were many of the examinations in those days. When they were returned, I was pleased to have a high grade. One of those highly competitive students only had a "B" on his paper. When he saw my grade, he wanted to see my paper to compare, and said he had all that same information and was going to see Dr. Volker to complain. He invited me to go with him, which I did. He showed the bluebooks to Dr. Volker, and made his complaint. Dr. Volker sat quietly studying the two bluebooks for a few minutes, and then looked up and said: 'Well, at least I could <u>read</u> Esther's paper!' His handwriting was awful, and I was glad to have turned out the winner!

Among our outside assignments by groups was time at the famous old Boston City Hospital. There I performed my first official tooth extraction. The patient was a skinny little 20-year-old, who was terrified. When I approached her with a smile, she said fearfully, 'Who is going to do it? I quietly said. "I am." Playing on those years of dental hygiene background began to pay off. I was beginning to gain confidence to practice dentistry.

From her early childhood, research and writing seemed to permeate Esther's experiences. Early in her second year at Tufts, October 1946, Esther's curiosity, search for knowledge, and quest to share information resulted in publishing an article in *Tufts Dental Outlook* entitled "Early Tufts Dental School Women Graduates," in which she investigated the women trailblazers at the then Boston Dental School. Little did she know she would top that list a few decades later.

"Lady Dentists" in 1946 are still as much a curiosity as they were when the pioneers started in the late nineteenth century. To be sure, the prejudices and attitudes of the general public

as well as of the male members of the dental profession towards women in this man's world have been altered somewhat since the early days. Women in dentistry may still be on the proving ground, but history shows their progress in making their own place in the dental field, a place which is unparalleled by women in all so-called "men's" professions. Today, about 1.5 percent of the practicing dentists in the United States, and nearly 5 per cent of those in Massachusetts, are women.

The Boston Dental School held its first graduation in 1869 and twenty-one years later graduated its first woman with the Class of 1890. Since that time, between the Boston Dental School and Tufts College Dental School, there have been but fifteen classes with no women.

First mention of a woman applying for admission into the Boston Dental School is found in the old Faculty Meetings' records in the minutes of the secretary, November 12, 1881, and reads as follows:

"A woman having made application for permission to become a student of the college for the present term: on motion of Professor Sharples. Voted—that the Dean be instructed to matriculate any woman as student but first informing her of the inconvenience that may occur to her and the circumstances with which she will be surrounded. On motion of Professor Wetherbee, it was voted that the subject of matriculating women students be laid on the table."

Perhaps the young lady who made the application was duly frightened by such terrifying references to surrounding circumstances and inconveniences. Whatever further action was taken on the matter is not included in these faculty records, but later in November 1887 we find Annie Felton Reynolds matriculating and then graduating with the Class of 1890, our first woman graduate. Dr. Reynolds, of Woburn, Massachusetts was 25 years of age on matriculation and a high school graduate.

The women students of the following year made the Dental School sufficiently co-educational that the Annual Announcement and Catalogue of the Tufts College Dental School for the first six issues read on its cover, "For Men and Women" (WILKINS, 1946, p. 2).

Esther conducted an interview with Dr. Agnes Kelley, Class of 1898, one of the only living women graduates from Tufts College Dental School and who was still practicing dentistry. The remainder of the article detailed other women graduates, including Dr. Jane Bunker, Class of 1904, who practiced orthodontia in New York; Dr. Marion Woodward, Class of 1891; Dr. Mary Gallup, Class of 1893; Dr. Ethel Grant, Class of 1906, who worked with the Red Cross in France during World War I (WWI); Dr. Anna V. Hughes, Class of 1909, who was made director of the Training School for Dental Hygienists at the Forsyth Dental Infirmary and then as director of the School for Dental Hygienists at Columbia University; and Dr. Laura B. Deane, Class of 1917, who

distinguished herself among her associates by serving as President of the Association of American Women Dentists in 1944 through 1946, as well as having been Vice President and President of the Massachusetts Branch of the American Society for Children's Dentistry.

The early women graduates of the Dental School proved their capability for success in dentistry, and secured the respect of all in the dental field. They well serve as an inspiration to all young women who might consider entering the dental profession. (WILKINS, 1946, p. 3).

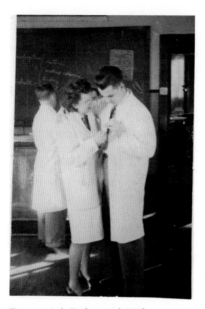

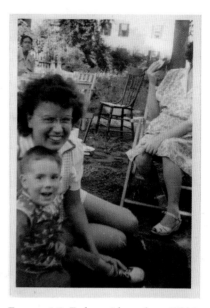

FIGURE 5.4: Esther with Tufts classmates, Biology Lab, 1946.

FIGURE 5.5: Esther with nephew, Rikki, 1946.

Esther's third year at Tufts began in the Fall of 1947.

> *At the start of our third year, Dr. Bibby was invited to become the Director at the Eastman Dental Clinic in Rochester, New York. Dr. Volker became our Dean. Then in our senior year, Dr. Volker was appointed to become the first dean at a new school in Birmingham, Alabama, and left before January. We were the only class in Tufts history to have three deans. And we were the last class to graduate from the "old school" on Huntington Avenue.*

In her third year, Esther published her junior thesis in *The Journal of the American Dental Hygienists' Association*, entitled "A Study of Oral Calculus" (Wilkins, 1948) in which she discussed from a clinical standpoint how calculus is related to all phases of dental care for the health of the oral cavity. She cited Drs. Bibby and Zander (Tufts professors). Of note in this article is Esther's early writing related to systemic influences, a topic she expounded throughout her career. Esther's conclusion in this 1948 article also foreshadowed her emphasis of the importance of reading the research and seeking new techniques: "Needless to mention the extensive research which yet must be done to correlate present knowledge and open new channels of discovery" (Wilkins 1948, p. 93). Esther was also very proud that her name appeared in 1948 as a contributing author in the *Journal of Dental Research*, along with Drs. Bibby, Wellock, Roberts, and Khenkeneurg on the effectiveness of various topical procedures using sodium fluoride and kindred agents:

> *The following year I was at the Eastman Dental Dispensary internship and then moved to Seattle, where I lived for over 12 years before returning to Tufts School of Dental Medicine to enter the graduate program in Periodontology. By that time, 1964, Tufts had*

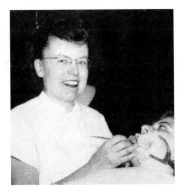

Figure 5.6: Esther with patient, Tufts Dental School, 1948.

moved downtown to Harrison Avenue. A few years later, when Tufts moved to the corner of Washington and Kneeland, the school on Harrison Avenue was now the "old" school, and the Huntington Avenue school became the "old, old" school."

Students were enrolled in seven classes in the first year, six classes in the second year, eight classes in the third year, and nine classes in the fourth year. Grades at Tufts College of Dental Medicine ranged from 100 to 70 (the minimum passing grade). Esther earned excellent grades, a 97 in Public Health and 95 in Dental History in her first year. Many noteworthy dentists were on the faculty at Tufts Dental School during the years Esther attended, including Drs. Volker, Marshall-Day, Christenson, Gavel, Glickman, Spector, and Zander. According to Dr. Robert J. Rudy, "As a student of Tufts College Dental School, from 1945 to 1949, Esther came under the pedagogical influence of Dr. Irving Glickman, the Moses of Periodontology. Dr. Glickman's public health vision for dentistry was the basis of Esther's inspiration. It underpinned her entire teaching career."

Esther attributed at least part of her success as a dental student to Gertrude (Trudy) Sinnett, who would have contributed hundreds of stories about her adventures with Esther through the dental school years, had this biography been written earlier. Trudy was a dental hygienist and practiced with Dr. J. Murray Gavel on Marlborough Street in Boston, who himself had achieved fame in the dental world. Trudy became part of Esther's life very early after Forsyth and was a member of Massachusetts Dental Hygienists' Association (MDHA), where she served on the legislative committee and as first vice president. She and Esther had met during an association (MDHA) meeting. Edna Bradbury, Esther, and Trudy served at the helm of the association for 2 to 3 years. Trudy was president of the Alabama Dental Hygienists' Association and became an associate clinical professor at Forsyth in 1974, and according to Esther, Trudy was *imaginative, ingenious, and had a delightful sense of humor.* Before her death in 1975, Trudy (Gertrude) contributed to *Clinical Practice of the Dental Hygienist* (*CPDH*) by writing Chapter 5, *Chair Positioning,* of the third edition. Esther wrote the obituary for her dear friend.

Esther finally earned her driver's license on June 19, 1948, at age 32 years when she was finishing dental school and was commuting to Rochester, New York, as an intern at Eastman Dental Dispensary. Esther's father tried to teach her to drive, *sitting with his hand on the brake!* Since she wasn't living at home at the time, they *never got practice sessions enough to prepare for the exam.* Her close friend, Trudy, brought her to take the driver's test in Roslindale in 1948 in Trudy's old wood-sided Ford station wagon, as she didn't want Esther driving to Rochester without a license; Esther passed the test the first time, *with only one little thing wrong. The examiner said to take a left, but I took a right!*

Dental school in many ways was an adventure for Esther. Her memories included pleasant as well as challenging ones, which she described as

> *fond and not so fond recollections. The principal lecture hall was on the fourth floor accessible by creaking wooden stairs for our daily 8 o'clock lectures prior to clinic at 9:00 as well as rats that occasionally ran through the locker room.*

One of the greatest challenges Esther faced in her first year was the death of her mother. She passed away in January 1946 in the middle of the week before end-of-semester examinations, so *Esther needed to make up examinations that first term of dental school.*

Esther was active in Tufts activities, having served on the staff of *Explorer* (Tufts yearbook) as managing editor. She also served as secretary of the Robert R. Andrews Society, the purpose of which was to "provide an opportunity for the members to meet and discuss their own endeavors or those of others in the field of scientific dental investigation. Members are selected on the basis of interest in research and are judged according to the caliber of their Junior thesis, scholastic standing, and professional attributes" (Tufts Dental College, 1949, p. 87).

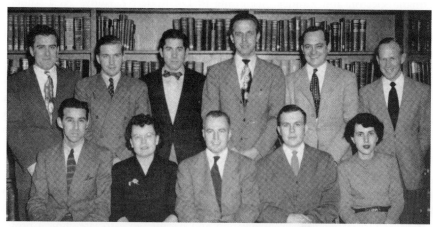

FIGURE 5.7: Members of the Robert R. Andrews Society, 1949.

Esther developed many new friendships at Tufts and remained in regular contact throughout their lives. Friend, Trudy, knew one of Esther's orthodontics professors very well *and grilled her on the exam questions for orthodontics so she would do perfectly.* The two friends went to Jacob Wirth Restaurant when there was something to celebrate.

The legendary "Jake's" opened in 1868 and is located directly across the street from Tufts Dental School. Jake's hasn't changed much since its early beginnings, according to Esther. The building looks pretty much as it did in the 19th century. *Back in the late 50's, the menu was similar, but of course the prices were much lower back then.* Jake's was one of Esther's favorite Boston traditions, and she especially enjoyed the German food, fish and chips, and the variety of dark beers they offer. She preferred getting there early and sitting in the corner booth, in front of the window facing the street and away from the bustle and noise. It was in that exact booth that she celebrated her 95th birthday. She insisted that Jake's was included in her biography, as it was an important place to her for many years.

During Esther's later years at Tufts (1948–1949), she achieved a student teaching fellowship in microscopic anatomy at Tufts. An option offered to the students in Esther's class was to take the Dental National Boards as a written exam when Esther was in her final year at Tufts. Esther's Class of 1949 was among the first to take the Boards. Only 10 students in her dental school class selected this option, and Esther was the only woman. *She studied and studied* all week and every minute until the exam, and she passed on her first attempt.

> *During our senior year the very first National Board Examination for dentists was given its trial run in selected dental schools across country, and Tufts was one of them. I took it, along with 6 or 7 of the men in my class. That first exam was an essay bluebook, and took all day, with a short break and a new bluebook every two hours. Perhaps my fatigue level reached an all-time high at the end of that day. The next morning was clinic as usual, and I was in the complete denture clinic with a difficult patient.*

Esther later commented that passing the boards was helpful when she applied for her license in the State of Washington.

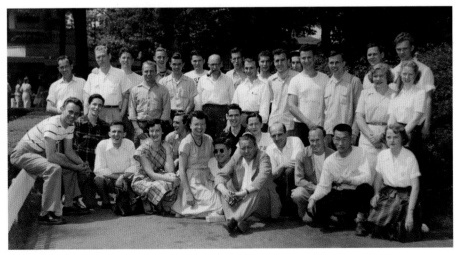

FIGURE 5.8: Tufts Dental School, class outing, 1949.

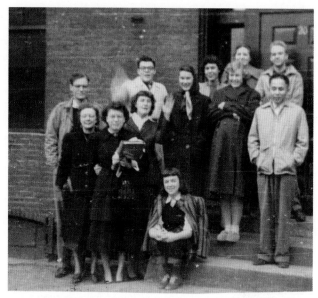

FIGURE 5.9: Members of Class of 1949 in front of door of Norfolk House, Tufts.

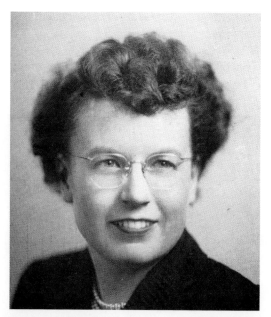

FIGURE 5.10: Esther's yearbook picture, Tufts Dental School, 1949.

❧ Esther Mae Wilkins, DMD ❧

Esther Mae Wilkins, DMD, graduated from Tufts College Dental School in 1949. Although she did quite well, she commented that she would have received more "*A's*" if she *hadn't had to work while taking classes.*

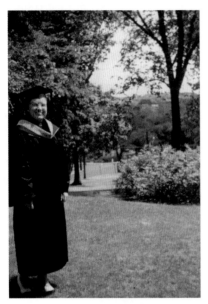

FIGURE 5.11: Esther's Tufts graduation gown picture on Tufts grounds.

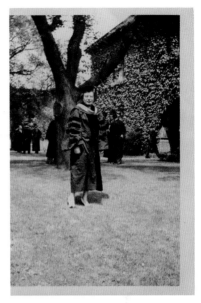

FIGURE 5.12: Esther's graduation, outside Ivy Walls of Tufts.

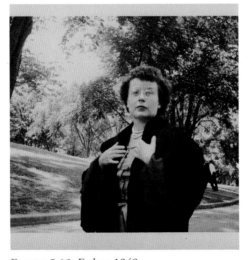

FIGURE 5.13: Esther, 1949.

Among her fellow graduates of the Class of 1949 were Drs. Algirdas Yurkstas, Thomas Quinn, James B. Gallagher (who was later to become an integral part of Esther's life), Arnold Vetsein, Albert Kazis, and Erling Johansen who became lifelong friends. Eight women graduated in Esther's class, including Hilde Tillman, who later taught with Esther at Tufts for many years, as well as four Norwegian women who were expected to return home to practice dentistry in Norway. These women were a part of a group of 22 students sent by the Norwegian government to fill the shortage of dentists in their country as a result of its dental school closing during WWII. The Class of 1949 included an unusually high number of women, as the class before hers and the class after hers had only two or three women.

Esther celebrated her degree with her family and friends at a reception held by the MDHA downstairs in the Hague auditorium at the Forsyth Institute. A classmate at Forsyth, Olive Nilsson, was president of the MDHA that year. Dr. Gavel was then president of the Massachusetts Dental Society and thus a special guest.

❝ On the beautiful Sunday afternoon of June the twenty-sixth the lecture hall at Forsyth Dental Infirmary was aglow with flowers, candles, beaming faces, and conversation. The happy event was the tea and reception given for Esther M. Wilkins by the Massachusetts Dental Hygienists' Association. Many of her friends attended in honor of her graduation from Tufts College Dental School. It was an occasion befitting the outstanding person for whom it honored. In a sense, there is no way the Association can ever demonstrate its heartfelt appreciation for all the time, effort and energy Esther has afforded for it—especially during these busy years while she was in dental school. Miss Olive Nilsson, President of the MDHA presided at the reception with usual ease and charm. The tribute in words she paid Dr. Wilkins in behalf of the Association graciously told of her many activities, attributes, and accomplishments. Dr. J. Murray Gavel brought the greetings of the Massachusetts Dental Association together with the gift of a bountiful bouquet of red roses.❞

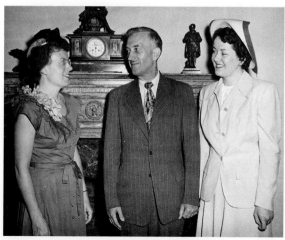

FIGURE 5.14: Tufts graduation reception at Forsyth, 1949.

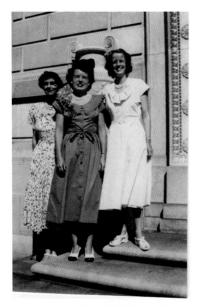

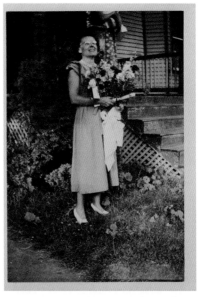

FIGURE 5.15: "Doc" Wilkins, Trudy, and Debby, June 26, 1949.

FIGURE 5.16: Smiling Dr. Esther Wilkins, with bouquet.

❝ Following this, Miss Nilsson read many telegrams, letters and greetings sent for the occasion; and presented Dr. Wilkins with the Association gift of a silver engraved cigarette box. Dr. Wilkins' thanks and expression of appreciation was moving to all present. Once again, Esta, the members of the Massachusetts Dental Hygienists' Association wish you happiness, success and satisfaction in your vocation" (Massachusetts Dental Hygienists' Association, 1949, pp. 2–3).

Included in this bulletin is a thank you from Esther:

To all of you who contributed in any way to make the Tea held on Sunday, June 26th, such a pleasant occasion, my sincerest thanks. The beautiful silver cigarette box and the memo book filled with greetings and autographs will remind me of that happy afternoon, and the friendships which the gifts represent are my dearest possessions of all. (p. 6)

Dr. J. Murray Gavel, Tufts Dental School Class of 1923, became a full clinical professor in the Department of Operative Dentistry and served as dean of the school in 1962 and 1963. "During 1967, Dr. Gavel became Trustee of the Forsyth Dental Center. Dr. Gavel watched and advised as the Center grew under Dr. John Hein's able leadership. With his wisdom and foresight, Dr. Gavel's advice was sought for 30 years as the Center evolved into the Forsyth Institute" (Tufts University, 2011, p. 1). His contributions to dentistry are extensive; his advice was sought by many in the profession. With dedication to the professions in which they were associated and kindred spirits with regard to fluoridation, Esther held Dr. Gavel in very high regard.

When Esther received the Gavel Medal in 2008, she brought with her a picture that had been taken of Dr. Gavel, Esther, and Olive Nilsson *from the early days*. Esther explained to the audience upon receiving this coveted medal:

> *This picture is such a great reminder of that lovely spring day at my alma mater where Dr. Gavel honored me with his words of welcome into dentistry, the profession he loved so much, and to which he devoted his long professional life.*

❧ EASTMAN DENTAL DISPENSARY ❧

When Esther graduated from Tufts, she determined that at least temporarily she did not want to become a private practice dentist, *as it required all that business end of things. Dr. Basil Clover Bibby suggested that I take the year-long program for Children's Dentistry at the Eastman Dental Dispensary in Rochester, New York, where he had been the program director since 1947.* Esther completed a 1-year internship at Eastman, during which she not only worked on fluoride research with Dr. Bibby, but *I was the one who applied topical fluoride and gave the children their fluoride tablets.* Esther continued as a clinical research assistant with Dr. Bibby at Eastman until June of 1950.

Dr. Bibby worked tirelessly toward investigating a formula for fluoride as a means for resisting tooth decay. Handelman and Zero (1997) described Bibby's fluoride journey, but important to this biography, stated that Bibby "created an environment that fostered intellectual curiosity and achievement" (p. 1623). As Esther's friends have reiterated in their stories, this intellectual curiosity certainly continued throughout her professional life. Esther carried with her a fascination and continual respect for fluoride, which was "one of the most successful preventive health stories" (Handelman & Zero, 1997, p. 1624) in the management of dental caries. Esther called it *one of the 10 most successful preventative health findings.* As she stated in her speech to new dental hygiene graduates:

> *NOW WE KNOW: the use of fluoride all one's life is important at all ages, especially drinking fluoridated water (letting the water pass over the teeth,) and used in cooking, every day, can guarantee a degree of dental and oral health throughout life that was never realized 50 years ago.*

She expanded on the importance of fluoride in an article she wrote in *Dimensions of Dental Hygiene* in December of 2008:

> *The era of fluoridation has profoundly affected the provision of oral health care. The introduction of fluoride into drinking water, dentifrices, and other fluoride application methods has significantly reduced the rate of dental caries.*

Most of the town worked for Eastman. George Eastman donated the funds on October 13, 1915, to build the Rochester Dental Dispensary; the University of Rochester Dental Fellows Program was developed in 1928, and the Rochester institution was renamed Eastman Dental Dispensary in 1941 (and changed again in 1965 to Eastman Dental Center).

Perhaps considering a career in teaching while working at the Dispensary (1949–1950), Esther enrolled in and successfully passed a 3-credit graduate course in "Principles of Teaching in Secondary Schools."

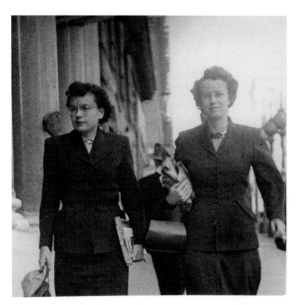

FIGURE 5.17: Esther and colleague, October 1949.

There were four opportunities at colleges which needed a new dental hygiene department chairperson: the Fones School (University of Bridgeport), The University of Vermont, the University of Oregon, and the University of Washington in Seattle. According to Wolff (1999), they "were courting her to join dental hygiene programs as director" (p. 16). Esther investigated all of them and flew to Burlington to interview at The University of Vermont. *That was my first flight in a small airplane, so I was able to look out the window of the plane to see how close the ground was. It was a new experience.* After considering her options, Esther chose the University of Washington, because it was a new program which she felt she could help grow and because she loved the mountains.

CHAPTER 6

Seattle and the University of Washington

"To Dental Hygiene Faculty: Thank you for your devotion to dental hygiene education. The future of a profession depends on its teachers. They show and tell, coax, referee, invent, develop, and especially provide role models."
(Esther's speech, Rhode Island Community College, May 22, 1990)

In July of 1950, Esther began an important phase of her life, taking the helm as the founding director of the new dental hygiene program at the University of Washington, in Seattle, "the first woman dentist to join the University of Washington faculty" ("Learning Dental Hygiene," 1950, p. 19).

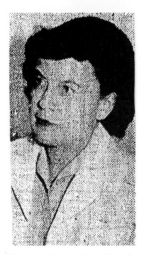

FIGURE 6.1: Esther, Seattle 1950, first week as director, *Seattle Times.*

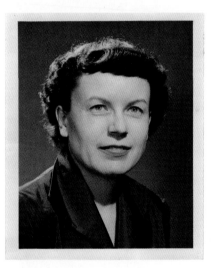

FIGURE 6.2: Esther, University of Washington, yearbook photo.

The next big adventure was the long Northwest Airline flight across country to Seattle, where on arrival it was snowing: a very unusual happening for Seattle. I was met by Dean Jones, who drove to the nice hotel in the University District. As he left, he told me to have

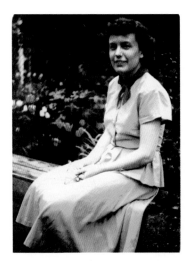

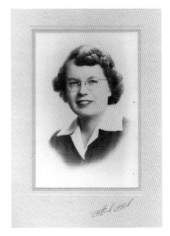

FIGURE 6.4: Esther, 1950,
professional photo.

FIGURE 6.3: Esther, 1950.

a good rest—he wasn't going to get up early. They would call me. The next day I had the tour of the dental school and met many faculty members. I also learned that one day while in Seattle I would travel to Portland, Oregon, to be interviewed for the position there. The two deans had planned together and each made a similar offer after the interviews.

Esther chose to accept the position as program director at the University of Washington, because she liked the mountains, because it was a brand new program, and because she thought she'd have fun there, *with its ideal climate and wonderful scenic view of Mt. Rainier and the Olympic Range across the Puget Sound. The principal reason I accepted UW was because it was a new program that I could build myself and make my own mistakes to be corrected.* That decision ultimately changed not only Esther's career for the rest of her life, but also her tenure at Seattle profoundly influenced the profession of dental hygiene.

With vivid remembrance of this new phase of her life, in 1950, at 34 years old, Esther M. Wilkins, DMD, became the head of the new Dental Hygiene School at the University of Washington. Esther had considered the program in Portland, Oregon, but the program was older and she really liked the idea of beginning brand new. In retrospect, she realized just *how naïve I was.* At this time, the dental hygiene program at the University of Washington (UDub, as the abbreviation of University of Washington is *UW. If you speak the letters, you'll say "you-double-you"*) was one of only 33 programs of dental hygiene in the United States, and it was 1 of only 3 baccalaureate degree programs in dental hygiene.

Esther reflected on her early days the University of Washington School of Dentistry, Seattle, in her address on February 2, 2008, at the Yankee Dental Congress in Boston, entitled *Dental Hygiene Educators' Challenges*:

You can all laugh with me when I think back on my naïve approach to accepting the Director's position in the new program at the new dental school. They had just graduated their first dental class, so we would graduate our first dental hygiene class with their third dental class.

A few years ago at Tufts when inviting another part-time faculty member to come one day for clinic, the department chairman made the remark, "Well, he's been practicing periodontics for 18 years, he ought to be able to teach it!!" Perhaps you that have been in "education" for a while can really appreciate that remark. Just what does it take to be an educator? Is experience on the top of the list?

Over the years many of our dental hygiene departments have had to take their recent graduates to help with the clinic coverage. Those part-time teachers were angels in disguise for clinic checking. But when it came to grading, testing, laboratory, and all the phases of teaching and education? Well—that's about where I was that first fall in Seattle. What did I know about educating? One of the first things I did was register up on the campus to start credits for my graduate degree in Education.

Perhaps I can call that one of my first challenges? That first course in Educational Psychology was nearly a disaster due to no time to do my homework. To finish that part of my story, I did take a course a semester. UDub let you spread your degree over 5 years, then they dropped credit for the oldest course on your record. Treadmill? It never was finished, of course, but I did gain a little bit of insight into what's behind experience when you are challenging yourself to become a real educator.

Enough on my big Challenges to arrange the schedules and find faculty. You can see that I had little time for the next level of challenges which I suggest may be some of your present day challenges in disguise. They include calibration of faculty for clinical checking and grading, as well as all department policies and preparation of a clinic handbook.

More important than all are the scientific facts, our knowledge, keeping up with the literature, research, and writing for the scientific literature.

The life of an educator can be overwhelming. Teachers—you are the future of the whole profession, because Dental Hygiene is a profession of Service.

In autumn of 1950, Esther began a full-time graduate program at the University of Washington in the masters of education program. She transferred 27 credits from prior college courses. Beginning with two courses, totaling 6 credits (Educational Psychology and Principles of Guidance), she continued the program by taking one or two courses per semester, including summers. Although she did not earn the degree, she spoke highly of the experiences and teaching skills she learned through the program.

Serving as founding director, teacher, and administrator, Esther's responsibilities also included recruiting and interviewing students for the program. *It was a Bachelor of Science program right from the beginning.* Students transferred into the program from other colleges, with the 2 years of prerequisites, came from 2-year programs, and entered as juniors. There were eight students chosen for her first class. Esther had little time to get everything ready, as she came to the University in July and the program began in September with the fall quarter.

One of the first challenges in this new professional adventure in Seattle was to

plan the curriculum for my 8 students. I had the Forsyth curriculum courses list from Louise Hord to go on. So what did they need first? Their BIG Basic Anatomy & Physiology course was held the first two quarters with the nursing students, so everything else rallied around that schedule. Dental anatomy fit in around the General Anatomy course. They had a professor who taught the dental students, and he gave them a similar course with lots of tooth carving! The first quarter I taught radiography, and Alberta [Beat Dolan] and I gave the Dental Hygiene 1 [Dentoforms for our instruments, etc.], and besides all that, we had a course for them to learn about dentistry. I invited the heads of the Restorative Department [who taught them how to roll gold foil], and Orthodontics Department to give 3–4 classes each year.

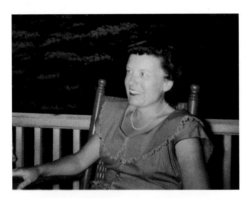

FIGURE 6.5: Esther, 1950, in "best dress."

One of Esther's students in the early years of the program was Astrid Odegard, who kept in touch with her former professor and director for over 55 years after her graduation from the UDub program:

❝ We were taught to be highly professional and yet to have empathy for each patient. There were times we were stressed with our roles, but in the long run, it was a great profession to be in. Esther taught us to instruct proper homecare and prevention for our patients. Before the advent of gloves and masks, we had to make sure our hands and nails were in good shape. Occasionally, our portable instrument cabinets were checked for neatness. Our Class of 1954 has had several reunions with Esther and we hope to continue our relationship with her in the future."

At UDub, there were second-floor clinics located in the same building, including two second-floor clinics originally designed for continuing education for the dental school. One of those clinics was dedicated for dental hygiene use. The school day was a long one for dental hygiene students, as clinic was held daily from 1:00 to 4:00 PM. The dental school moved downtown, so the lower level of the clinic then became part of the dental hygiene program. Esther was *pleased that no one else could use it.*

Esther's office as director was on one floor, and the dental hygiene faculty offices were on another. Esther developed the curriculum, led the dental hygiene faculty, and at first taught many of the courses herself, guided by both her dental hygiene and dental education and training. According to many former students, Esther completed her tasks with the same energy she had throughout her whole life.

Peg Ryan, a member of the Class of 1956 and later UDub faculty, said Esther did not

❝ walk the halls of the Health Sciences Building, she scurried. When she encountered me as she was scurrying, I would hear her, 'tsk tsk bobby socks,' as she went by. The Dental Hygiene Student Dress Code stipulated that we were to wear nylons whenever we were in the building. In the 1950s, only 'nerds' wore nylons on campus. My misdemeanor was frequently identified on my quarterly evaluation." Peg also noted that "there would often be a 'buzz' in the students' locker room on Monday morning after Dr. Wilkins had been sighted dancing at one of the pubs near the campus. It seemed too out of character for Dr. Wilkins, the task master we knew!"

Esther related herself that on Wednesday nights, she went to Scandinavian Folk Dances in a crowded hall held up the street where she lived, and *there was no charge.*

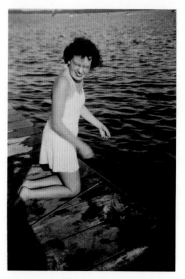

FIGURE 6.6: Esther, 1951, in bathing suit.

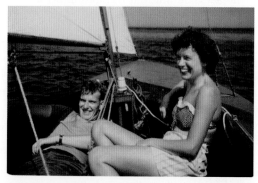

FIGURE 6.7: Esther on boat excursion, 1951.

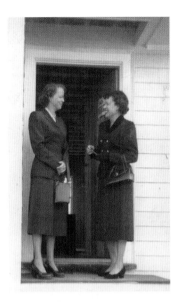

FIGURE 6.8: Esther in doorway, 1951.

Students in dental hygiene at the University of Washington while Esther was director attended all classes together, taking all the same courses on the same schedule, and there were very few elective choices. Esther described being

The largest class in the dental hygiene program included 14 students. Alice Tronquet, Class of 1956, reminisced about entering the program at the University of Washington.

    ❝ I was 13 years older than the other 12 students in the fourth Dental Hygiene class at the University of Washington and was interviewed by Dr. Wilkins,

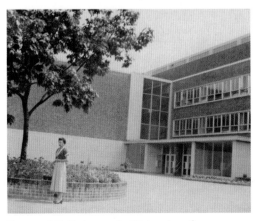

FIGURE 6.9: Esther at the University of Washington Dental School.

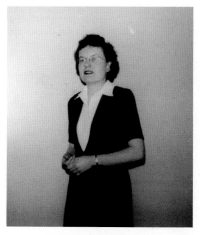

FIGURE 6.10: Esther, 1953.

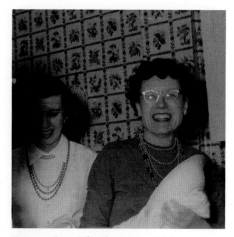

FIGURE 6.11: Thanksgiving, 1954.

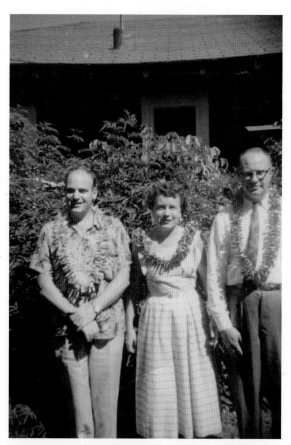

FIGURE 6.12: Esther and colleagues, Seattle 1958.

Department Head, and Dr. Hickey, Dean of the Dental School. Both were courteous and helpful in explaining the required courses in the four year program."

As a student in the program, Alice said that

❝ Esther was very demanding that we students be professional at all times. We thought she was being overbearing and she was. We had to wear our full uniform [from white hose to cap], even when a few Girl Scouts came to visit. Inasmuch as very few people then knew the difference between the educated dental hygienists and the office trained assistants, we students soon appreciated Esther's professional attitude and were proud to be part of the small [we felt elite] cadre of hygiene students."

Upon graduation, Alice joined the faculty, teaching radiology during Esther's tenure as director.

Peg Ryan, Class of 1956, went back in time and described the teaching materials used, the "embryonic stage" of *Clinical Practice of the Dental Hygienist* (*CPDH*):

❝ At the beginning of each lecture in the two year clinical dental hygiene course series we received mimeographed pages of outline formatted text on the topic of the day. The material was either new or a revision of material we had received earlier. We would open the metal straps of the notebook size binder and insert the pages. We were expected to have what was then titled "The Syllabus" with us for each class. By the time we graduated, the Syllabus [now called the Bible] was at least four inches thick."

One of Esther's secretaries in her Seattle days said she "dittoed so much she ended up with purple ink on her underwear" (Wilkins, as cited in Wolff, 1999, p. 16). Peg said they had no idea at the time that this syllabus would become the "major text for dental hygiene students through the country for the next 52 years and beyond!"

Sheila Reid, Class of 1955 and later faculty, remembered her days as a student under the tutelage of Dr. Wilkins and the dental hygiene faculty:

❝ The courses were well organized and all encompassing, as there was no textbook, such as *Clinical Practice of the Dental Hygienist*. For us, there was much competition for reference books in the Health Science Library among classmates and dental students. This led to many painstaking hours of copying notes in the library."

Sheila described how back in the old days when a faculty member became pregnant, she would be asked to resign her position. "Esther kindly allowed me to continue working throughout most of that time." Sheila related a story of a dental hygiene student being interviewed on the street by the daily newspaper who was asked what her favorite book was. Her answer was *CPDH*; Sheila said it was special to be able to later relate the story to Esther.

Esther's reputation as a pioneer dates way back in her career and continued with vigor at the University of Washington. As Peg Ryan remembered,

" In the 1950s, principles of ergonomics did not receive much attention in dental and dental hygiene education and practice. However, in the preclinical laboratory sessions, the manikins were attached to dental chairs and we were to sit on adjustable stools with very hard wooden seats. We worked from a seated position throughout all clinic sessions. At that time, students in other programs learned clinical procedures on manikins which were attached to tables. Students stood beside their manikins during laboratory sessions and beside the chair during clinic sessions."

Once again, Esther, the trailblazer, was training future dental hygienists in processes that were not truly fine-tuned until many years later.

Esther remembered that fluoridation was a *hot topic* during the time she was in Washington. A student raised her hand in class and asked, "Are you going to talk about fluoridation all day today, too?" For those who knew Esther, the profound impact of fluoridation on oral health care was a passionate topic for her. She often reminded anyone who would listen to her that you should drink water from the tap, not from a bottle.

The introduction of fluoride into drinking water, dentifrices, and other fluoride application methods has significantly reduced the rate of dental caries. Fluoridation was proclaimed one of the top 10 public health measures of the 20th century, a list that also included the vaccine for poliomyelitis.

Esther had an extensive collection of documents outlining the development of fluoridation from its early beginnings.

The promotion of fluoridated drinking water became Esther's favorite soapbox speech since its foundation in 1945. She related a story many years later, 1995, in her keynote address to Student American Dental Hygienists' Association (SADHA) in West Virginia:

When I was a dental hygiene teacher in Seattle, our students were involved in the campaigns for getting fluoride passed on the public ballot. It took three elections in Seattle to get fluoridation passed. Even after I left, before the 3rd balloting that DID pass, I would hear about the efforts from my former students. One enthusiastic hygienist wrote on a Christmas card that I would be proud of her. She had gone all through a large parking lot and removed all the anti-fluoridation propaganda from the windshields and replaced it with the favorable publicity!!!

An even greater challenge than developing the curriculum and recruiting students at UDub was Esther's search for new faculty.

Notices to the other dental hygiene programs and the ADHA Journal brought one or two possibilities. Helen Newell, with her 18 years or more clinical experience, came from Minnesota. She worked part time while completing her degree before she could join the

University Faculty. After Helen had been there one year, Alberta Beat Dolan was invited to Chair the new Department at the University of North Carolina. After Helen completed her degree that next year, she was invited to be the Director at the new program at the University of Iowa.

Esther compared the challenges of directing a dental hygiene program to being on a treadmill that doesn't stop. She felt she just didn't have enough time for what she called *the next level of challenges*, and she suggested throughout her entire life that these challenges are similar to those faced by educators today: *clinical checking and grading, department policies, preparing and updating a clinical handbook, and keeping up with the literature and research and writing for the scientific literature. The life of an educator can be overwhelming!*

Alice Tronquet was in private practice when she received a telephone call from Esther, asking if she would be interested in joining the faculty: "I was thrilled and will never forget my response: 'Who, me?' I was able to participate in many of her advanced ideas and was privileged to proofread much of the first *CPDH* as she and her friend, Pat McCullough Wagner, were writing it."

Esther felt she was not *really good at assigning jobs to staff.* She *many times asked for help* on something during dental hygiene faculty meetings but ended up doing it herself, as *they were all so busy with courses to teach, as well as clinic hours.* Alberta Beat Dolan had already been employed at University of Washington, responsible for the dental clinic at the child health center, when she began teaching part-time as a clinical instructor from 1950 to 1952 in the dental hygiene program under Esther's direction. "The experience was very valuable to me when I left Seattle in 1953 to direct a new dental hygiene program at the University of North Carolina in Chapel Hill." This is another example of the rewards received by those professionals who had the fortunate experience of working under Esther's mentorship. During these early years of teaching, Esther was cautious to make sure she treated all students equally, not showing affection to any in case another would feel she *played favorites.* She attempted to do the same with her faculty, trying not to meet socially with any of them, so the others would not *view her leadership as favoritism.*

Several former students of UDub in the early years commented on Esther and her faculty and their commitment to professionalism.

> ❝As students we did not realize how advanced Esther and her faculty were in the curriculum they developed and in teaching methodology. The first commitment was reflected in the content and rigor of the curriculum. The latter was reflected in the professional conduct she required of students. As students we met monthly as an organized extension of the Seattle component of the State Dental Hygienists' Association" (Peg Ryan, Class of 1956).

Peg later served as a faculty member and shared the reality and humor of working under Dr. Wilkins:

> ❝Esther spent the better part of most weekends at her desk in the Dental Hygiene Department. When the faculty arrived on Monday morning, we would find notes on our desks giving us assignments or reminding us of something we

were to do. If we were lucky, there would be only 3 or 4 notes. Soon after our arrival, we would hear Esther calling us one by one to discuss the progress we had made to follow up on her directives. One of the faculty members would wad the notes up and throw them in the wastebasket when she arrived. When Esther called her, she would hastily grab the notes from the basket and smooth them out before going in to Esther's office."

Professionally licensed only in Massachusetts, Esther was required to take the Washington Board Exams. The dean of the dental school, Dean Ernest Jones, *showed Esther his films in preparation for her exam.* That first year she studied, employed a tutor, took the weeklong boards in January 1951, and passed on the first try. Esther then became an active member of the Washington State Dental Association.

The West Coast Educators' meeting was held in the fall in Portland, Oregon, for which she *splurged and bought a dress.* But, it was one of those really hot fall days. There was no air conditioning. *I was so hot, I took the jacket off.*

Although Esther was extremely busy in her position at UDub, she continued to publish on topics dear to her heart and make presentations at annual meetings. She long advocated for the importance of the contributions of each member of the health care team, active membership and leadership in health care organizations, new research prevention, and patient care.

Esther enjoyed relating the story of her friend, Fumiko "Fumi" Saito, also a dental hygienist, who had relocated to the Boston area after World War II. She had been in a Japanese relocation camp during the war and could choose where to go to college in the United States. She chose Boston and the Forsyth School, Class of 1945, and lived with a family while attending school. An opportunity came to go to Hartford, and she obtained her first dental hygiene position at the Hartford (Connecticut) Institute of Living, where she met Esther. They became lifelong friends. On Louise Hord's recommendation, Esther became a substitute for Fumi when she returned to California for a month to see her family, during the summer of 1946. Esther said that Dr. Willis couldn't accommodate her all summer, so this short-term appointment worked out for her. *It did not pay well, but it was interesting.* Esther's friends, Trudy and Debbie, drove her down (*more angels,* Esther said) and delivered her to the Institute; she stayed in the dorm where the help staff stayed. Although she had never met Fumi before, she was just impressed with her from the very beginning. *I knew in a minute she was a talented lady.*

Fumi later practiced dental hygiene with the U.S. Public Health Service in Seattle and reconnected with Esther, who later hired her as a dental hygiene clinical instructor at the University of Washington, where Fumi completed her bachelor of science degree. According to Fumi, Esther said, "Help me with the clinical teaching" (Massachusetts College of Pharmacy and Health Sciences [MCPHS], 2008, p. 31). Fumi taught at the University of Washington with Esther until 1955.

Although they enjoyed a trip through the Panama Canal, Esther said she and Fumi were *terrible roommates.* They shared *the Costa Rica hot, muddy land tour into one of the villages. It started in Miami and ended upon the other side. I just went for the Canal part. Fumi had the connection through her elderly residence in Washington State, and I asked if I could go.* They remained close friends who traveled together, visited each other, and exchanged correspondence for nearly 70 years. Esther reflected on her long-time friend who passed away in 2009 as *a kind, helpful, amazing lady.*

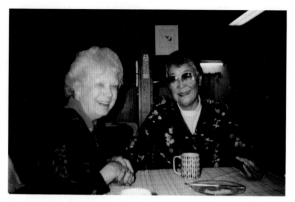

FIGURE 6.13: Esther and Fumi.

Esther had bowled (candlepin) in the women's league in Manchester-by-the-Sea, but when she went to Seattle, *they had BIG balls,* so she had to take lessons before joining the league there. As the YMCA was close by, it provided other activities for Esther. Few people came to visit Esther in Washington, as *it was a very long way.* She got a little apartment near the college and could walk to class, but she would take a streetcar downtown on occasion. The apartment had very little furniture, one room with kitchen/bedroom and a bath. The double bed swung out of a closet. She had a couch and she *picked up a few other pieces of furniture here and there.*

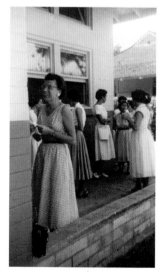

FIGURE 6.14: Esther, 1954.

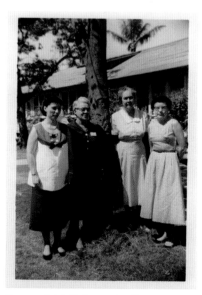

FIGURE 6.15: Esther and colleagues, 1955.

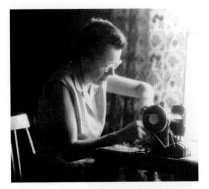

FIGURE 6.16: Sewing, Seattle, 1956.

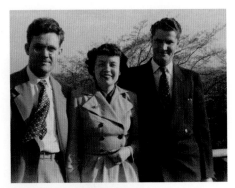

FIGURE 6.17: Esther and friends, 1956.

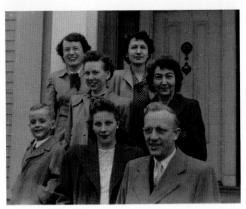

FIGURE 6.18: Esther and group, 1956.

With the precision of a surgeon, for every single year Esther was in Seattle, she kept detailed records in a small, black spiral notebook, every play and movie she saw and which theater, every concert she attended (primarily symphonies), every ballet, as well as every book and poem she read with the author or poet noted. It is a comprehensive diary of what she did with her spare time outside of the university. She held the past in the palm of her hand through the keepsakes she stored in boxes all her life.

There was an old-fashioned market nearby where Esther lived in Seattle, at 1415 N.E. 52nd Street. From lobster Newburg (frozen tails from Africa), pork chops, and pot roast, to a few other favorites, Esther entertained and loved to cook for herself and others. There was a boyfriend, but no details about him were discussed.

Esther enjoyed her tenure at UDub and bought her first car her last year or so in Seattle, a Rambler. She was so proud of that purchase that she kept the receipt for both the car and her first insurance policy all her life. She wrote in an email in 2012,

> *Since the car has been an important part of my life I think it's appropriate to save the original car receipt, and put that in my bio. I thought I'd warn you this way. I am very sentimental about that first little car.*

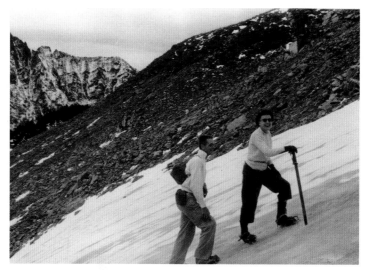

FIGURE 6.19: Mountain climbing, 1957.

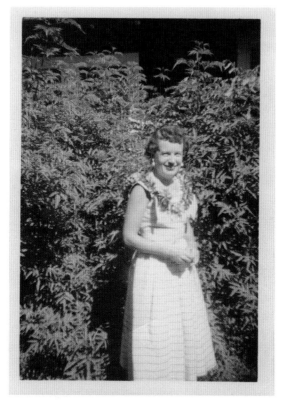

FIGURE 6.20: Esther, 1958.

Esther didn't get back home too often, but her niece, Betsy, recalled that Esther returned East in the early 1950s, when Betsy was in elementary school.

    “I remember that my mother was excited and told us we had to have a special menu of things that Esther could not get in Seattle at that time—coffee ice cream and swordfish! Esther still keeps coffee ice cream in her freezer for dessert!” Betsy also recalled that “when Esther was in Seattle, she always sent us holly [at Christmas]. My mother was always happy to see the holly come and she used it all over the house.”

It was in Seattle that “The Book” was conceived, essentially a compilation of the handouts made into a clinical manual that Esther and her colleagues utilized for instruction at the University of Washington (see Chapter 7, “‘The’ Book”). Ann Dinius related a story of how she came to be introduced to “The Book” and to take over Esther's position at the university after Esther left Seattle in 1964 to continue her education:

    “My introduction to Esther Wilkins' now world-renowned text was at Christmastime 1961 in the United Airlines passenger lounge at O'Hare Airport, Chicago. I was returning to San Francisco where I was working as a dental hygienist in private office practice. Waiting for the same flight was a Michigan classmate who was going back to her faculty position at the University of California-San Francisco. She was carrying the textbook UC-SF was currently using to teach clinical dental hygiene, *Clinical Practice of the Dental Hygienist*, and she eagerly shared her enthusiasm for this text with the unique format. Little did I know that by 1965, I would be the dental hygiene clinic coordinator on the faculty at the University of Washington where I not only inherited Esther Wilkins' desk copy of her first edition with her name in it but also the wooden desk and chair that she had used as founding chairman of U-W's Department of Dental Hygiene.”

Ann said that her career developed, as did her friendship with Esther after she actually met her in 1969:

    “It continued through the ADEA meetings, IFDH Sessions, ADHA annual sessions, and wonderful social occasions with colleagues in many parts of the U.S. and Europe.”

Esther kept in contact with many students who became dental hygienists under the great influence of the University of Washington's Dental Hygiene Program founding director. Emily Jean McCleary recalled with fondness her days as a student in 1954 and said that they would meet each other after her graduation, at the Washington State Dental Hygiene Meeting, state conventions, and “even a San Francisco national.” They remained friends for over 50 years. When Esther was back in Boston in 1967, Emily and her family, major Red Sox fans, visited Boston. They went to dinner with Esther and her husband, Jim, and Esther took them around to all the *city historical sites plus all the universities*. When they were leaving, Esther, of course, gave them a copy of *Make Way for Ducklings*. Emily's University of Washington Class of 1954 looked forward to “seeing Esther whenever she comes back to Seattle.”

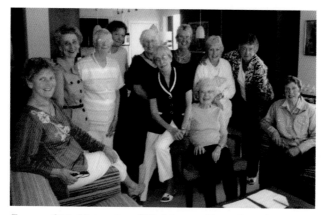

FIGURE 6.21: University of Washington Class of 1954 reunion.

Esther was an honored guest at the Washington State Dental Hygienists' Association's 90th anniversary gala in April 2011 in Lynnwood, Washington. She was acknowledged as founder of the dental hygiene program at the University of Washington and author of the definitive text in dental hygiene and "who remains active as a lecturer, mentor, and advocate" (University of Washington, School of Dentistry, 2011, p. 1)

Gail Hatley, a University of Washington alumna and Esther's former student, admired Esther's choice of curriculum for her new dental hygiene program. "Her choice of courses in anatomy, physiology, nutrition, and radiology, were so useful in my professional as well as my personal life." Barbara Posner Sommer was also a student of Esther's at University of Washington in the new dental hygiene program when she entered the program in 1953. She remembered, "Before the book, we 'toted' a syllabus—bulky and heavy, which we carried everywhere." Kumiko Homma Hasegawa, a student of Esther's at the University of Washington in the Class of 1957, stated, "The high standards we all learned and practiced still remain in our lives. One example is that we all taught each patient how to dental floss in clinic and it did not become common in dental offices until many years later." Barbara, who called Esther a "dynamo," recalled being struck by Esther's professionalism, her perfectionism, and complete dedication to her students and to the dental hygiene profession. "It was the 1950s after all, and she had to buck the 'old boys' cliché of the dental school in order to have dental hygiene recognized and respected—she accomplished both!"

Gail Hatley recalled with great excitement her long-time association and friendship with Esther.

     ❝ Years ago Esther was in Seattle for the State Dental Convention, or perhaps giving continuing education classes, I invited her to my home for lunch. She accepted. My husband came home for lunch that day, as he had met and enjoyed Esther at previous functions. While we were enjoying our lunch together, I shared the information that Esther was writing her 5th or 6th edition of her book on dental hygiene. My husband had a quick and enjoyable sense of humor and immediately said, 'What's the matter with you, Esther, can't you ever get it right?'"

Esther continued to tell that story many times during her life (and she insisted it be included in her biography).

In the dedication of *CPDH* 12th edition, Esther paid homage to the early classes at the University of Washington.

> *A very special recognition goes to the students of the first 10 classes in dental hygiene at the University of Washington in Seattle for whom the original "mimeographed" syllabus was created. They are remembered with much appreciation because their need for text study material made this book possible in the first place.*

Among the many envelopes of keepsakes at Esther's Tremont Street condo were letters to and from the early class members at UDub. Esther and these women kept in touch for 60 years, their lives shared. She kept 3 × 5 cards for each of them, noting the exchange of holiday cards since 1951, marriages, births of children, and other major events in their lives, until one by one they passed away, duly noted on each card. Her devotion evidenced how deeply Esther's students meant to her and their lifetime respect for Esther.

Esther completed her tenure as director of dental hygiene at the University of Washington in September 1961, at which time she worked for 3 years as a dentist in private practice for Dr. J. H. Losh in Seattle, until her entrance into the 2-year course in periodontology at Tufts University, graduate and postgraduate studies division in 1964. The dental hygiene program at UDub closed in 1985. In 2016, UDub Professor Emeritus Norma Wells said, "Over the years we have given thanks to her in many ways as she brought dental hygiene education—an emerging profession then—to Seattle. We can be forever thankful to her willingness to come West to work with the School of Dentistry and for having such talent in our midst" (University of Washington, School of Dentistry, 2016, p. 1).

CHAPTER 7

"The" Book

If you are a dental hygienist you surely know her name.
She's the author of a textbook that has brought her much acclaim.
"Clinical Practice of the Dental Hygienist" is the book she wrote,
And with each new edition it becomes more difficult to tote (Biron, 1997).

The birth of *Clinical Practice of the Dental Hygienist* (CPDH) is quite exciting, even for those not employed in the dental hygiene field. What began in the 1950s as a collection of mimeographed handouts distributed by Dr. Wilkins and her faculty to students in classes at the University of Washington has become the Bible for those currently practicing or aspiring to enter the dental hygiene profession. The Book, as it is referred to by students and faculty alike, is a point of pride mentioned with major emphasis by several contributors to this biography. Caren Barnes recalled, "As a student, I just couldn't imagine who this brilliant woman was. I was in awe of her then as I am now!" Lois Barber, who crossed paths with Esther while working for Teledyne Waterpik, was so impressed with Esther's credentials as a registered dental hygienist (RDH), doctor of dental medicine (DMD), periodontist, faculty member, and author that she dreamed of meeting her someday. Mindy Adshead (as cited in RDH, 2001) said that she knew she wanted to become a dental hygiene educator "ever since I was knee-high to a Wilkins textbook" (p. 2).

❧ PRELUDE TO THE FIRST EDITION ☙

In 1950, Esther became director of the newly founded dental hygiene program at the University of Washington (UDub). At that time, there were very few books or even guides for teaching dental hygiene that dealt specifically with clinical techniques for dental hygienists. (Dr. Alfred Fones wrote the first book for dental hygienists, and Esther used his fourth edition while training as a dental hygienist at Forsyth; others included Pauline Steele, Dr. Russell Bunting, and Dr. Dorothy Hord.)

According to Esther's assessment, *there was an obvious need for a clinical dental hygiene text with more detail, more emphasis on total care, especially patient assessment.* Hence, Esther and two of her faculty members created their own handbook, a mimeographed dental hygiene tome, with *dangerous metal claps that cut you when you opened or closed them.* This handbook consisted of a series of outlined study sections for each part of the clinical program at UDub.

Unbeknownst to many in the dental hygiene field, The Book was informally distributed a year before its official printing in 1959. At the time, it did not occur to Esther that she might publish the manuscript. According to Esther,

> *The three authors [Esther Wilkins, associate professor and director; Patricia A. McCullough, instructor; and Claudette Stickels, instructor], decided to assemble the mimeographed student handbook into a book form in 1958. We made a cover page, a table of contents of the 42 chapters, and an Appendix for a "First Aid Reference Chart." It was a huge book, nearly 2 inches thick, bound with a brown cover and metal clasps that cut you when you opened or closed them. We mailed a copy to each of the dental hygiene programs of study in the United States. There was a favorable response of appreciation.*

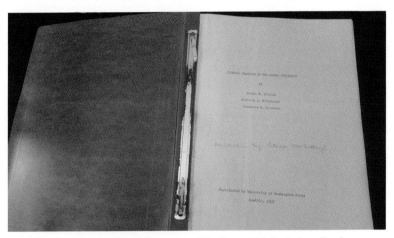

FIGURE 7.1: Original *Clinical Practice of the Dental Hygienist* handbook with clasps.

The early version of the handbook was typed on a typewriter, with carbon copies made and distributed. It was 431 pages, separated into 7 parts, with 42 chapters. The Preface outlined for the reader the rationale for the book:

> *There has been no book exclusively devoted to the techniques of the clinical practice of the dental hygienist. The present volume is the result of a five-year project in building a syllabus for the pre-clinical and clinical courses for dental hygiene students at the University of Washington.*
>
> *The stimulus and incentive to prepare this revision of the "Syllabus for Dental Hygiene Practice" came from requests of graduates, as well as faculty members of dental hygiene curricula in other universities, to make our material available for their use. The book is primarily written for the use of the dental hygienist in the private dentist office, but the clinical techniques described apply wherever the dental hygienist performs clinical services, whether in private practice, public or school health programs or in a special clinic. The book would be valuable for postgraduate or refresher courses since it is planned in concise outline form.*

The expressed purpose of the book: *is to provide the student and practicing dental hygienists with a comprehensive outline of the clinical procedures and theories of procedure required in the oral prophylaxis appointment* (see Figs. 7.2 and 7.3, Preface to the CPDH handbook).

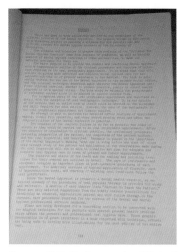 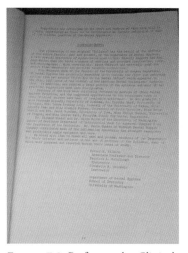

FIGURE 7.2: Preface to the *Clinical Practice of the Dental Hygienist* handbook, first page.

FIGURE 7.3: Preface to the *Clinical Practice of the Dental Hygienist* handbook, second page.

Acknowledgments for contributions to the mimeographed handbook listed in the original copy included the entire faculty, past and present, of the Department of Dental Hygiene, including special acknowledgments to Jean McCann Quam, Mrs. Beverly Leggett, and Alice Tronquet; Margaret Ryan from the University of Oregon Department of Dental Hygiene; those professionals from other dental hygiene schools who provided critical reviews of the book, including very well-known names in dental hygiene, Miss Gertrude Sinnett (University of Alabama), Dr. Dorothy Hard (University of Michigan), Miss Lorna Bruning Long (University of Texas), Miss Alberta Beat and Miss Eleanor Forbes (University of North Carolina), Miss Helen Newell and Mrs. Janet Burnham (University of Iowa), Miss Evelyn Hannon (University of Oregon), and Miss Louise Hord (Forsyth School for Dental Hygienists). In addition, Dr. Richard Riedel and Dr. Alton Moore (University of Washington School of Dentistry, Department of Orthodontics) and Mr. Earle Choate (Midwest Dental Supply) were thanked for their assistance with specific information and review on occlusion and equipment.

The "Acknowledgments" section concluded with the following statement:

We would also like to thank all past and present students of our department for their interest and patience in the use of the sections of the syllabus, many of which were prepared and inserted during their years of study.

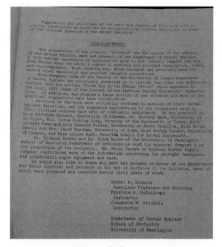

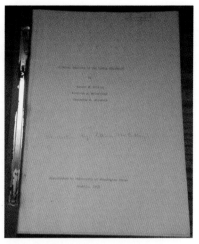

FIGURE 7.4: Acknowledgments page, *Clinical Practice of the Dental Hygienist* handbook, 1958.

FIGURE 7.5: Title page, *Clinical Practice of the Dental Hygienist* handbook, 1958.

Kumiko Homma Hasegawa, a student of Esther's at the University of Washington in the Class of 1957, was eager to relate that she and her classmates "used the original version of the Handbook written on purple 'ditto' ink and mimeographed pages." She exuded pride in having been attuned to the developments in her profession with Esther as her teacher.

In perusing the documents stored by Esther in her many boxes of treasures through the years, a short article was located in the January 1959 edition of the *Journal of Dental Hygiene*:

❝ Clinical Pratcice [sic] of the Dental Hygienist by Esther M. Wilkins, Claudette M. Stickels, and Patricia A. McCullough. This book, reviewed in the July *Journal*, has been revised to include a large new section (13 Chapters) describing the Applied Techniques for Patients with Special Needs. The book is available from the University of Washington Press, Seattle 5, Washington, for $5.00" (American Dental Hygienists' Association [ADHA], 1959, p. 47).

✣ THE FIRST EDITION—1959, TEAL BLUE, ✣ 39 CHAPTERS, 463 PAGES

In fall of 1958, Mr. Hudson, who represented the West Coast for the Philadelphia publishing company, Lea & Febiger, *came as he did each year* to the University of Washington, to show new books. Wearing a bow tie and starched, stiff-collared shirts, Mr. Hudson was in Esther's estimation *the very essence of a perfect company representative and ever the old-fashioned gentleman in every way. Our department secretary loved to see him coming—he really charmed her.* Esther related that she trusted him.

While they were chatting, Esther told him that she thought there should be a book on dental hygiene. Prepared with her mimeographed handbook on her desk, she moved it toward him and said, *You might want to take a look at this*. While he was reading, *quietly turning the pages*, the big fat handbook in his lap, Esther admits that she *kept her mouth shut for once*! He very quickly determined that they should publish the manuscript, and Esther very quickly replied, in what she called a stunned state: *I think that's a good idea*. He then asked her if she could have it ready by fall, and as Esther later recalled, *and therein was the beginning of the rest of my life.*

Esther then asked the teachers in the department if they wanted to work on a book, based on the handbook they had developed. Claudette Stickels declined, so she and Patricia A. McCullough, one of the members of the first graduating class from the UDub dental hygiene program, now an instructor of dental hygiene, *shaped it up, filled in the spaces, and put things into sequence.*

During this period, other faculty members covered Esther's classes; she deliberately worked in a space with no telephone in order to remain focused. The work was laborious without the use of computers or other office amenities. She confined herself to a small office in a lab in the dental school. When the first draft was complete, she went to the main clinic, where there were no students and which had the only air conditioner, and she read the manuscript *until the school closed.* Esther recalled she had the assistance of several secretaries who helped with the book, but she thinks she exhausted them. In recruiting the last one, Esther insisted she have one with more skills, *who was up a grade*! By the end of a hot July of 1959, she had proofread all of her material, line by line, comma by comma, a practice she continued for the next six decades.

The first edition of CPDH went to press in November of 1959. The chapters were arranged in six parts, the order of which agrees with the logical order of the different steps used to treat patients. The manuscript was credited to Esther M. Wilkins, DMD, and Patricia A. McCullough and published by Lea & Febiger, the oldest medical book publishing company in the United States and the same company which had published Alfred Fones's *Mouth Hygiene* in 1916.

The Preface to the first edition included acknowledgments to those who helped with the handbook, the many members of other dental hygiene programs who provided a review and feedback to the original handbook, consultants who provided assistance in the preparation of specialty areas, the dean of the University of Washington, and her talented artist. The Preface concludes

all past and present University of Washington dental hygiene students have helped make this book possible. Their interest and patience in the use of sections of the original syllabus and, more recently the mimeographed edition, have provided a continued stimulus and challenge to modify and improve materials. The authors will feel amply rewarded if Clinical Practice of the Dental Hygienist *helps dental hygienists to better understand and meet the oral health needs of their patients* (ADHA, 1959, p. 5).

The first printing of The Book was priced at $9.50 and sold out by the end of the year; Esther's publisher provided her with a list of schools as they adopted her manuscript. There were 37 dental hygiene schools in the United States, and Forsyth was one of the early adopters.

Esther knew all those who worked at the publishing house and travelled to Philadelphia several times for meetings. She thought very highly of these gentlemen and enjoyed working with them until Lea & Febiger was sold to Lippincott in 1985. The 7th, 8th, 9th, and 10th editions were published by Lippincott Williams & Wilkins (the Wilkins is no relation to Esther). Those following the 11th edition were published by Wolters Kluwer Health/Lippincott Williams & Wilkins.

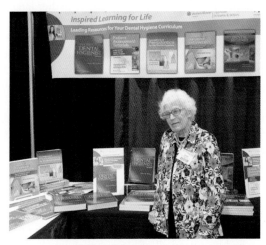

FIGURE 7.6: Esther at the Wolters Kluwer Health Booth, American Dental Hygienists' Association, Annual Meeting, Boston, 2013.

Esther remained in touch with a few of her original publishers with whom she worked on her masterpiece, and they maintained their mutual respect and admiration for her. In 1999, Bussy sent Esther a copy of his book detailing the history of their publishing company with an inscription that read "this book has sold as many copies since its publication in 1985 as your textbook sold in the past two weeks!" The first edition had a reprint in 1962.

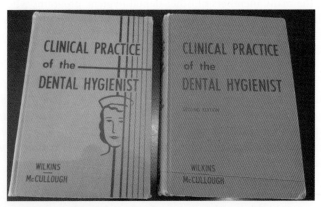

FIGURE 7.7: Photograph, first and second editions, *Clinical Practice of the Dental Hygienist.*

In keeping with Esther's keen sense of humor and her incredible sense of timing, in a speech in April 1986, she recalled that first edition:

Back in the Teal Blue days, we had all the answers!! Since then, the questions have been changed . . . We all need to be accepting of change and contribute to it.

❧ THE SECOND EDITION—1964, ORANGE, ❧ 41 CHAPTERS, 536 PAGES

The second edition of CPDH was published in 1964, again authored by Esther M. Wilkins and Patricia A. McCullough. It included two Prefaces, the original first edition Preface, as well as a half-page new Preface, which outlined the aim of the second edition and an explanation for the essential need for periodic revision,

since scientific research continually is providing new or improved concepts and techniques. In this edition, material has been brought up to date, the original text has been improved, and new technical data and bibliographic contributions have been added (CPDH, 2nd ed., Preface, p. 3).

The second edition included a new chapter on radiography. "Acknowledgments" section was included as the final paragraph of the new Preface:

Acknowledgment is sincerely given to the many friends and colleagues who have contributed unselfishly of their time and specialized knowledge to offer constructive suggestions for the improvement of the text. Their critical evaluation has resulted in the correction of errors or misinterpretations, in clarification of specific areas, and in supplementation for more thorough coverage. It is hoped that such critical evaluation will continue in order to provide a text which includes the most generally accepted concepts of the clinical practice of the dental hygienist (p. 3).

The second edition had reprints in 1966 and 1968.

❧ THE THIRD EDITION—1971, YELLOW, ❧ 42 CHAPTERS, 529 PAGES

For the first time, an ISBN was assigned to CPDH; the first and second editions had a Library of Congress Catalog Card Number.

Esther's name appeared alone on the third and subsequent editions, as she and Patricia McCullough agreed that Esther should continue without her as coauthor. Since then, she was solely responsible for constantly renewing the definitive source book for an entire profession, and she was justifiably proud of this feat.

Esther explained, *it wasn't until the third edition that the style became the two columns that all the book pages are now.*

In the Preface of the third edition, the major purposes of the book were outlined, and new chapter material was presented.

Patient care by the dental hygienist is a component of total dental care, and the services to be performed should be coordinated with the other services specified in the total treatment plan. This concept has been brought into focus in the revised Chapter 2, Planning Dental Hygiene Care (p. v).
As in previous editions, the material is divided into sections so that principles, procedures, and techniques are considered first, followed by suggested applications for patients with special oral or general health problems (p. vi).

A new Part III entitled "Pretreatment Patient Evaluation" was added in the third edition. Included in this Part III is the preparation of study casts, and clinical oral exfoliate cytologic procedures were added to the oral inspection chapter.

Esther included a statement that CPDH has been useful not only to dental hygienists but also to dentists who *found it helpful preparation for employing dental hygienists* and dental students who *have used various chapters as an introduction to clinical techniques* (p. vi).

"Acknowledgments" section is part of the Preface, which concludes with thanks to a list of professionals for their *specialized expertise and unparalleled advice for the betterment of the text.* Esther provided a special acknowledgment to former coauthor, Patricia McCullough Wagner.

Esther was still working on the third edition in 1969, as Jim (husband, James B. Gallagher) commented

❝ was shades of 1964 all over again!" In 1970, Jim related about the year: "If we do think of our proudest accomplishments, for Esther, completing the third edition of the D.H. book, which is almost certain to occur before 1971 (though maybe not until 11:56 New Year's eve at the present rate)." Finally, in 1970, he said, "The third edition of the book did get finished and on the market in March. That sigh of relief was short-lived, as just before Thanksgiving the publishers called for minor corrections for a reprinting . . . never ending, for sure."

The third edition had reprints in 1972, 1973, and 1975.

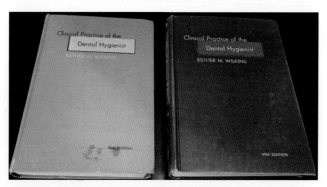

FIGURE 7.8: Photograph, third and fourth editions, *Clinical Practice of the Dental Hygienist.*

❧ The Fourth Edition—1976, Blue ❧ with Red and White, 54 Chapters, 799 pages

The Preface of the fourth edition outlined the changes since the third edition, including new chapters, acknowledgments for those who made suggestions and constructive criticism, and for those who reviewed chapters before publication. Esther made a special *note of gratitude goes to Mrs. Anna Pattison, University of Southern California, for specific contributions to Chapters 11 and 12, as well as many other chapters,* in addition to a list of several other colleagues for their reviewing of chapters. She added lastly, *Dr. James B. Gallagher, Tufts University School of Dental Medicine, for patiently reading all newly prepared drafts, for reviewing material on care of removable dentures, and for countless practical suggestions related to format and illustrations.*

New chapters for the fourth edition include *material on vital signs, dental and periodontal indices, dental hygiene treatment planning, sealants, periodontal dressings, and sutures. There are new chapters on the care of patients with complete oral rehabilitation, acute necrotizing ulcerative gingivitis, and oral cancer.* In addition, there was new content added to previous chapters.

Jim and Esther's Christmas letter of 1975:

❝ As time goes by and we try to recall an event which occurred during this past year, it probably won't be associated with 1975 specifically, but instead will be remembered as happening during the year of the 4th edition. Our activities this year have necessarily been subject to Esther's confinement in preparation for the arrival in 1976 of the new edition of her dental hygiene text in a spanking bright red, white, and blue cover (hopefully the publisher will agree to that idea)."

Charlotte Wyche, a contributing editor of later editions of CPDH, said this edition was published on the 200th anniversary of the United States and the edition she used herself in school:

❝ I did indeed keep it in my treatment room for many years so I could consult if I had a question about anything. I still own my original book today, as well as a copy of every other edition."

I asked Esther when she realized she had reached a status of both name recognition and "famous." She responded that it was when her students, once they became directors of programs, began ordering the subsequent editions of CPDH for use by their students. Esther related that the book was the one they knew, so that was the one they ordered. Esther estimated this came with about the fourth edition or so, about the mid 1970s. Her students became faculty and began ordering the book for their schools or began new schools. Esther became thrilled, not because of her notoriety, but because students then began inviting her to their campuses to see their displays and to meet her. Students were awestruck to realize they are in the midst of the guru of dental hygiene, their idol.

The fourth edition had reprints in 1977, 1979, 1980, and 1981, "which speaks to the expanding sales and use of the book with each edition" (C. Wyche, personal communication, August 1, 2017).

❧ The Fifth Edition—1983, Green, ❧ 58 Chapters, 913 pages

The fifth edition was the first to have both a Preface and an "Acknowledgments" section. It represented 25 years since the first edition and *noted changes in the scope of dental hygiene education and practice.*

The first objective of this book is to make available comprehensive information and major reference sources fundamental to clinical dental hygiene practice. The second objective is to present practical material about patients with oral, systemic, physical, and other problems that require special additional knowledge and adaptation of basic techniques (p. v).

The separate "Acknowledgments" page included an extensive list of individuals who generously gave their time to reviewing the individual chapters of the book, both general and in the areas of special needs, removable prostheses, edentulous patient, oral surgery, intraoral and extraoral examination, and epilepsy.

The large new chapters on care of patients with disabilities was initiated by members of the staff of the Tufts Dental Facility at the Belchertown State School. The final acknowledgment read *and finally, thanks to my husband, Dr. James Gallagher, whose patience is amazing and measureless.*

Several chapters were rewritten, and additional information was provided, although the overall general format did not change.

It is hoped the approach to dental hygiene used in this book will increase understanding and sensitivity as the dental hygienist engages in the most challenging and rewarding of tasks, namely helping patients to cope with their own oral health problems and providing safe and effective individualized professional care (p. vi).

In a letter in 1979 when working on the fifth edition,

I have just declared a moratorium on programs and speaking assignments, unless they are already firmed upon the calendar . . . Why? I am officially into my book revision and even with making the big sacrifice, I know I will barely reach the proposed final printer's date-line next summer. In fact, by spring I will probably be crawling the walls.

In 1980, Esther's courses took her to several cities in the United States, but according to Jim, "the rest of the time she spent on the eventually forthcoming somewhere over the rainbow fifth edition of CPDH, but we won't talk about that!"

In their Christmas letter of 1981, Jim shared, "finally the 'last word' [Index] of the bright green with gold letters cover arrived last week; it seemed almost true that the fifth edition of CPDH would at last become a reality." His update in 1983 "celebrated the day in January when CPDH [Esther's fifth edition] finally made it out on the market after the long struggle." The fifth edition had reprints in 1983, 1984, 1986, and 1988.

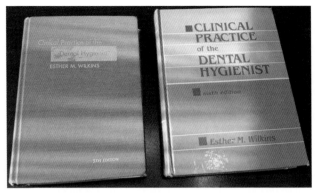

FIGURE 7.9: Photograph, fifth and sixth editions, *Clinical Practice of the Dental Hygienist.*

❧ THE SIXTH EDITION—1989, PURPLE, ❧ 60 CHAPTERS, 802 PAGES

The sixth edition marked a change in the dimensions of the book. The first five books measured 7 ½ by 10 ½ in. The sixth and subsequent editions measured 8 ¾ by 11 ½ in, a much larger book, resulting in a reduction of the number of pages.

In the Preface of the sixth edition, the objective of the book is stated as

> *the sixth edition of CPDH has as its main objective to make available comprehensive information in a concise manner. The new chapters included one to describe debonding, and the other to assist the practitioner in the care of the patients with alcoholism. New and improved sections within existing chapters include information on transmissible diseases and infection control, contributing factors to periodontal diseases, probed attachment level, tooth fractures, microbiology of bacterial plaque, and new indices, particularly the Community Periodontal Index of Treatment Needs (CPITN) of the World Health Organization. In the area of prevention, new topics include the care of space maintainers and dental implants, eating disorders and fluoride toxicity and safety.*

Additions included new terminology, new illustrations, tables, and a pronunciation guide for words listed in the Glossary. The Preface concludes with the statement:

> *A principal goal of this book is to help each dental hygienist provide instructional and clinical services that will assure quality control for high standards of professional practice* (p. vi).

The "Acknowledgments" section of the sixth edition is extensive, outlining specific professionals with specific contributions to the sixth edition. Appreciation was also expressed for the artists of the sixth edition and to the people and the publisher, Lea & Febiger: *The publication of* Mouth Hygiene *by Alfred C. Fones in 1916 gave dental hygiene its first textbook. Since then, Lea & Febiger has retained leadership* in publishing dental hygiene books. The significant impact of these books on dental hygiene and, hence, on the dental hygiene profession is acknowledged with gratitude.

In 1986, Jim reported, "Now that the sixth edition and next edition of the Book is hanging over like a little dark cloud, things are pretty tight." The sixth edition had reprints in 1991 and 1993.

❧ THE SEVENTH EDITION—1994, PINK, ❧ 61 CHAPTERS, 893 PAGES

In the Preface of the seventh edition, Esther began with emphasis on the value of the dental hygienist *as a change agent with opportunities to influence the attitudes toward, and habits of the personal oral health of many individuals.* She expounded, not only in her book but also in speeches, publications, and conversations with anyone who could listen the crucial importance of prevention, as well as the need for professional education, *both for the new student preparing for practice and for the practitioner seeking renewal and continued proficiency.* The changing research and advances in medical care necessitate advancing education.

The objective of the seventh edition mirrors the objectives stated for all the previous editions, *to make available, in a concise manner, comprehensive information essential to the professional practice of dental hygiene.*

New illustrations and tables were included in the seventh edition, as well as a table of key words, which were placed at the beginning of each major chapter. One new chapter was added for the seventh edition, Chapter 56 on mental disorders, which Esther indicated was *an area of limited coverage in many dental hygiene curricular in the past.* New material/topics were included: universal precautions, information about HIV infection, periodontal screening and recording (PSR), cumulative trauma, anticipatory guidance for parents and infants/toddlers, and exercises and procedures to prevent carpal tunnel syndrome and related problems.

The Acknowledgments pages list those specific individuals who contributed in a variety of ways and those who edited specific chapters. Esther concluded these pages with a special thank you:

The illustrations for this edition reflect the work of a talented artist, Marcia Williams of Newton, Massachusetts. Much appreciation is expressed for her personal interest and patience in preparing the new educational drawings and updating many from the previous editions.

Through every edition, Esther sought comments and suggestions, as she had a constant quest for correctness and excellence. She took pride in the high standards she demanded for each new edition. In response to an August 1994 letter she received from the director of a dental hygiene program in Kansas, shortly after the "pink" seventh edition was published, she wrote,

Thank you for your comments on the CPDH-VII format. The color does give a little "class" I think!! Let's hope the content doesn't get old too soon. Please ask your faculty to watch for typos, or any little corrections, as time for a reprinting will come only

too soon (usually in 2 years) and I need help—sometimes I can't see trees and leaves for forest. And, of course, you and your faculty should be alert to changes for a new edition—1999??

With about 1 year to go before the seventh edition, in 1991, Esther wrote

Special mention of interest and curiosity for some of you is the brand new FRENCH translation of the dental hygiene text—and while I am on that subject, the 7th edition will hopefully be about completed by the time I write to you next year. The following Christmas letter, 1992, described Esther's technical progress: *Last year you may recall that I finally joined the 20th century but on making a survey. I don't seem to have progressed much farther than I was a year ago. Now people tell me I need a "scanner." What will that do for me? Well, you're supposed to be able to run this gadget over a page (such as a page of my book that is underway toward a 7th edition) and it will print the page right into the MAC . . . then I take that page and make the revisions right on it!! So, I am thinking of it quite seriously and maybe will have advanced that far into HIGH TECH by the time for the 8th edition!!!*

In a letter to a colleague in 1993, during the writing of the seventh edition, she commented,

To update you on the 7th edition, I finally finished my corrections and additions about September 1st. It took me much longer than I had hoped, but I worked as fast as I could. Some days this summer I started by 6 a.m. and stopped only for meals. Some days I would go to the library to check the references and readings—going over about 4 p.m. and back by 8 to 9. Now at this point I am waiting for the editor's reading of the manuscript, then after that phase, it goes to the printer. Another phase will follow to read the printed galleys and page proofs.

Editing for the seventh edition was described in her 1993 Christmas letter.

The real truth is that this has been the year of the 7th ed. of CPDH and not a lot else has been going on. I am still not out of the woods—Phase 5 will be coming up soon after the first of the year. (Phase 5 means pages in print to proofread!) The seventh edition was completed in 1994, celebrated by Esther in her annual Christmas letter: *On a scale of 1 to 10, no doubt the biggest event of the year happened when the pink book "came out"—sounds like a debutante?—who knows, I might even have the courage to shoot for the 8th in 1999?? In the meantime, I am still picking up after the last episode. So now "think pink" and understand why this Christmas letter is on pink paper!!*

Esther used a typewriter but began using a computer for the seventh edition, although she continued to use the two-finger method. Publishers sent Esther about five cases of books after each new edition was published, and she gave these away, almost always signed in the appropriate color pen, to dignitaries and friends. The seventh edition had a reprint in 1995.

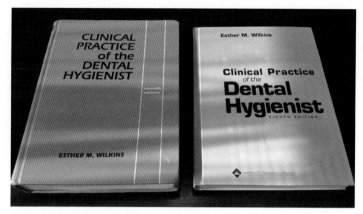

FIGURE 7.10: Photograph, seventh and eighth editions, *Clinical Practice of the Dental Hygienist*.

❧ THE EIGHTH EDITION—1999, AQUA, ❧ 61 CHAPTERS, 990 PAGES

In previous editions, those individuals who contributed content or reviewed material were listed in narrative form in a separate Acknowledgments page. For the eighth edition, an alphabetic list of 29 contributors, placed before the redesigned Preface, was included. The Preface of previous editions was one narrative, in paragraph form.

The "Objectives" and "Organization" section stated the objective of the book. As with previous editions, Esther then stated that all chapters have been reviewed and updated *to ensure that the material reflects current information and developments.* In this section, the reader is introduced to Parts 1 to 6, which corresponds to the sections in which the chapters are presented. New chapters included Chapter 22, "Prevention"; Chapter 27, "The Patient Who Uses Tobacco"; Chapter 31, "Anxiety and Pain Control"; as well as several chapters that were completely revised.

The "Challenge" section of the Preface is short and highlights the importance of personal integrity, competence, and ethics.

It is hoped that this book will facilitate learning and, by preparing knowledgeable ethical dental hygiene practitioners/clinicians, the dental hygiene care and instruction for each patient will be the best possible, and the image of dental hygiene will continue to be elevated.

The "Acknowledgments" section included a statement of thanks for the students, faculty, and practitioners around the world who *influenced the preparation of this eighth edition*; contributors of the chapters; a special note of gratitude to several people who carried the book through development during the merger of Williams & Wilkins and

Lippincott-Raven; Marcia Williams for her illustrations and patience, and Patricia Cohen, her friend, chapter contributor, and *numerous contributions to the progress and mechanism of this major undertaking.*

> *Edition VIII of CPDH is beginning to crystallize—will take me to the Land of Oz for a while!* (1996 Christmas Letter) followed by the 1998 letter: *So maybe I don't have any exciting news right now (just dull stuff like proofreading) but you wait until MAY and THEN the balloons will fly!!! The 8th edition should be out by then and we hope there won't be any typos or other goofs!* and followed yet again in 1999: *I wrote, the 8th edition should be out by then, and that is just what happened!! Then they sold so many that I was proofreading the whole book again by August in preparation for the reprinting!!*

Release of the eighth edition Italian translation of CPDH was in 2000:

> *How does it look when it is written: La Pratica Clinica dell'Igienista Dentale?*

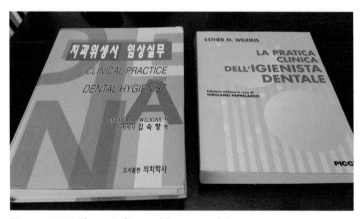

FIGURE 7.11: Photo, Italian and Japanese editions.

Caren Barnes related the story of the dedication of the eighth edition:

> ❝ I contacted each of the contributors and they agreed with me that we should dedicate the eighth edition to Esther, which we did. All I had to do was contact the publisher and they were delighted with the idea."

Thus, the eighth edition was dedicated:

> *The Contributors to the 8th edition of* Clinical Practice of the Dental Hygienist *lovingly dedicate this book to Dr. Esther Wilkins in honor of her lifetime of devotion and service to the dental hygiene profession.*

❧ THE NINTH EDITION—2004, BLUE/AQUA, ❧ 66 CHAPTERS, 1,189 PAGES, 45TH ANNIVERSARY EDITION

With the publication of the ninth edition came Connection, a free companion Web site to CPDH. For the first time, the chapter names and numbers were printed on the inside cover. Esther made a very special recognition for the ninth edition of CPDH:

The ninth edition of Clinical Practice of the Dental Hygienist *is dedicated to all past and present students who have studied from the eight preceding editions. Also to their teachers in the many different dental hygiene programs around the world, for their leadership in, and devotion to, dental hygiene education. A very special recognition goes to the students of the first ten classes in dental hygiene at the University of Washington in Seattle for whom the original "mimeographed" syllabus was created. They are remembered with much appreciation because their need for the text study material made this book possible in the first place.*

The alphabetical list of contributors was listed on a separate "Contributors" page, now totalling 30. The Preface again lists the objectives of the book, information about changes and additions to the ninth edition, and four new sections were added: "Textbook Sections," "Dental Hygiene Ethics," "Student Workbook," and "Instructor's Website."

New chapters included are Chapter 24, "Protocols for the Prevention and Control of Dental Caries"; Chapter 46, "Pediatric Oral Health Care: Infancy through Age 5"; Chapter 57, "Family Abuse and Neglect"; and Chapter 62, "The Patient with a Respiratory Disease." Other chapters were combined or divided.

The "Textbook Sections" outlined for the reader how the ninth edition was organized. "Dental Hygiene Ethics" describes the addition of Everyday Ethics. The "Student Workbook" section introduces the reader to the accompanying workbook, the first for CPDH. "Instructor's Website" section introduces the Web site new to the ninth edition that *provides case studies, quiz questions, PowerPoint slides that provide lecture notes and slide images, and active learning exercises.*

The Preface again included an "Acknowledgments" section thanking Donna Homenko for Everyday Ethics, Charlotte Wyche who *added a new dimension to teaching/learning capacity of the textbook* through the *Student Workbook*, Rhoda Gladstone and Cheryl Westphal and other New York University faculty for the teacher Web site, and Marcia Williams for art.

Esther's own constant review of the literature provided substantive information to her in the various topics presented in her chapters. She sought to learn and include new ideas, as evidenced by the invitation to readers through the publisher to help build the ninth edition by sharing what new tools and innovative features they felt should be included, suggested features, how to make learning more enjoyable and help students learn better. Caren Barnes explained,

❝ Everyone knows that Esther was the first to highlight 'selective' polishing. No matter that polishing research is one of my areas of expertise—her instructions were to write about polishing and I was not to forget one minute about including selective polishing! I was not to write a negative word about it. Of course, I respected her request."

New charts were introduced in the ninth edition, now called Documentation Boxes, which are intended to provide examples of how to document various instances of patient care in the patient record. New chapters for the ninth edition were sealants, dental caries, pediatric oral health, family abuse and neglect, and the patient with a respiratory disease, as well as extensive revisions to many of the chapters. For the first time, the ninth edition text included full text and new photographs and illustrations, and the workbook was developed. A comprehensive text bank was included, as well as critical thinking and case-based exercises, PowerPoint lecture slides, and an image bank. It is with the ninth edition that Everyday Ethics was added at the end of each chapter, which included ethical dilemma cases.

This is the year of the 9th edition of CPDH. All I can say is that this book writing' ain't like the good old days. But if I were to live it all over again, I would learn how to do computers when I was in the 4th grade or before like the kids nowadays (Christmas Letter, 2003). Excitement came when the 9th edition of DH book landed on Earth in June, but topping that was the day the Red Sox Super Bowl paraded by under my balcony. Already my next 2 years are plotted out for me because talk for the 10th edition started before the kettle that cooked the 9th had even gone through the dishwasher (Christmas Letter, 2004).

And you ask the same question as so many others. Why did I take on the next edition of CPDH? As one cousin would say "Give it up and smell the roses!" (I just have different roses). Well, 9 was such an odd number to end on. Ten sounded so much more complete. Whatever, this is an exciting time in the history of dental hygiene. I just didn't want to get caught in a bathrobe warming my feet by the fireplace.

For the ninth edition, Everyday Ethics was created by Donna Homenko, who contacted Esther to suggest that there was a need for ethics education across the curriculum in dental hygiene. They met in Boston in a "quaint little pub," Donna recalled. "[We] spent the afternoon talking about ethical situations that happen every day in the dental office. The result: EE's [Everyday Ethics] were born. We re-wrote Chapter 1 of the text and added ethics information to each of the introductory sections of the book. The 9th edition contained 66 chapters and I devised, while Esther revised, an Everyday Ethics [EE] scenario with critical thinking questions for every chapter. There were days, a few Sundays referred to as 'Black Sundays' when we worked on the EEs from morning until night—connected to each end of our computers and the telephone to meet the publisher's deadline."

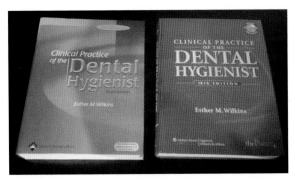

FIGURE 7.12: Photograph, 9th and 10th editions, *Clinical Practice of the Dental Hygienist.*

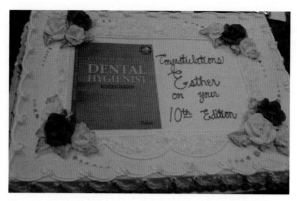

FIGURE 7.13: Celebration of the 10th edition cake.

❧ THE TENTH EDITION—2008, RED, ❧ 66 CHAPTERS, 1,197 PAGES

In addition to a bright red color, the 10th edition included a CD-ROM, stored in a plastic pocket inside the front cover of the text. On the opposite side are instructions for using the Web site link to the Point, which contains resources for students (video clips, quick bank and board-style questions, and audio pronunciations) and resources for instructors (PowerPoint slides with lecture notes, image bank, test generator, and supplemental clinical images). For the first time, Esther listed not only her Tufts University affiliation but also Forsyth School of Dental Hygiene, Massachusetts College of Pharmacy and Health Sciences (MCPHS) on the title page.

The contributors to the 10th edition number 29, again listed in alphabetical order and included affiliations. The Preface is a comprehensive listing of the plan of the textbook, the eight major sections, a statement indicating all chapters have been updated, and one new chapter was added, Chapter 43, "Whitening Teeth." The "Acknowledgments" section also named several other contributors to the 10th edition: Donna Homenko, Barbara Bennett, Janet M. Lampi, Pamela Bretschneider, as well as Marcia Williams.

An added section to the Preface was "Additional Resources," separated by the subheadings, Students and Instructors, in which Esther explained the resources available to adopters of the book, including interactive quizzes, clinical video collection, and Stedman's audio pronunciation guide for students and Brownstone test generator, PowerPoint presentations, image bank, supplemental clinical image collection, WebCT, and Blackboard ready cartridge.

Esther described in a speech the changes for the 10th edition:

> So what is different inside the text [10th edition]? Lots of color. The boxes, tables, everyday ethics, and factors to teach the patient are all in colors. Still 66 chapters, with one more appendix—now including the Code of Ethics of the IFDH [previously already had codes of United States and Canada]. What's new in the text?

*New Section Dividers—balloons of the DENT HYG. Process of Care—are illustrat-
ed on the dividers and there are now eight sections—one wholly new chapter: on Teeth
Whitening—every chapter has been "touched"—some with more revision than others partly
dependent on the new research. Chapter 1 has a new section on Cultural Competence [and
when I saw the ADHA resolution in our HOD program for this meeting, I now will want
to check our definition to see if we are in harmony].*

*Throughout the book I attempted to find spots where something culturally oriented could
be plugged in. Such as*

- *History taking and intra/extraoral exam—we tucked in a question for the Lady wearing head covering—asking about giving her a complete head/neck exam . . . would she
mind letting down her shawl.*
- *About "normal" gingival color? Yes, the lovely pink tones have always been "normal"!
But around the world we have a variety of normals.*

*Some chapters had a lot of revision: Much time was spent on the Fluoride chapter—
you'll like that. We still emphasize manual scaling.*

- *We believe it encourages the development of sensitivity and thoroughness.*
- *But our ultrasonic/sonic chapter has had quite a lot of editing, too. But you still need
that final check with fingertip sensitivity of a fine probe or explorer.*
- *And we built in a description of the endoscope—I want to believe there will be a
comeback—and it will be available so that dental hygienists can all have the satisfaction of seeing the periodontal pockets come back to health with no bleeding on probing.*

*There is a second edition revised Student Workbook by Charlotte Wyche [Detroit/Mercy]
on its way which you teachers will be pleased to see—We hope it will be ready at the same
time as the book—March 2008 they tell us.*

Chapters added for the 10th edition included whitening teeth, cultural competency,
home visits, and street drugs and chemical dependency, as well as new indices for early
childhood caries and root caries.

It was during the writing of the 10th edition that Esther broke her hip after a fall
during a continuing education trip to South Carolina (see Chapter 12). Confined to a
rehabilitation hospital while she recuperated, Esther's niece, Betsy, FedExed chapters so
she could continue to work. As Esther described,

*Everything went at the usual pace for the 10th edition . . . that was until September. I
stubbed my toe, down I went, and changed everything (Christmas Letter, 2006). The book
revision was behind whatever schedule it was supposed to be on, and stayed behind all year.
I finally sent the last of the proof reading two days before Thanksgiving. So now—the big
paper chase has started (Christmas Letter, 2007). Probably the big thing of the year was
finally finishing the 10th edition of the textbook.*

Esther described the "balloon system" (a special graphic developed by Esther to il-
lustrate the Dental Hygiene Process of Care) for the 10th edition, changing set up and
sections. She said she really liked that and had a special artist, Marcia Williams, who drew

some of the illustrations by hand. When Esther decided she wanted pictures for her book, she went to the Tufts Art Department. She used a few early art from Tufts staff back then, but Marcia later touched them up. Esther was very appreciative of Marcia's talents and acknowledged her major contributions to CPDH:

> *The illustrations of this and previous editions have been the work of our talented artist, Marcia Williams of Newton, Massachusetts. Her personal interest and patience in preparing new, revising previous, and adding color to enhance the line drawings, is acknowledged with sincere gratitude* (CPDH, 10th ed.).

The 10th edition was quite special, as it represented the 50th anniversary of the first edition. As Bennett (2005) concluded in the review of the 10th edition of CPDH, "It would be hard to imagine a well-rounded dental hygiene library without this book" (p. 1393). *Dimensions of Dental Hygiene* (n.d.) announced that *Dental Hygiene Legend Releases New Edition!* Colgate and *Dimensions of Dental Hygiene* sponsored the 10th edition book signing with a celebration at the ADHA convention in Albuquerque, New Mexico, an invitation-only event held in June of 2008 *to celebrate and honor my contributors. I wish I could attach a picture of the beautiful cake with the red book cover reproduced in the frosting!! Unbelievable!* (Christmas Letter, 2008).

It is at this convention that Esther attended an event at which Debbie Reynolds was the guest. Esther, seated purposely in the front row, was called to the stage. She was later compared by Charlotte Wyche as the "icon" of her profession to the icon that Debbie represented to entertainment. The flashcubes were active for those few minutes, as Esther grinned from ear to ear, primarily to be on stage with Debbie Reynolds, not to be acknowledged by the hundreds in the audience as an icon in her own right by all her adoring fans. Esther shared the stage once again with Ms. Reynolds during the 2013 ADHA convention in Esther's home town of Boston.

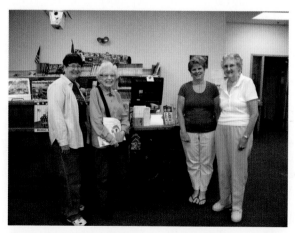

FIGURE 7.14: Donating a copy of *Clinical Practice of the Dental Hygienist* to the Tyngsboro Library, 2010.

❧ THE ELEVENTH EDITION—2012, ❧ MULTI-BLUE, 69 CHAPTERS, 1,147 PAGES

Charlotte Wyche became a contributing editor for the 11th edition, and she provided assistance to Esther with the task of a new, expanding edition. Charlotte's assistance was very much needed and appreciated, as Esther was 92 years old when she began work on the 11th edition. On the inside title page, Charlotte's name and title were placed directly under Esther's.

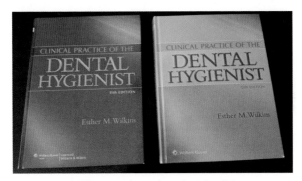

FIGURE 7.15: Photograph, 11th and 12th editions, *Clinical Practice of the Dental Hygienist.*

I was so sad not to send out a Christmas Letter last year. I was overwhelmed by the 11th edition of the dental hygiene textbook and that continued almost to Thanksgiving this year. So I wouldn't have so much of the book to do myself, I enlisted another person to be a contributing author along with Charlotte Wyche in Michigan. Sadly, that third person became ill and had to drop off. Charlotte and I were left with her Chapters as well as our own to finish. There is also a Student Guide which Charlotte has done exclusively, so she had a very busy year doing her own book and answering all my questions. She earned a medal of honor. The scope of the dental hygiene profession, as well as the enormous increase in research and information, has changed the whole perspective of the needs of our textbook—now over 50 years old (Christmas Letter, 2011).

There were 33 contributors for the 11th edition, again listed in alphabetical order, and a page was added entitled "Reviewers." Charlotte Wyche explained, "These 22 dental hygiene professionals listed here provided peer review for Esther's book by reviewing chapters before publication and offering suggestions for changes based on their areas of expertise."

The Preface expanded both in content and length, with headings Objectives, with a bulleted list of four aims for the 11th edition; The Textbook Plan, Features of the New Edition, which included a detailed outline format, chapter outlines, key words boxes, Everyday Ethics boxes, factors to teach the patient, and new emphasis on the Process of Care Documentation; Student Workbook; Additional Resources for both instructors and students; and an "Acknowledgments" section in which Esther thanked her contributors, as well as Other Appreciation to K. Vendrell Rankin, Marcia Williams, Pamela Bretschneider, Marie V. Gillis, Gail Shoomaker, The Community College of Philadelphia (the students and faculty of whom appear in the video), and our readers.

Highlights of the 11th edition included new chapters "for orientation to clinical practice describe Evidence-Based Dental Hygiene Practice (Chapter 2) and Effective Health Communications (Chapter 3)."

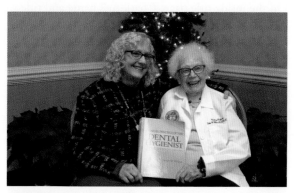

FIGURE 7.16: Esther and Linda Boyd, 12th edition

❧ THE TWELFTH EDITION—2016, ❧ LIME GREEN, 69 CHAPTERS, 1,251 PAGES

Esther began work on the 12th edition in 2012; she was 96 years old.

So now what else do I do with my time? Working on the 12th edition of the dental hygiene text? You thought I said I wasn't going to do another one? Someone told me that I said that back a few years about the 11th edition. And maybe the one before that? (Christmas Letter, 2012).

With the 12th edition, Charlotte Wyche continued as a contributing editor and Linda Boyd joined the team as contributing editor. Esther's name is on the front cover; Esther and the two contributing editors' names are all on the inside title page.

Esther, Charlotte, and Linda held the first planning meeting for the 12th edition in September 2012. Linda recalls not entirely realizing what she was getting into as the book organization, chapter contributors, and deadlines were discussed by Esther and Charlotte, because she had previously only been involved in preparing individual chapters for various textbooks.

❝ Esther had very specific guidelines for contributors to follow in revision of chapters. Early on in the process, Esther worked diligently to review chapter submissions on the computer and I went to her condo in downtown Boston often to assist her. Esther poured over every word in every chapter draft no less than three times before she saw them in proofs. Charlotte and I tried to talk her into just two reviews, but she would have none of it! As time progressed, it became apparent Esther could not meet the publisher deadlines because of computer challenges, so in 2014 I began enlarging the font and printing paper copies for her to edit. The copies were delivered and picked up from Esther on a regular basis by my Forsyth staff and myself. I made regular visits with Esther to work with her on revision of her chapters and ultimately was asked to take the lead on the periodontal chapters."

Linda continued to reflect on the process of participating in the writing the 12th edition.

❝ Probably the most stressful thing I ever had to do was submit the first revision of the periodontal chapters to Esther. I had published many chapters and articles before, but this felt very high stakes, as Esther's approval meant everything to me. Esther was tough and had very high expectations of herself and others, so she held back nothing when commenting on chapter drafts. Esther remained a 'force of nature' throughout the book revision and at each meeting had found new literature and suggestions for improvements."

❝ She was incredibly forward thinking even in her later years," Linda said. "She loved a 'spirited' discussion about periodontal topics. Emails from her would come to me, Charlotte Wyche, and contributors all in capital letters when she got excited about something. She often signed her emails 'Esta.' It was very surreal working with Esther on the 12th edition. Thinking back to sitting in class with my 4th edition in 1976, I could never have imagined I would be working side by side with the 'rock star' of dental hygiene."

Esther relied on both Charlotte and Linda for much support, especially with the revision and editing processes. Charlotte observed that "Linda's help was indispensable, because as she aged, Esther was much less able to get out, and Linda generously came to her with whatever was needed to keep the work moving forward." There were challenges in reviewing the proofs, because the font couldn't be enlarged enough for Esther to read them easily, with increasing issues with her sight.

Contributors for the 12th edition numbered 42, including Esther. The number of reviewers expanded to 59 professionals. The Preface again was extensive, primarily with the same headings and subheadings, with Objectives, Textbook Plan, Features of the New Edition, Student Workbook, Additional Resources, and Acknowledgments to Marcia Williams, Pamela Bretschneider, Anna Pattison, Elizabeth Ioakimidis, and "our readers," as well as an added section called "Individualized Review" (obtained by purchase), *an adaptive, formative quizzing program that remediates to the book. PrepU helps students identify where they need to spend more study time and provides instructors with real-time data for maximizing class performance.*

There were no new chapters added for the 12th edition, but several chapters were expanded. The 12th edition was the last one written by Esther Wilkins. She passed away the year the 12th edition was published.

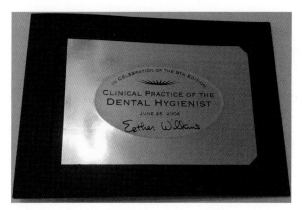

Figure 7.17: Signed Bookplate, ninth edition.

❧ The Thirteenth Edition ❧

On November 24, 2015, Esther sent an email to Linda Boyd with the subject line *THANKSGIVING with Congratulations*. The first sentence said, *MY sincere congratulations and best wishes as you officially become Chief Editor of CPDH 13th edition!!!!!!!!* Linda related,

❝ Esther went on to note that we should be reading the 12th edition as soon as the first copies arrived to look for errors in preparation for reprints, so she was already moving on to her next steps. She ended the email in bold font: '***Best wishes ALWAYS. It has been wonderful working with you—and I am thankful and grateful to you for your patience and kindness to me personally and for the betterment of the textbook!! Love, from Esther.***'

By this point, 2015, Esther was approaching her 99th birthday. Linda responded by asking Esther if she was sure this is what she wanted. Esther responded, *"It is exactly what I want. . . . "* In occasional meetings with Esther the following year, Linda said,

❝ She started a list of edits and changes for the 13th edition and in October 2016, shortly before she passed, she said she thought we were behind on getting started with the next edition. The textbook was the center of her life and she put incredible thought, care, and energy into each and every edition."

❧ Edition Colors ❧

Esther chose the color of each of the editions of the book, usually at the end of the revision process.

It was hard to decide—I thought over all the colors and variations. We started out with the teal blue book with the outline drawing of a dental hygienist with a cap. And the colors went from there—the orange, yellow, blue with the touch of red, white, and blue for 1976, green, purple, pink, aqua, another shade of blue, and now here we come to the 10th edition—so what color shall we use. SUDDENLY, it was all decided for me when I was participating in the Colorado State Dental Hygiene Association meeting. Linda Wilkinson had made this beautiful red scarf for me. When she pointed out the colors of the book scattered through—I said, that settles it—the next book will be red!! And so indeed it will be. I hope you like the idea!

Esther began to investigate different "reds." She wanted fire-engine red, and it didn't come out exactly as she wanted. Essentially, the publisher has full control and it resulted in more of a neutral red, but Esther was happy with it. Then, when she signed books, she dressed in the color of that edition of the book and signed with a pen to match the book color. She said the blue for the ninth edition wasn't what she wanted, either; *they do what they want.* Flaherty (2012) noted, "even as the first copy arrived on her desk, she cast a critical eye, right down to the cover, which looked to her like a dark blue. She wrote back to the publisher: *We wanted purple. Is it too late?*" (p. 29).

Esther received the official first copy of each new edition of the book, followed by her contributor copies. For the earlier editions, she knew more about how many were printed. The first copy, Esther described with excitement, is gold leafed, there is only one and she got it!

In an interview with Flaherty (2012), Esther explained the importance of the edition colors:

   ❝ The cover's hue is more than trivial among hygienists, it is a secret handshake of sorts" (Flaherty, 2012, p. 29). "Every edition is a different color, you see. When I ask a dental hygienist what year she graduated, she'll say, 'Yellow Book.' So I'll know immediately it had to be between '71 and '76" (Wilkins, as cited in Flaherty, 2012, p. 29).

❧ CLINICAL PRACTICE OF THE DENTAL ❧ HYGIENIST WORKBOOK

A few years ago, Esther recommended a workbook of student study exercises to accompany CPDH and immediately thought of her friend, Charlotte Wyche, to write it, as Esther knew her writing capability. Charlotte recalls that the first time she met Esther was through Victoria Tondrowski, who taught dental hygiene at the University of Michigan from 1936 to 1969:

   ❝ Vickie was my father's aunt. In the mid-1980's, she asked me to drive her to the Detroit airport to meet Esther. I was excited because this was my opportunity to meet the person who wrote the textbook I used when I was a dental hygiene student and someone I really admired" (Wyche, as cited in Gwozdek, 2006, p. 82).

Not only did Esther and Charlotte keep in touch, Esther asked her to write chapters for the 8th edition of CPDH. Charlotte recalls that she feels she must have made a good impression because not only was she asked again to work on the 9th and 10th editions but also collaborated with Esther as a contributing editor on the 11th and 12th editions.

Esther was delighted when Charlotte accepted her request to lead development of the *Student Workbook for the Clinical Practice of the Dental Hygienist* to accompany the 9th edition, although Charlotte said she wasn't sure what she was getting herself into. The workbook was developed and has been published to accompany each subsequent edition of the textbook! For the 12th edition, Jane Halaris became a team member to help revise the workbook.

❧ BOOK SIGNINGS ❧

Book signings, sessions of "meet the author," and meet and greets, or celebrations in her honor continued for years after each edition. One of the book signings was in celebration of the ninth edition of CPDH at the ADHA Annual Session in 2004. Esther was very happy, as she was for any event, and kindly agreed to send a signed book plate for those who could not attend a book signing.

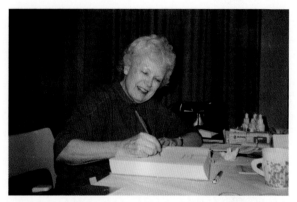

FIGURE 7.18: Esther signing books, 1990s.

Esther especially enjoyed events that involved visiting students at their colleges, signing books, and answering student questions. Marilyn Rhodes invited Esther to present to graduates of Chabot College in Hayward, California: "Her presentation to our graduates inspired us all to do what she outlined in her textbook—deliver quality dental hygiene care." Esther enjoyed my telling her that one could buy a copy of the old editions for 75 cents each on online auctions, but a first edition copy was a rarity indeed. People don't part with those! Never forgetting her roots, Esther gave a first edition copy of CPDH to the Littlefield Library in Tyngsboro, where her cousin Christina Clarke Bell said, "I was the librarian!"

Esther enjoyed the book signings and, according to friend Lana Crawford, she would sign any edition and has "the perfect color pen for each textbook," regardless of the color. She often wrote notes inside the books she signed and enjoyed conversations with the requesters.

❝ I will never forget how she engaged in conversation and eye to eye contact with so much sincerity and interest. A few people shed tears as they marveled at Esther when they were waiting in line to have her sign their books," Lana Crawford remembered.

Mary Dole, close friend of Esther's since the 1940s, received one of the original mimeographed copies:

❝ I was very fortunate to receive, from Esther, a mimeographed copy of that first book and still cherish it. With all the book signings of CPDH, I realized in 2007, Esther had never signed this copy for me, so on her 91st birthday, she signed this book."

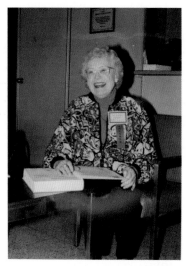

FIGURE 7.19: Book signing, 1996.

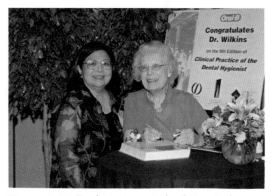

FIGURE 7.20: Book signing, ninth edition, Esther and Anna Pattison.

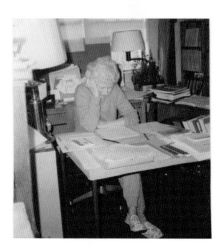

FIGURE 7.21: Esther editing session, 1983.

In 1999, at the new clinic dedication at Palm Beach Community College, Esther related in her speech a story of the longest line of autograph seekers during a Florida Dental Hygienists' Association Meeting:

> *I can never forget that lunchtime when lines of students were either at the buffet, or lined up with their books for me to sign—and then they were eating, and the line kept coming. When I signed the last book, all had finished eating, and were gone over for a tour in the school and clinic! It must have set a record for the number of books signed in one session!! (I had all the delicious left-overs for my lunch!!)*

Once, Esther received a request from the president of MCPHS to come to a private book signing at the college for a representative, who had a young dental hygiene student from his country with a special request from her idol, Dr. Wilkins. I understand the student was thrilled with her privately signed copy. Esther was excited, also, when she received a letter from Fiji: "I'm writing on behalf of our association, the Fijian Hygienists Association, just to say thank you very much for a wonderful work done in writing the books on dental hygienists. Currently, we are using this book, namely the *Clinical Practice of the Dental Hygienist*, to teach our hygienists students." They found Esther's contact information in the *Israeli Dental Hygiene Association Journal*.

❧ THE CONTRIBUTORS ❧

With a new edition often came the need for new chapters due to expanding information. The book grew from 39 chapters in its original edition to 69 chapters in the 12th edition. Esther brought together a group of colleagues who would eventually be known as Esther's chapter contributors. Caren Barnes explained that many of the contributors wrote sections of the book prior to being formally recognized, which didn't occur until the eighth edition, at which point the identities of Esther's group of colleagues were finally revealed.

> ❝ It had always been kept a secret," said Caren. "And when she first started acknowledging contributors, she forgot and left my name out both times—I tease her and never let her forget it."

Esther insisted that her chapter contributors kept up to date on new research and changes in terminology, including taking courses. *Our new research outdates the old paradigms, things people used to assume about their teeth.* She was meticulous, especially about citations and spelling, and had a keen instinct for choosing the right word. *In a precise profession such as ours, there is no room for mediocrity.* Every single reference was reviewed, regardless of who wrote or assisted in writing the chapter. As Charlotte Wyche said,

> ❝ Esther [was] very involved in reviewing virtually every word in every chapter of every edition. The book [was] much better because of her hands-on approach. I've never known anyone like her. She [was] amazing" (Wyche, as cited in Gwozdek, 2006, p. 83).

A contributor once found an error on a name and address that was in the book, and Esther said, *She was right!* Enjoying the advantages of the electronic form, she proofread every single word after the contributors proofed it. Then, she proofread it again. She did tell a story about a typo that she missed over three editions until a teacher from one of the colleges told her about it. *She said she was sorry to tell me because she knew I would fix it and spoil her fun telling her students about it!* Some contributors Esther said are *very conscientious about writing their chapters.* Others she had to work with more closely. She appreciated the contributions of each and every one of her authors.

The dental hygiene professionals, all dental hygienists (or former, such as Esther herself and Karen Ragalis), who serve as chapter contributors are, according to Bennett (2005), "well-respected experts in their fields who add breadth and depth to the scope of the book" (p. 1393). Esther considered many of her contributors as close friends, who had insightful comments on what it is like to work with Esther as a chapter contributor. Jan Selwitz-Segal wrote,

> ❝ I was honored when she asked if I would be interested in writing a chapter in her book. It turned out to be one of the most challenging projects I ever attempted. Esther's help with arranging the material and personal involvement was invaluable. I enjoyed our email discussions of how best to present the material."

Esther admired many of her contributors, and commented,

> *Jan had just received my email about the book chapter and was already getting warmed up to work on it. She has been just the perfect contributor and loves it. She has been saving references ever since the other edition was finished!*

Contributors are not paid financially for their contributions, and the publisher remained neutral over Esther's choice of authors of her book chapter. Esther shared that their rewards are *notoriety and the honor of being included.* Caren Barnes noted she was so honored to be asked to contribute as she was doing something to help Esther out. Nancy Sisty LePeau said her experience as a chapter contributor was "stimulating and allowed for growth in my ability to teach new students by developing with Esther the content of the chapters." As Caren Barnes reflected on her association with CPDH and with Esther,

> ❝ Seriously, there is no honor greater than to be asked by Esther to contribute to her book. I am sure that she never imagined that what started out as a clinic manual would become the all-time, best-selling dental hygiene textbook and not only for an edition or two—but now, 11 editions and 50 years of being the major influence on dental hygienists throughout the world. And after all these experiences with Esther, I don't overuse references, and I think I've finally mastered the use of outline form!"

Occasionally, chapter contributors decided not to continue with the revisions, and in those instances Esther sometimes took over a chapter previously written by someone else. She once said she didn't give away any of the chapters:

> *They are still all mine!* In most cases, Esther sought out other talent to take over for them. *There is so much new literature to cover, and we need to find people with special expertise. We still only let dental hygienists be contributors. Kathryn Ragalis and I get away with it because we started out as dental hygienists!*

Of utmost importance to Esther was that every chapter contributor must be an RDH. Seeking fresh ideas, Esther was delighted when a new author joined her team. On more than one occasion while attending a dental hygiene conference, she acknowledged someone for their expertise in a specific area, approached them, and asked them to write for her. It was considered a great honor to become a contributor to CPDH.

Karen Raposa's mother once commented to Esther that her memory was amazing. Karen said she will never forget Esther's response: *Well, why do you think I keep writing this book; it keeps my mind working!*

❧ THE PROOFREADING AND ❧ EDITING PROCESS

Quite a bit of hoopla ensues when a new edition of CPDH comes out. In Bussy's (1985) history of Lea & Febiger, he indicated that CPDH "led the list" of the books the company sold in 1985 (fifth edition). Esther didn't remember the year but remembered her book was the 17th best seller for the whole company one year.

Esther occasionally shared the challenges of writing a textbook. It often consumed her, because as soon as one edition was published, she began work on revisions and the next edition. When Jim and Esther moved to Tremont Street, she not only liked to look out over Boston Common out her large picture window but she also had a room devoted solely to CPDH.

I have a bigger room to spread my book around in, and what a mess of piles of paper it is!!! Jim is away at a dental meeting this week, and I have spread parts of the book out over the living room!! I shall have to bring it back in before he gets back . . . there is a limit after all, and he has waited so long for me to finish. He is most helpful at reading sections and offering good notes on inadequate writing, as well as questions about the dental aspects (E. M. Wilkins, personal communication, March 20, 1981).

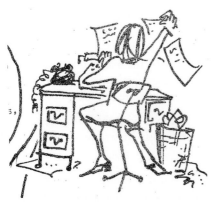

FIGURE 7.22: Jim's pen drawing of Esther's editing process, 1977.

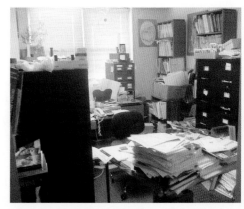

FIGURE 7.23: Organized chaos, Esther's Tremont Street home office.

The following table represents the exhaustive efforts of Esther and her many contributors to constantly improve their own work and match the pace of an ever-evolving profession. CPDH is a highly respected authoritative source for dental hygiene, often called the Bible of dental hygiene, and occasionally referred to as a "tome," a mainstay, and an essential tool for any dental hygienist. With each new revision, Dr. Wilkins sought improvement in any way if it clarified information that dental hygienists could utilize in their practice.

Clinical Practice of the Dental Hygienist

Book Editions

Edition	Date	Color	Chapters	Pages	Publisher
1	1959	Teal blue	39	463	Lea & Febiger
2	1964	Orange	41	536	Lea & Febiger
3	1971	Yellow	42	529	Lea & Febiger
4	1976	Blue with red and white	54	799	Lea & Febiger
5	1983	Green	58	913	Lea & Febiger
6	1989	Purple	60	802	Lea & Febiger/Williams & Wilkins
7	1994	Pink	61	893	Lippincott Williams & Wilkins
8	1999	Aqua	61	990	Lippincott Williams & Wilkins
9	2004	Blue/aqua	66	1189	Lippincott Williams & Wilkins
10	2008	Red	66	1197	Lippincott Williams & Wilkins
11	2012	Multi-blue	69	1147	Wolters Kluwer Health/Lippincott Williams & Wilkins
12	2016	Lime green	69	1251	Wolters Kluwer Health/Lippincott Williams & Wilkins

Special Book Editions

Edition	Date	Color	Chapters	Language
4	1976	Pink, purple, or white	54	Japanese
6	1989	White	30	French Canadian
7	1994	Pink	61	Korean
8	1999	Aqua	61	Italian
9	2004	Light green or white	66	Portuguese (South American)
9	2004	Blue	66	Japanese

The work for each new edition began immediately after the publication of the previous edition. For example, immediately after following a book signing in Albuquerque, for the 10th edition, Esther contacted contributors to ask them if they wanted to continue and to let them know the writing for the 11th edition was to begin *now! There are lots of articles being published in their areas. I want them to start right away, but they don't, as they are tired and the last edition just came out.*

At the beginning of the revision process, Esther met with the project manager from her publisher (one is assigned for each edition), and together they reviewed the plan for The Book. *Misprints and typos are embarrassing—as hard as I work at the proofreading—they happen!* Large sheets were utilized, so right side marginal notes could be made, a process that Esther enjoyed, despite how time consuming it could be when compared with more modern techniques for editing, such as "tracking" in Microsoft Word. She preferred being able to see the whole scope of the pages, although she acknowledged that it was antiquated and caused eye fatigue.

Esther insisted on excellence, although it was a time-consuming process. Esther did not succumb to modernizing her editing techniques until the 11th edition. In some ways, Esther missed the long sheet process, as she could see the order of paragraphs, could mark them up and review edits, and as she could go back to review the changes she made. For the 11th edition, Esther began using the National Library of Medicine (NLM) citation style for referencing and citations, abbreviating titles of journals according to the style used in the Index Medicus. For the 12th edition, the change to American Medical Association (AMA) style was implemented. When asked her preferred citation method, Esther responded, *the Esther M. Wilkins Format!*

There was never in her life when Esther just sat around and relaxed. She had an unparalleled work ethic. When one task was accomplished (and never done hurriedly or not complete), she had others added. Yet, regardless of the length of her "to do" list, she always submitted material in time for due dates, with the exception perhaps of a few chapters of her book, as she waited (not patiently) for contributors to submit their material. She researched everything and did not miss a period or comma. Once a book edition was submitted to the publisher, Esther waited: As she wrote to Mary Rose Pinelli in 1998, *About next week, I can expect the page proofs—then I will be back to the slavery again!!!* Book submissions usually go *right up or over the deadline established by the publishers, so they end up hounding you!*

With the diligent and consistent efforts of her chapter contributors, Esther was able to make great strides, especially in the 9th, 10th, and 11th editions. The workbook was developed as well as a comprehensive test bank, PowerPoint lectures; photographs and illustrations were added alongside critical thinking and case-based exercises. Changes were warranted in various forms for each new edition, sometimes minor, others more far reaching. And of course, new chapters were added as needed.

For the last several editions, *contributor guidelines* were developed and utilized to guide contributors with the writing, editing, and submission processes. A Preface explained to contributors the organization of the guidelines, a list that *will be helpful when updating any cross-references to other sections of the book that are included in your chapter*, as well as readers (the three primary authors) assigned to their chapter(s). It also included a complete list of contributors, contact information, and chapters assigned.

Book chapters have been rolling in and out and there are three reviews waiting as I talk to you. I wish all this busy-ness for me meant more were finished and sent, but time will tell that! (email to author, 2006). Editing a chapter in Esther's book is no simple journey, for either herself or her contributors. *I got quite a lot of book done this week—well, most of what I worked on was the tail-end of 3-chapters that now are ready to send in—so that is always good. Today I am reviewing a long one for the first time and am weary of it! So am working hard to finish this review* (email to the author, 2005).

Caren Barnes recalled,

❝ The chapter on ultrasonic scaling was completed by Peggy Waring and me. Esther nearly killed us with requests to change things and we agreed she has no qualms about making demands or last-minute changes. And, she will do anything to find you if you are writing one of her chapters—she will fax, FedEx, call, email—night or day, weekday, or weekend. No matter, we always ended up laughing hysterically about how she never failed to find us and never missed a minute thing that we may have gotten wrong—whether we really got it wrong or she didn't agree with the way we wrote it!"

Esther's filing system for a new edition was entirely unique to her, using a personally developed "chair" and "box" system. There would be a box for each chapter. As new journal articles, reports, sheets for mark-up, and research were identified for a particular chapter, it went into the appropriate box for easy retrieval and referral. Esther was fond of referring to her system with a term her sister used frequently: *organized confusion.* All furniture was utilized during the process, including organized "stacks" on the couch. According to Betsy, if Esther was using a journal as a reference, she would put the journal in the chapter box with a bookmark for the article. Proper referencing and citation were important to Esther, and she assured completeness by keeping every single reference on 3×5 cards—a separate box for each edition. Esther had two bedrooms, but one acted as an office in perpetual dedication to The Book, also filled to the brim with mementos and paper, and a complete wall of filing cabinets.

Anna Pattison, who worked with Esther at her apartment on Chapter 44 of the 10th edition of CPDH, commented in her Editor's Note in *Dimensions of Dental Hygiene* that she shared a kinship with Esther, that of clutter and organized chaos. "Our workspaces are filled with countless piles of articles, books, journals, and stuff that appear to be disorganized heaps to others but for us, they are our personal, precious, eccentric, carefully chronologically placed filing system. Every pile is an archeological treasure of recent dental hygiene history. God forbid that some well-meaning person like an industrious housekeeper should touch our piles of paper" (p. 10). Anna and Esther agreed that "the gravest offense is when someone actually throws something away because he or she assumes it is old and insignificant" (p. 10).

Esther said, *many suggestions for terminology and content have come from all over the world.* She said that *oral inspection* used in early editions grew into using *examination and assessment* which were less military. *When we changed [the words terminology from] plaque to biofilm last edition [eighth edition], it became something of a game to see who could find the most.* Other changes Esther has noted are *operating room* and *operator* have been changed

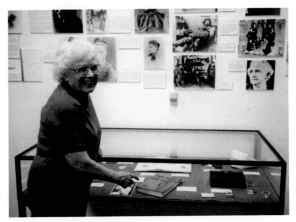

FIGURE 7.24: Esther with first edition *Clinical Practice of the Dental Hygienist* in case in Museum of Dentistry, Baltimore.

to *treatment room and clinician*; *oral physical therapy*, which she used from her days at Tufts, have now been changed to *plaque control*. Esther suggested that proper terminology will elevate the profession of dental hygiene.

❧ THE IMPACT OF *CLINICAL PRACTICE* ❧ OF THE *DENTAL HYGIENIST*

CPDH is a highly regarded authoritative source on dental hygiene, and Esther Wilkins was a highly respected author, educator, and experienced clinician. According to ADHA, more than 90% of the dental hygiene education programs in the world include CPDH on their syllabi. Esther (as cited in Ray, 1996) explained that "the language of the book is geared to first-year dental hygiene students, explaining terminology and philosophies in easily understandable terms" (p. 8). Many practicing dental hygienists reflected on how Esther thought out of the box.

    "She was ahead of the curve in promoting new ideas, which then became standard practices. One that comes to my mind immediately is that she first promoted the use of safety classes for the patient way back in the fifth edition (1982) on page 52. Safety glasses for the clinician are first illustrated in the third edition (1971) on page 31," Charlotte explained. Gladstone and Garcia (2007) commented that "it [The Book] contained many concepts that are still correct today. Other chapters, such as the one describing the ergonomics of standing correctly since practicing in a seated position, was [sic] rare at the time" (p. 14).

Many of Esther's former students and colleagues submitted letters and statements which confirmed that The Book is still of paramount importance to them and still present in their daily lives. Lynda McKeown described Esther's endeavor as "enterprising" and "fearless." She aptly stated, "[Esther] saw a need and she filled it." Carol Griffin continues to use The Book as an immediate reference point for settling professional debates and "for clarity of the basic theories in the practice of dental hygiene." Tonya Smith Ray admitted that The Book "was my date on many late nights and my companion during two spring breaks, and was there when I studied for my Boards. I often wondered who was this 'Queen of dental hygiene'" (p. 8).

Wouldn't it be incredible to know just how many students of dental hygiene have learned their craft through the influence of Dr. Wilkins's Bible? How many students have fallen asleep, and as Teresa Duncan described,

> " found The Book lying beside her the next morning. This is not to imply that Esther's book was boring, but as all who have lived through the dental hygiene curriculum know, school was exhausting. When I heard she was speaking in Atlanta, I was surprised. I can't explain why, but I thought she was dead. Most famous authors I'd read, Twain, Shakespeare, and Alfred C. Fones, had passed away years ago and after writing such a large textbook, I didn't think anyone could survive. When I and several classmates attended the course at Clayton State College, we found she was very much alive!" Teresa continued, "Like all good dental hygiene students, we had our 'Red, White, and Blue' edition signed and posed for photos with Dr. Wilkins."

As Lynda McKeown observed, "The Book is a work of love, which requires constant tending and incredible networks, so the knowledge and terminology remains current and relevant for dental hygiene education." For this reason, The Book continued to grow and adapt with each edition, and as Esther recalled, eventually *it became the feature of one of the Christmas party skits—where a student came in hauling her handbook on a workman's moving cart.*

Esther gave a copy of the first edition of CPDH to the National Museum of Dentistry. It would not surprise those who knew Esther that when in 2009, Lana Crawford visited the museum in Baltimore that not only is a copy of Esther's early editions (third, fourth, and eighth editions) displayed but, according to Lana, Esther's voice in the audio tour (#404) is also "giving information about the benefits of fluoride." Lana reported that the eighth edition the museum holds was owned by Wilma Motley and dedicated to her by Esther, signed May 5, 1999.

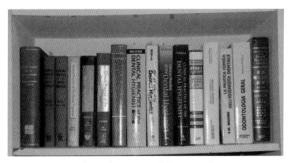

FIGURE 7.25: *Clinical Practice of the Dental Hygienist* editions on shelf.

Many of the reflections presented in this biography discuss the importance of CPDH long after dental hygienists used it in their training. They continue to review the lessons to keep up to date, to refer to it to help them in their practice. Esther and CPDH have become what Lynn Hunt Nunn described as

> " a profound influence on my life in terms of helping train me to become a health professional. In so doing, she has assisted the many patients whom I have seen over the years to obtain a better state of oral health."

❧ Esther's Perspectives of ❧ Clinical Practice of the Dental Hygienist

CPDH continued to be a significant part of Esther's life. She was proud of her accomplishments but prouder of the influence it has had in educating dental hygienists of the next generations. She sought to provide students with the most up to date, scientifically based, and accurate information. Her greatest fear was to discover something was wrong in the book, that *students would then be learning the wrong things*. She felt that it was rather frightening to have that much responsibility.

CPDH has been translated into five different languages, two editions in Japanese, as well as French Canadian, Italian, and Korean. Her collection of editions, each one in pristine condition, including a copy of the original mimeographed handbook, were always prominently displayed in her home and moved with her to her assisted living facility many years later. Her story of how she was able to complete this collection was one of her favorites to tell:

> *In the late 1970's I was invited to present a continuing education course at Temple University in Philadelphia. The chairperson of the Dental Hygiene Department, Betsy Allen, greeted me on my arrival and I had barely enough time to take off my coat when she grabbed my arm and said, "Come on down to my office, I have something to show you." We went down a long hall and into her office, and she reached up on a bookshelf to take down a large, brown-covered book and handed it to me. It was the first bound copy of the old mimeographed handbook that I had ever seen! Of all the exciting, precious moments of my life, this can be recorded as one of the greatest. I was spellbound, with tears cresting in my eyes, as I gently opened the familiar pages. She knew I was surprised, impressed, and I told her how honored I was to see it in bound-book form.*
>
> *Fast forward about 10 years. Betsy Alden retired about the time Temple University decided to close the dental hygiene department. At some time later, when I obtained Betsy's address, I wrote and asked her where that big book had gone when she closed her office. She said she supposed it went into the college library with other books from her shelves.*
>
> *When I called the librarian and asked about it, she told me that yes, indeed it was in the library, and would I like to have it? Of course, I accepted. It will always be a special treasure and serve as a fond memory of the years in Seattle at the University.*

Esther still had that original bound manuscript, the prefirst edition, proudly displayed on her shelf with the other editions.

Many people have asked Esther why she wrote a dental hygiene book, and her response was frequently *you go with what you know!*

There is one sentence that is included in many editions of the book. Esther said it represented the objective and dedication of the book to the profession *and to the perfection, responsibility, and passion we all want to see in our students and practitioners.*

Very early in her career, Esther shared her belief in the importance of keeping up with both the literature and in professional publishing, which *does not stop with articles for members of our own profession* (Wilkins, 1960, p. 4). In advising new dental hygienists, she stated,

Dental hygienists are responsible for providing patient care rooted in current and strong evidence-based therapies. She felt it was the moral obligation of the professional person to contribute to the body of scientific knowledge and publish such information for the benefit of the other members (Wilkins, 2008, p. 1). *We cannot reach that goal alone. We need to work together with members of other health professions to keep them informed of current oral health research* (Wilkins, 2008, p. 12).

Expounding on the value of published literature, both reading and writing: *We ask, what has the new research found that is necessary to know about and apply for the benefit of our patients and community groups. For our knowledge of the newest research, we must watch to find, then read and apply. With each new year, more research will be reported to provide us with more detailed explanations* (from a speech given by Dr. Wilkins, 2009).

Well recognized for her continuing education presentations, Esther also was a prolific writer and practiced what she expounded throughout her professional life, publishing not only 12 editions of CPDH but also a significant number of professional papers and peer-reviewed articles (see Appendix L, Esther Wilkins' Publications, accessed via the online eBook).

CHAPTER 8

The World of Dental Hygiene: American Dental Hygienists' Association and International Federation of Dental Hygiene

"The dental hygienist's obligation is to see that no patient needs special rehabilitative dental or periodontal services because of any condition which could have been prevented by dental hygiene care"
(Esther Wilkins, *Clinical Practice of the Dental Hygienist*).

Every profession has its idols, and dental hygiene has Dr. Esther Mae Wilkins.

"In the world of dental hygiene, I would say she is the most well-known, most respected and most loved person" (Hempton, as cited in Camire, 2006, p. 1).

Esther's world encompassed dental hygiene. She loved its history, its growth and development, and especially the students who are training to practice in the field. Esther defined the registered dental hygienist as

a licensed, professional oral health educator and clinical operator who, as an auxiliary to the dentist, uses preventative, therapeutic, and educational methods for the control of oral diseases to aid individuals and groups in attaining and maintaining optimum oral health.

The profession has come a long way since dental hygienists were considered prophylactic operators and patient educators in dentists' offices; they are now an integral part of the health care team. One cannot imagine this evolution without the significant influence of Dr. Esther M. Wilkins.

In *The Evolution of Dental Hygiene: Looking Back at 70 years of Dental Hygiene and Envisioning What the Future Holds* (Wilkins, 2008), Esther reflected on her own career, beginning with a description with pride of her first dental hygiene position with Dr. Frank Willis in Manchester-by-the-Sea, at 8 Union Street. She realized how fortunate she was that her first professional dental hygiene position was in a learning environment, a helping environment, with a dentist who valued her and the help she provided to her patients. She recalled her 6 years in this little coastal town in light of the changes that have occurred since she boiled water to sterilize instruments, but she viewed it all with an emphasis on progress that is being made and that will be made in the future: *from the profound impact of fluoridation on the dental world, to required standard infection controls, to dental hygienists administering anesthesia and practicing nonsurgical periodontal therapy.*

❧ AMERICAN DENTAL HYGIENISTS' ❧ ASSOCIATION

I am a proud member of the American Dental Hygienist's Association and like to participate. I am proud because we are an active organization, that we can use our hearts and heads to plan and develop efforts for the stability and growth of the profession.

Esther looked forward to the annual American Dental Hygienists' Association Meeting, held alternatively on different coasts or section of the country. From the 27 young ladies who Wilma Motley (1986) described as the first dental hygienists in the world who had graduated from the Fones School in June 1914 (where classes were held in the evening in Dr. Alfred C. Fones' office reception area), and the first dental hygiene license awarded to Irene Newman in 1917 (her license bears the Number 1), the professional organization of dental hygienists (American Dental Hygienists' Association [ADHA]) now has over 100,000 members.

The first association was formed in 1914 in Connecticut, followed by other states, such as Massachusetts and New York, but it was California dental hygienists, according to Motley (1986), who first proposed through resolution to form a national organization. Although discouraged by Dr. Fones who thought it was too soon to join together, the dental hygienists persisted in their "grand experiment" (Guignon, 2007, p. 2). The ADA responded with support to a second resolution, a constitution and by-laws were drafted: "to all known dental hygiene organizations and alumni 'with well-known merits and high standards,' asking for their comments, and inviting them to join the new organization" (Motley, 1986, p. 5).

The rest, as they say, is history, chronicled with great detail in Dr. Motley's *History of the American Dental Hygienists' Association* (Motley, 1986). Included is the story of dental hygiene, the formation of the organization, lists of officers over the years, a photograph of eight dental hygienists in 1923 in Cleveland, Ohio, at the newly formed organization's first meeting, as well as a description of the evolution of dental hygiene training programs. "Survival of the Fittest: Dental Hygiene's Future Evolves from Its Past" (Helm, 1993) and "75 Years of Commitment to Care," published in the *Journal of Dental Hygiene* (1988) also provide documentation of the evolution of the profession.

The *Journal of the American Dental Hygienists' Association* (*JADA*), a quarterly publication, was published for the first time in January of 1927. In 1971, the first bimonthly issue was published, and it became *Dental Hygiene* in 1972. In addition to publishing many articles in the *JADA*, Esther was a strong advocate for the need for members to communicate and be kept abreast of changes in the profession of dental hygiene.

We have resolutions presented to this assembly which recommend regular newsletters to our active and junior members, newsletters that are spicy and stuffed with facts, prepared in an easy-to-read form, will be read. The more contact with our members the more they will develop and maintain a desirable image of the Association and be aware of current events and trends (Wilkins, speech, 1962, Philadelphia).

The mission of ADHA is to "lead the way as a unified force, the ADHA works to support dental hygienists throughout their career lifecycle and advance the dental hygiene profession by developing new career paths, expanding opportunities for care, and providing the latest training and information" (ADHA, 2017, p. 1). The organization's headquarters is located in Chicago, Illinois, and is organized under an executive director. It is structured around an executive office, member services, education, research, government affairs, communications, finance and management, information systems, and an institute of oral health.

The Oath of the ADHA is taken seriously by dental hygienists, especially Dr. Wilkins. It is a solemn oath to render health service and teach the public, especially children and young people, the value of dental health and to broaden knowledge in order to share information in this special field, which was sought by Dr. Alfred Fones, himself the son of a dentist, founder of the dental hygiene profession (Furnari, 2012).

In 1995 in Philadelphia, in a speech for dental hygiene graduates, Esther highlighted the importance of ethics in the dental hygiene profession:

This year ADHA will vote on a new Code of Ethics, which the committees have been studying and writing for 4 years. The Code of Ethics will be important to you as you start your practice and identify with the professional world.

When the final draft of the ADHA Code of Ethics appeared in ACCESS in 1995, Esther encouraged every dental hygienist to read it. *We endorse and incorporate the CODE into our daily lives.*

Esther also encouraged ADHA to be ethical about the finances of the organization. In a speech she gave in 2000 at an installation of the ADHA Finance Committee:

Be sure to keep the total membership in mind when you review the previous budget and develop the new one. Remember that the money has come from our hard-working, sincere, devoted hygienists who trust you to disperse their contributions frugally and wisely with only the best interests of all dental hygienists in mind . . . All members want a fair budget and honest use of their funds. The same challenge goes out to those elected and appointed officers of the Association to check their choices for use of the appropriated funds to ensure that each move is honest and truly necessary.

Esther became involved with the ADHA, primarily due to the influence of Isabel Kendrick, who was President of ADHA when Esther was President of the MDHA. Upon Isabel's encouragement, Esther became involved on the national level, as District I Trustee, a position she held even while attending her first year of dental school at Tufts. Esther was a strong believer in the importance of all dental hygienists becoming members of the ADHA.

This is a highly significant time for all dental hygienists to join hands to strengthen the power of the ADHA—their professional organization. Membership and participation in the ADHA support efforts that are in the interest of the individual dental hygienist and, therefore, the entire united profession (Wilkins, 2008, p. 14).

Esther was an invited speaker at many ADHA annual sessions, as well as at individual state conventions, where she often advocated for banding together and membership in professional organizations, especially ADHA. In a speech in 1962, she explained her position:

The House of Delegates is challenged with making the policies, clarifying and updating previous policies, defining our objectives in the light of today's needs, and programming to meet these objectives. We've worked at this for 38 years—and we are big girls now. Our meeting is short and the year long—3 ½ days is scarcely enough for our group to gain a cohesion which will allow group decision through effective problem-solving techniques.

We want to make mountains out of the proper molehills—in order to see our forest for our trees. Our forest is defined in the objectives stated in our Constitution: cultivate, promote and sustain the art and science of dental hygiene; represent and safeguard the common interests of the members; and contribute toward the improvement of the health of the public.

A tremendous amount of imaginative leadership is required if our hopes for increased membership participation are to be fulfilled.

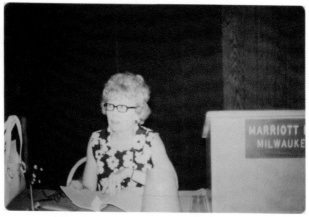

FIGURE 8.1: Esther, American Dental Hygienists' Association 1973 District VII workshop.

Throughout her career, Esther continued to share her belief in the strength of numbers as a collective voice. In a speech in 1976 at a student event at ADHA, Esther advised students after graduation to join state dental hygiene organizations:

You will become officers, delegates, and you will find satisfaction in contributing to the advancement of the profession. Get involved at the national level. There are junior dental hygiene activities. In 1992, she told students she would meet you at MDHA and ADHA meetings. Perhaps some of you are ready to leave next week for Louisiana. Wonderful! The Association is where the action is—participate.

Esther's voice, advocating for ADHA membership continued all her life: *Our American Dental Hygienists' Association is OUR professional organization; you will need it as much as it needs you. Hold hands and stick together, and say this often: I am a dental hygienist and I am proud of it.* At the ADHA 75th Annual Session in 1999, Esther stated, *Dental hygienists get farther and accomplish the most when they do it together!*

As a strong proponent of volunteerism for the dental hygienist, Esther related to Christine Hovliaras-Delozier (2008), *No man is an island, and many dental hygienists work alone. They may not have another dental hygienist in the practice that they can talk with, so volunteer. There are many opportunities to volunteer in your local dental hygiene association and in community health. Join the fluoridation cause for yours or a neighboring community* (p 35).

After dental school, Esther was not eligible to serve as president of ADHA, as she was no longer practicing dental hygiene. During her many years in dental hygiene, Esther had the pleasure of meeting many of the presidents of the ADHA, including *some of the early ones*: Cora Ueland, A. Rebekah Fisk, Frances Shook, and Margaret Bailey. Esther served as installing officer at ADHA in DC in 1974.

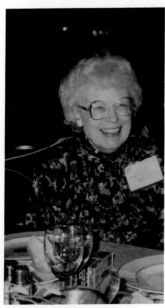

FIGURE 8.2: Esther at American Dental Hygienists' Association Meeting, 1989.

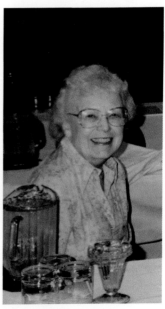

FIGURE 8.3: Esther at American Dental Hygienists' Association Meeting, 1994.

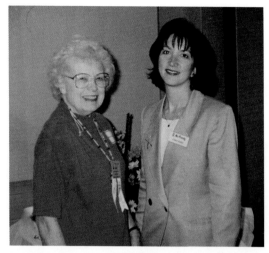

FIGURE 8.4 Esther and Karen Neiner, American
Dental Hygienists' Association Meeting, 1995.

In addition to attending many professional sessions offered at ADHA conventions, in 2008, in Albuquerque, New Mexico, Dr. Wilkins celebrated the publication of her 10th edition of *Clinical Practice of the Dental Hygienist* (CPDH) with book signing, parties, and celebrations. Anticipating an opportunity to get out on the dance floor:

> *I walked over to the President's Reception, an annual event at ADHA and this year our President was Jean Conner from Massachusetts, where there were dancing 1,000 female dental hygienists all out on the floor at once. Everyone often dances "by herself" as it gets too hot out there! I danced with all four male dental hygienists; I've danced with them for years and years!*

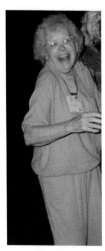

FIGURE 8.5 American Dental Hygienists'
Association Meeting, Esther dancing, 1991.

127

Many dental hygienists who wrote about Esther commented emphatically about her love for dancing. Winnie Furnari said, "As a student, I immediately was taken with Esther as we danced at a student conference." She is always the life of the party, outdancing many of them. Not one friend of Esther Wilkins said that anyone they knew could keep up or outlast her on the dance floor. Susan Polydoroff described that Esther danced until "the last song was played." At midnight, she was still going: The Eveready bunny had gone to bed hours before! Mary Kelleman, who has known Esther for over 40 years, recommended that if you "want to meet Esther, you have to dance!"

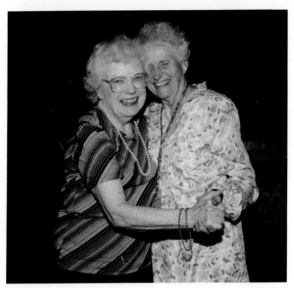

FIGURE 8.6: American Dental Hygienists' Association
Meeting, Esther and Wilma Motley dancing, 1998.

During an ADHA annual session held in Boston in the 1980s, Pat Ramsay related a story about Esther's ability to pretty much control any situation with skill and perhaps cunning. "We enjoyed an evening on a Boston Harbor cruise and we were all returning to the headquarters hotel on a charter bus. Esther in her usual way managed to get the bus driver to drop her off at her apartment. As the bus stopped and the door opened, the entire bus broke out in a rendition of 'Goodnight, Esther!' Of course, she loved it!"

In Washington, DC, in 2009, the author had the pleasure of accompanying Esther at the ADHA convention. The challenge was keeping up with Esther! When Esther thought she'd like a break from the many meetings and activities at the ADHA convention, one of her most favorite meetings of the year, she suggested a bus tour of the city in *one of those buses with upper decks*. Although we were concerned the ride would be too long to last without facilities (as we decided to see all the stops and not get off), not only were we successful in that regard, but Esther negotiated her way to the two best seats on the upper deck, without needing to "take turns," as directed by the tour bus operator. Esther enjoyed seeing the monuments once again.

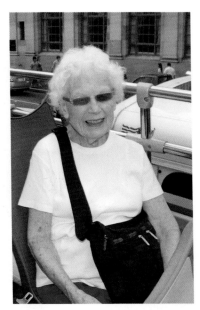

FIGURE 8.7: Esther on top of the double-decker bus, Washington, DC, 2009.

Janet Lampi said she was hard pressed not to join her students "in their shy reserve when meeting the extremely affable Dr. Wilkins." Pat Cohen added, "it is a sight to behold. At the ADHA conference in Washington, DC, in 2009, I witnessed this phenomenon. We had come into the hotel lobby after dinner and Esther was not even down the stairs from the door into hotel when the glances, giggles, and wide eyes of amazement began from all corners of the room. Pens in hand and equipped with anything they could have signed, they began shyly at first, slowly moving closer to Esther to see if it was okay to approach her, then slowly jockeying for position, waiting to ask for that enviable autograph and to meet their 'star.'"

Dental hygienists and dental hygiene students were quite mannered and respectful of the time Esther spent with each person, as they waited their turns, all the while chatting and giggling with each other with anticipation of what was about to happen. It actually took almost 2 hours for Esther to complete conversations with her awaiting court and for the room to clear, only to have little minisessions begin with other adoring fans as she made her way back to her room. You'd think Dr. Wilkins would get tired of the attention, but she seemed to actually thrive on it.

Karen Raposa had known Esther since 1986 and is a contributor to CPDH. She made a point of making a date to go out to dinner with Esther during the Annual ADHA convention in 2006.

❝Going out to dinner with Dr. Esther Wilkins always proves to be a memorable event. She is a celebrity in her own right and no matter where you are, if there are hygienists in the vicinity, they are coming by for photo opportunities and autographs.❞

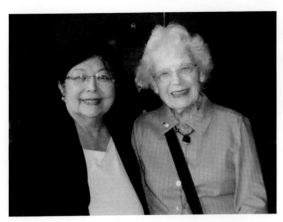

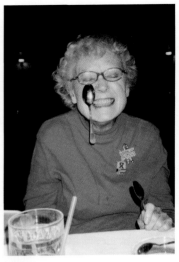

FIGURE 8.8: Esther and Anna Pattison at American Dental Hygienists' Association, Nashville, 2003.

FIGURE 8.9: Esther at American Dental Hygienists' Association, spoon on her face, 2002.

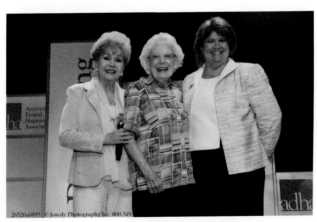

FIGURE 8.10: Esther, Debbie Reynolds, and Jean Conner, American Dental Hygienists' Association, 2008.

During the next ADHA Annual Convention after Esther's accident (in 2007), Karen again arranged to have dinner with Esther. She related,

❝ I had not seen Esther since her surgery and was fortunate to get some time on her calendar for a dinner on the night that she arrived to the meeting in New Orleans. I'll never forget seeing her come barreling into the hotel lobby, through the revolving doors with her cane, which Esther fondly called 'her shadow' and luggage in tow, never hesitating or stumbling, not even for a split second.

She proceeded to the counter, gave her room request/orders, we trudged on up to her room to drop off her bags, and proceeded to dinner. All the while I'm thinking to myself, I hope I grow up to be just like her!!"

When she had her fall in 2012 and was in a rehabilitation hospital, Esther was disappointed she could not attend the ADHA Annual Session. She was able to send a video to attendees:

Hello Everybody, this is Esther calling from a Rehab near Lowell, Mass. I am getting well. I miss not being with you because ADHA Annual is one of my very favorite places to be. I've been to almost all of them for over 60 years. I look forward to seeing you all in my home town Boston next June as we celebrate 100 years. Have a great time this week.

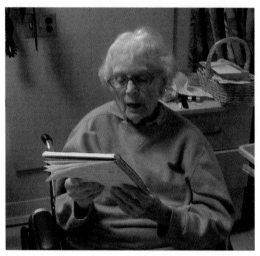

FIGURE 8.11: Esther in rehab, reading her speech to American Dental Hygienists' Association, 2012.

❧ AMERICAN DENTAL HYGIENISTS' ❧ ASSOCIATION ANNUAL SESSION, NEW ORLEANS, 2007

Rhoda Gladstone enjoyed recalling the ADHA meeting in New Orleans in 2007:

    "We pre-planned to take a tour of the city. She was always very specific in what she wanted to do, and Esther wanted to take the Katrina tour. She said she must sit in the first seat. We got to the line too late for two empty seats in the front. Since there was one available, she took that and I moved to a seat about four rows back. The driver started to pass through the bus to collect the tickets. I realized I didn't have the original ticket. When the driver came to me and I offered to show the stub, the driver replied, 'don't worry, your mother already gave it to me.' We both had a good laugh about that!"

Rhoda was fascinated with Esther's insistence on taking one little grey wheelie-less suitcase she cherished. She carried that favorite gray little suitcase trip after trip when everyone younger traveled with "wheelie" bags. She seemed to take it as a badge of courage that she could fit everything in and carry it with no difficulty. "It finally gave way in 2009 and she replaced it."

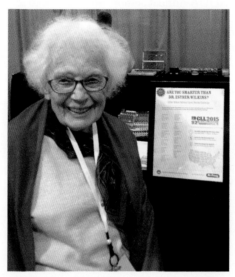

FIGURE 8.12: Are You Smarter Than Esther Wilkins, 2015.

❧ ARE YOU SMARTER THAN ❧ ESTHER WILKINS

The inaugural year of "Are You Smarter Than Esther Wilkins" event was 2008 in Albuquerque, New Mexico, a part of the student program of the ADHA convention. Students have flocked to the game-style program for all subsequent years. Students compete together in groups by ADHA district, which Hu-Friedy, sponsor of the event observed "fosters comradery and teamwork" (Friends of Hu-Friedy, 2017, p. 1). The event lasts approximately 2 hours, an hour of which includes questions on topics, such as pharmacology, nutrition, and oral pathology.

Esther and Anna Pattison asked the questions and explained the logic behind the answers when they were provided, along with advice for test-taking strategies for the board exam. A photo session followed with Esther, along with an ice cream bar and refreshments. When Esther could not attend, a life-size poster was available for students to pose for photographs. Winning teams "left with bragging rights and exclusive, limited-run tee-shirts with Esther's image, and all participants left with gift bags and autographed bookplates from Esther Wilkins herself" (Friends of Hu-Friedy, 2017, p. 1).

It was at ADHA in Washington, DC, that the author experienced first-hand this popular student event. Evident was a tremendous amount of enthusiasm on both the students' and Esther's part during this exciting and special student event. "Runners" brought answers to the group of tally volunteers in the back of the room who kept records of the correct number of answers reported. The students truly enjoyed the experience, especially Esther's active involvement in the process and the humor she inevitably shared with the students. They were mesmerized that their idol was spending time with them, helping them to learn. Evident was the mutual admiration throughout the whole process, as well as any other event in which students were involved; she loved them and they admired her. As Linda Boyd has observed firsthand on many occasions:

❝ When she is with students her eyes light up. She talks to the rest of us, but it is not with the same gleam in her eyes."

Esther looked forward to this student event every year, although she forgot its actual title and often called it "Are You Dumber than Esther Wilkins!" After Esther passed away in 2016, the event in 2017 went high tech, and students answered questions using clickers.

Most important to Esther was future dental hygienists of the world; she lit up when she talked with students and always had time for a photo, an autograph, or an offer to visit the many dental hygiene programs that sought her always energetic presentations. As Pat Ramsay related,

❝ attending an ADHA meeting with Esther can be quite an experience. It is difficult to get through the hallways at the meeting site, since the attendees are anxious to stop to have few words with her. I have walked through many hotel lobbies with Esther and heard students or dental hygienists whisper, 'there's Esther Wilkins!' No matter how many times this occurred, Esther always graciously stopped and shared a bit of her time."

❧ STUDENT AMERICAN DENTAL ❧ HYGIENISTS' ASSOCIATION

Esther was dedicated to and attended conferences of the regional Student American Dental Hygienists' Association (SADHA). Attendees found her presentations informative, exciting, and useful. Dr. Laura Mueller-Joseph related her student experience at the Northeast Regional Student Dental Hygiene Conference where she was "mesmerized by her presentation on treatment protocols. Meeting her was very exciting and highlight of my educational experience." She continued that, after the meeting, "Esther danced the night away!" Esther was admired by students, faculty, and administrators in the field and served as what Laura called "the role of advocate for the profession of dental hygiene," and who Tessei Lamadrid Black (Colgate Oral Health Advisor) described as "the greatest dental hygiene advocate in history"

Esther returned to her roots in 1996 when she gave a speech at the closing of the SADHA in Lowell, Massachusetts. It was held *in the very same auditorium* as her own high school graduation. Esther felt SADHA

> *is full of opportunities for learning, fellowship, and making new friends from dental hygiene programs from way down east in Maine to way down south to Virginia. We have attended and been inspired in a variety of ways by talks, discussions, table clinics, mini courses, and just plain visiting!*
>
> *We have learned leadership and about our mother organization and how as a group we are working to advance the profession of dental hygiene.*

❧ PHILANTHROPY ❧

Esther was admired for her willingness to support ADHA and other professional organizations in many ways, not only for the example she continuously set for excellence, but also her generosity and support for the Association. Helena Gallant Tripp related,

> " More than 20 years ago, when Warner Lambert first partnered with the American Dental Hygienists' Association to present the Excellence in Dental Hygiene Awards, Esther was in the first group of recipients—not a surprise to anyone. The well-deserved award, presented at ADHA's Annual Meeting, included a crystal obelisk and a check. Just a few weeks later, in my role as Forsyth Alumni Association treasurer, I received a check from Esther for one thousand dollars for the scholarship fund to be listed in the records as 'a donor'—no fanfare, no special recognition—just Esther's commitment to dental hygiene education."

Esther's support was continuous. Helena wrote that she approached Esther in 2006 about establishing an Institute scholarship in her name—one that would focus on dental hygiene educators. If she would make a donation, the most important aspect of the scholarship drive would be that ADHA could use her name for the fund raising necessary to reach the $100,000 level and start distributing the scholarships. Esther agreed immediately. However, before ADHA could even start fundraising, Esther contacted her again and said that she did not want to wait. She knew how critical the shortage of educators had become. She would fund the entire $100,000 herself so that the scholarships would not have to wait for the fundraising. "Her generosity spoke volumes of her devotion to the profession of dental hygiene," agreed Marie Cole. Jane Weiner wrote that Esther helps encourage those in the profession to be active. According to Daughn Thomas, "She has continued to share her vast knowledge of dental hygiene to thousands of dental hygienists [including me] and paved the way by bringing dental hygiene into the 21st century."

The Esther Wilkins Education Program, America's ToothFairy, through the National Children's Oral Health Foundation, provides eligible members with a ToothFairy 101 Community Education Kit, the aim of which is to provide oral health literacy through outreach activities. The kit contains a display board, magnets, and a giant toothbrush, used to share preventive strategies improving for oral health from pre-natal through young adult learning levels. An online portal provides access to bi-lingual curriculum and other resources. Esther served as Program Honorary Chair of America's ToothFairy:

> *I am so proud to have been able to launch the Esther Wilkins Education Program to engage children and their caregivers in preventive, smile-saving practices. The ToothFairy 101 Community Education Kit enables dental hygienists and students to share important health messages about germ transmission prevention, nutrition and oral hygiene* (National Children's Oral Health Foundation, 2016, p. 1).

Esther Wilkins worked with the National Children's Oral Health Foundation to launch a movement to rescue children worldwide from preventable pediatric dental disease with the Esther Wilkins International Education Program. Dr. Wilkins commented,

> *I have been fortunate to be involved with exciting oral health advancement throughout my career, but nothing has equaled this opportunity to forever change the lives of countless innocent children.*

It became apparent from a review of the many letters submitted in the quest to tell Esther's story from the perspective of friends that Esther gave of herself in a myriad of ways, seemingly small sometimes, but with remarkable impact on others. Claire Silk, who had been friends with Esther for 35 years, since Claire was president of the Ohio Dental Hygiene Association and Esther was the keynote presenter, shared many conversations with Esther related to ethical issues facing dental boards. "Esther was always supportive and knowledgeable in assisting me to deal with these issues."

In a conversation in April 2010, Esther called the author to ask if the author could locate an older version of her textbook which was located on one of the online book sites. She delighted in telling in her story of why she needed the book. A dental hygiene student from Longview, Texas, Angel Lazenby, had written to her; she and her classmates wanted to surprise their dental hygiene teacher with a signed copy of the edition of CPDH that she had used herself as a student, as she, unfortunately, no longer had it, lost in a fire. So Esther sent the book, inscribed to the students' teacher, Ms. Davis. A letter followed from Angel who had written to her after receiving the book for her teacher:

> ❝Dear Dr. Wilkins: We gave Ms. Davis the book. We had signed the inside and she started to read the inscriptions. We smiled and told her to turn the page. Her eyes became wide and she started to cry. 'Oh, look at her handwriting, and it's in purple!'"

The letters abound with comments from her friends describing Esther's generosity, not only her expertise. Lois Barber fondly remembers,

> ❝this is a woman with a heart. Among all the special kindnesses that she provided to me, none has brought me to tears the way her donation did after I lost my home to Hurricane Frances in 2004. She was one of my generous contributors that helped me get my life back on track." She concluded, "I dream of having a life as fulfilling, a smile as beautiful, and a heart as giving as my dear friend and mentor, Dr. Esther M. Wilkins."

There are several awards given in Dr. Wilkins's honor through the ADHA: The ADHA/Hu-Friedy (formerly ADHA/Oral-B) Esther M. Wilkins Future Leader Award "was created to recognize dental hygienists who exhibit a strong commitment to the dental hygiene profession and have demonstrated leadership in ADHA within five years of graduation" (ADHA, 2016) and is awarded annually at the opening ceremonies of the ADHA's annual session.

❧ Advanced Education ❧

Esther considered herself primarily an educator, and she felt education was the means to achieve greater things in any profession. When she began at the University of Washington in Seattle, she was not confident about her teaching abilities. She knew dental hygiene and dentistry, but what about grading, testing, and

> *all the phases of teaching and educating? Well, that's about where I was that first fall in Seattle. What did I know about educating. One of the first things I did was register up on the campus to start credits for my MS in Education. I gained a bit of insight into what's behind the experience when you are challenging yourself to become a real educator!*

For dental hygienists, Esther advocated strongly for not only the bachelor of science degree but also the master's degree and advanced dental hygiene practitioner. Taking any opportunity to convey her message and her own experiences as education, Esther said,

> " I didn't originally know how to teach, and I'll never forget my first lecture ever. Anyway, I was terrible. I was scared, but once you get up there, you have to forget yourself and think only of your audience" (Wilkins, as cited in Hovliaras-Delozier, 2008, p. 34).

It seems Esther certainly grasped the concept and skill of teaching throughout her career, and she suggested to others that they *read, read, and read some more [health care is always changing]*, join ADHA to learn and collaborate, volunteer in local community health organizations and in local dental hygiene organizations, and study the current research and literature in their field *to keep updated with new information that can help our patients.*

Esther willingly gave of herself, even if it was just small advice to Mary Kellerman, then president of MDHA, who was nervous before a speech. Mary asked Esther how she would be able to get up and speak in front of everyone. "Esther told me to go to the Toastmasters as she did; I did enroll and found it was helpful, thanks to Esther." Esther was a member of the Boston local chapter of Toastmasters International in the early 1990s.

The importance of patient education had been a career-long topic for Esther. As early as 1961, Esther stated in an article in *The Dental Assistant,*

> *The prime objective in education is to develop sound attitudes and habits which will motivate people to obtain and maintain good oral health. Dental personnel apply this objective throughout the practice—to make better informed, more appreciative patients who will*

understand the purposes of the services rendered, be more cooperative, and follow through in the program for continuing care; who will do their part personally in daily care for the preservation of the oral tissues and restoration.

Patient education as foremost in the myriad of responsibilities was a frequent topic for Esther in many continuing education programs and published articles:

Motivation of individuals to apply the basic preventive measures and incorporate them into their lifestyle habits throughout their lifetimes is our objective. All of our future educational curricula need special teaching emphasis in how we can reach and motivate our patients. People need to learn how they can protect themselves from dental caries, periodontal infections and oral cancer. Because, after all, that is our major objective—to have people realize that the responsibility is theirs.

As such, Esther felt the obligation of the patient is to keep all appointments and to be on time, or the dental hygienist's schedule is impacted the rest of the day, as well as his or her other patients. Catherine Murphy (Simmons, Class of 1938) related that "one day my little granddaughter, Leslie, told me that she had to go to the 'gentle hygienist.' I repeated this to Esther, who replied, *Of course, they are all gentle!*"

Esther felt strongly that dental hygienists must seek higher education in order to meet the challenges of the profession, including taking a research course so they know how to use the databases:

Education is an essential consideration for the future of dental hygiene. At all levels, leaders with higher degrees will be required. A drastic shortage of teachers for our professional schools exists, and the creation of many new schools has increased the demand. All of the bachelor's and advanced degrees will need more advanced periodontal subject matter, both from the new research of recent years, and from the newest in clinical care.

The ADHPP [advanced dental hygiene periodontal practitioner] will need new and review skills for nonsurgical periodontal therapy using the latest ultrasonic and manual instruments including those used with an endoscope. The ADHPP also will need increased education to accommodate the advancing knowledge relating the periodontal infection inflammation as a risk factor for systemic conditions, especially cardiovascular and cerebrovascular diseases, respiratory diseases, diabetes mellitus, and adverse pregnancy outcomes. Teaching lifestyle modifications for oral health is a new area where dental hygienists can contribute to lifesaving habits, including tobacco use control. The feature for a dental hygienist has always been the specialist in prevention of oral disease. Esther felt the future of dental hygiene was in the *hands and minds of each individual dental hygienist.*

One of Esther's favorite presentations to continuing education audiences, dental hygiene meetings, and presentations to student/faculty groups, was on biofilm. Carol Griffin related a story about this lecture: "Esther was the keynote speaker at the Georgia Dental Hygienists' Association 2003 Annual Session in Atlanta. She also presented a lecture on biofilm to students from our state. Her rendition and artistry on a transparency was impressive to all and we asked her to allow us to submit it to our Silent Auction fundraiser that same day, which she quickly agreed. Needless to say, it was the biggest sales item, of which I am proud to be its owner!" Essentially, when Esther teaches about plaque, it includes her overhead projector and the following story:

> So there are families, houses of plaque, sticking together like glue; when a person brushes, a few gullies are made, bumping a few houses. So the plaque sticks together and tries to fill in the new gaps. But when the dental hygienist uses her tools properly, she goes deeply into their village and does major damage to the plaque buildup.

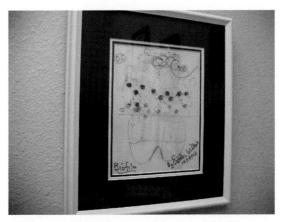

FIGURE 8.13: Framed photograph, Esther's biofilm drawing, 2003, Atlanta.

Suzanne Box, who met Esther when she was teaching at Forsyth, described her amazement that Esther "could take one slide, find and describe details in it for at least an hour and never repeat herself." It is comments like these that kept Esther going, kept her driven, kept her happy—the consummate educator. Nancy LePeau's tribute expressed the impact Esther has had in her role of educator:

❝ She is the consummate teacher who challenges and opens your mind to new ideas. She has the ability to work with students and colleagues alike to quickly identify strengths and limitations, to show respect and to encourage and to gently guide for growth toward achieving full potential. That is the definition of a teacher."

Esther was presenting with Anna Pattison in 2008. Mary Kellerman, an attendee said,

❝ Esther at age 91 was up on the podium using advanced overhead technology, drawing dots of bacteria, telling the most up-to-date story of bacterial periodontal infection. She has advanced with the times."

Frieda Pickett was one of the few who actually learned dental hygiene in 1963 using the first edition of CPDH. She described Esther as the ultimate educator:

❝ Esther set the standard for thoroughness and excellence in professional work. My goal has been to meet the standard she set. She taught me the importance of referencing information in professional communication, rather than repeating what one may have heard in other lectures. As a young educator, I wasn't very interested in reading clinical studies or research. Dr. Wilkins challenged me to verify information I included in my professional activities. She encouraged me to rise above mediocrity." Frieda continued to explain how she now expects the same eagerness from others in the health professions: "I expect them to search the literature to find answers, just as Dr. Wilkins had that expectation of me. She is a legend in the dental hygiene profession."

❧ Mentor ❧

Today a dental hygiene educator contacted me for advice. In my opinion, that is the ultimate compliment for a mentor!

According to many resources, a mentor is someone who facilitates growth and development for another by sharing expertise, experiences, and knowledge. It includes partnerships between individuals that include faculty, students, librarians, administrators, staff, and peers. It is evident from the many dental hygienists who have worked with Esther as a book chapter contributor, or who attended a dental hygiene continuing education program that she presented or copresented, or as a long-time hygienist or one just starting out, Dr. Wilkins was a mentor to at least thousands of inquiring minds who have learned from her in a myriad of ways. Teresa Duncan said that the highest honor of her dental hygiene career was the opportunity to be a copresenter with Esther at a continuing education course.

Reference to Esther as mentor began as early as her days at the University of Washington, where both former students and former faculty expressed thanks for her tutelage in those early years.

    Esther encouraged students to consider working in public health or teaching, as well as clinical practice," recalled Peg Ryan, UDub Class of 1956 and later faculty. "Esther was responsible for my entering dental hygiene education shortly after I graduated, and she encouraged one of my classmates to pursue a career in public health. She was and continues to be a mentor. I believe she has had a profound impact on dental hygiene education practice, not only in the United States, but also other countries. She promoted the development of dental hygiene education and practice in Nigeria and other countries as early as the 1950s."

Many of the letters received for this biography included at least one passage about Esther's mentorship and her influence on dental hygienists' and dentists' practices so much so that "they model many of her ways," said long-time friend, Jane Weiner. "She has been an inspiration to ever so many people and students throughout her life. She is a model role model and exemplary professional."

One of the greatest honors someone can bestow on someone else is to emulate them, to follow in their footsteps, to learn from "the consummate teacher," and to grow from the experience. Yet, Esther was the first to say that she felt mentoring was mutual, that she often felt mentored herself. In 1971, she wrote to a colleague,

> *When I was at the University of Washington dental hygiene program, we had close and pleasant relationships between our departments, and the Dean of Nursing was an inspiration and provided guidance for me during the formative stages of the program.*

Esther expounded on the importance of mentoring in a 2008 article in the ADHA *Access*:

> *I have mentored a lot of people, Christine, which included students at all different levels, educators, clinicians, and pre-dental hygiene people who are considering dental hygiene as a career. I am also mentoring practicing dental hygienists who may be thinking of going to dental school. I do not intend to discourage them, but I want to be sure of their objectives before encouraging them. I tell them of the many opportunities in dental hygiene especially related to the Advanced Dental Hygiene Practitioner credential* (as cited in Hovliaras-Delozier, 2008, p. 35).

Pat Cohen, in her many years of association with Esther, during many trips together and teaching together, she has learned,

❝to always learn, get things done, be energetic, to explore and question, meet new people, keep in touch: to do, to be, to enjoy. These are the lessons she has taught me by her words, her actions, and her reactions. Esther is a gift to me." Olga A. C. Ibsen, recipient of the 2017 Esther M. Wilkins Lifetime Achievement Award, stated, "my goal as a professional has been to make a difference in the lives of patients, students and colleagues. Esther led the way. She was a dear friend, colleague, and mentor" (*Dimensions of Dental Hygiene*, 2017).

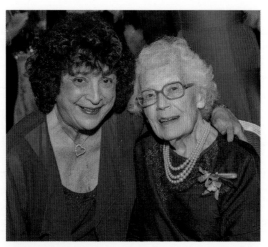

FIGURE 8.14: Esther and Olga Ibsen, American Dental Hygienists' Association.

Linda Boyd is Dean of the School of Dental Hygiene at Massachusetts College of Pharmacy and Health Sciences (MCPHS), coauthor of CPDH 12th edition, and future editor of CPDH subsequent editions, as appointed by Esther herself.

❝ Esther is the voice in our head pushing us to be the best dental hygienist we can be and continue to advance our profession.”

The letters from friends, colleagues, and students are filled with themes of learning from Esther, to delight in what Kathy Bassett called "jabbering with the master," who, according to Nancy Sisty LePeau, "challenges and opens your mind to new ideas." Teaching was Esther's primary love, and she was extremely skilled at the profession.

❝ She has the ability to work with students and colleagues alike to quickly identify strengths and limitations, to show respect and to encourage, and to gently guide for growth toward achieving full potential.”

Esther was truly a dental educator. When Mark Hartley (2006) posed in *RDH Magazine* the question, in the last 100 years of dental hygiene, "Who are our da Vincis?" the top 10 list placed Esther in distinct company; the list included Irene Newman, Irene Woodall, Wilma Motley, and Esther Wilkins, as she "has been a motivational role model to several generations of dental hygienists" (p. 1).

As Lana Crawford described,

❝ Esther is a sage, who is always there to advise. In the early days of our profession, most dental hygienists practiced in schools teaching children prevention. It was Esther's vision to raise the bar for us to see ourselves as preventive specialists also in clinical practice. She inspired us to probe more, scale meticulously, and give patients preventive care.”

Shirley Stenberg (Forsyth Class of 1956) described how dental hygiene had changed through the years, and "Esther's own academic background gave credibility to these transitions, making her a possibility thinker for all dental hygienists."

Winnie Furnari's reflected,

❝ she continues to impress me each time I interact with this fabulous lady, a true professional who has mentored thousands of dental hygienists and dentists to strive to be as brilliant and professional as she is." Friend Marie H. Cole was impressed that Esther was "willing to share her wealth of knowledge with a fledgling educator." Jane Weiner felt Esther was an inspiration to many people and students throughout her life, "a model role model and exemplary professional." She inspired others, related Kathy Bassett, to share what you know, to give back to dental hygiene, to help dental hygienists "to become more knowledgeable and astute in their positions" (Hovliaras-Delozier, 2008, p. 35).

Anna Pattison, expressed when Esther received the inaugural Lifetime Achievement Award from *Dimensions of Dental Hygiene/Colgate*:

❝ Whenever I feel the need for professional motivation, I pick up the phone and even a short conversation with her inspires me to put forth that extra effort that has been a hallmark of everything Esther Wilkins has done during an illustrious career that has immeasurably enriched the profession of dental hygiene" (*Dimensions of Dental Hygiene*, 2010b, p. 18).

In 2002, Janet Lampi asked Esther to sit on her doctoral dissertation committee and

❝ was amazed and astounded when she replied with a tremendous amount of support and encouragement, but declined to be a committee member. Imagine my incredulity when she explained, ever so humbly, that she did not feel qualified!! As she had never sat on one before, she felt she was not experienced enough to do me justice. I explained that, as my topic was dental hygiene related and I needed a 'content expert,' she was not only qualified, but if she were gracious enough to agree to sit, she would indeed be the *most* qualified among my committee. Bless her heart, she agreed and was of inestimable value in my progress."

Janet said that Esther was the first one to call her doctor. The stories number in the hundreds of those who have not only been mentored but inspired by Esther's words of encouragement, guidance, direction, example, and support. Yet, when you told her she was mentor to you, she often responded, *oh, no, dear, you are a mentor to me!*

According to Mary Rose Pincelli Boglione, Esther has always been a mentor, as well as a friend. Wana Milam considered Esther, with her "winning smile," a gracious and kind person "who captures all with her winning smile and also who shows great love for our profession and can express it, in a manner which inspires us to return to our individual offices and try to make each day a better one." She gave her and thousands of others a pat on the back and encouragement to continue forward. Sometimes, Esther just was Esther.

❝ I happen to be going back to the room from a presentation and Esther was walking alongside me and she took my arm and we walked together," remembered Connie Croffoot. "It was a special moment, one I will not forget."

Jane Weiner reflected on the impact that Esther has had on her and others; "I have learned from watching her present and actually model many of her ways with such respect." But as Jane related, not only do dental hygienists and future dental hygienists consider her a major influence on their professional lives, they also consider her a friend. "Whenever I need an answer to something, she is there for me. She encourages me to keep on going with my endeavors."

Jane met Esther face to face for the first time in Florida at the annual meeting. Jane was in a bar with a friend and

❝ who should stroll along but Esther Wilkins herself and of course we asked if she would like to join us [never thinking that she would] and lo and behold it was the beginning of a beautiful friendship. We had such fun, laughing, joking, and even getting a big serious, but what a wonderful way to get to know someone as special as Esther M. Wilkins."

A close friend, on whom Esther had a great influence, is Pat Cohen who assisted Esther in the clinical course she taught at Tufts. Pat, who calls Esther an "unforgettable character" and "fireball of energy," recalled that Esther is "a real force to be reckoned with," positively, of course. It became obvious from the many stories told by Esther's friends and colleagues that Esther not only valued education but also encouraged others to use their talents to continue to challenge themselves and pursue as much higher education as possible.

The letters from her friends frequently cited Esther as one who has taught them so much, including the value of the profession of dental hygiene, of teaching, and the importance of growing and questioning and exploring the unknown.

❧ DENTAL HYGIENE, ❧ AN EVOLVING PROFESSION

Esther enjoyed reflecting on the progress that has been made to the patient's benefit, since she began in the profession in 1939. She considered the greatest change in dental hygiene to be the patient's overall health and the role of the dental hygienist in educating the patient to be responsible for his/her own regular dental care (which, of course, includes flossing and brushing frequently). Esther often related that the original role of dental hygienists to "clean teeth" has evolved into a role of educator and patient advocate who focuses on the whole patient's mouth and body. She cited research that

> extended the possibilities for prevention, control, and treatment of both dental caries and periodontal infections. Educating patients about the connections between oral and systemic health is now a routine responsibility of the dental hygienist, including examination of all oral tissues to detect signs of various early pathologies-particularly oral cancer—and taking the patient's blood pressure (Wilkins, 2008, p. 12).

Esther wondered how to get people to stop using the term *cleaning teeth* when the patient must clean the teeth every single day with a toothbrush, floss, and other dental aids.

In a speech given in 1998 to the Pennsylvania Dental Hygienist's Association, Esther said,

> As one of the oldest constituents of the ADHA, you carry pride and responsibility. You are as old as DHA—their 75th celebration was this year too. Dental hygiene has jumped through many rings of fire on the way to being classified as a full-fledged profession, and although progress may seem slow, we know that we're part of a huge continuum in the prevention of oral disease and the promotion of oral health.
>
> Over the past 75 years, and especially in the last 50 years, research advancements and practical application of preventive measures have brought a decline in the debilitating dental, periodontal and other oral conditions that were widespread in the past. . . . Challenges? Many. The future is exciting to think and dream about.
>
> Personal integrity, continuing competence, and a devoted belief in the worthwhileness of what we are doing—those are the keys to our professional quality control and professional growth.
>
> We must believe in what we are doing!!! Professional growth requires the loyalty and unity of the whole of us together. Keep the light from the 75th birthday candles burning bright—dental hygienists get farther and accomplish the most when they do it all together!

International Federation of Dental Hygienists

The International Federation of Dental Hygienists (IFDH), founded in 1986 in Norway, is an international, nonprofit organization, not affiliated with any government agency, dedicated to the promotion of dental health around the world. Its purposes include an exchange of knowledge, promotion of access to quality oral health, public awareness of oral disease prevention, discussion of dental hygiene issues, professional alliances, and the advancement of the profession of dental hygiene.

Esther was nominated for life membership in IFDH in 1989. "Life membership is reserved for those who have made a significant contribution to the development of the IFDH and its members" (personal communication, IFDH, September 6, 2010).

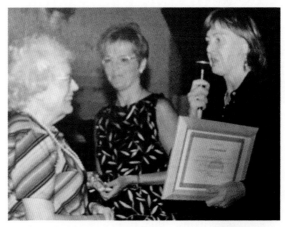

FIGURE 8.15: Esther receiving life membership plaque:
Mary Rose Boglione, Esther, and Inger-Lisa Bryhni, 2010.

The organization meets every 3 years in conjunction with the International Symposium of Dental Hygiene hosted by various countries. The Symposium has been held in several countries since the first symposium in 1970; Esther attended in Stockholm, Sweden; Brighton, United Kingdom; Ottawa, Canada; Hague, The Netherlands; Tokyo, Japan; Florence, Italy; Sydney, Australia; Madrid, Spain; Toronto, Canada; and Edinburgh, Scotland.

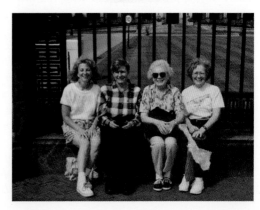

FIGURE 8.16: The gate of the
Peace Palace, The Hague, 1992.

144

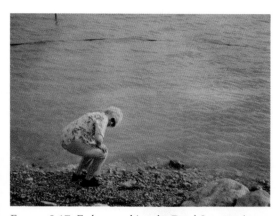

FIGURE 8.17: Esther touching the Dead Sea, 1994.

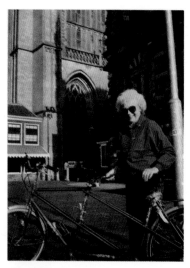

FIGURE 8.18: Esther with bike, Haarlem, The Netherlands, 1992.

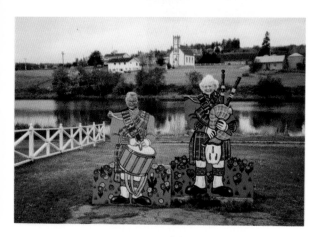

FIGURE 8.19: Esther and Fumi, North Glasgow, 1995.

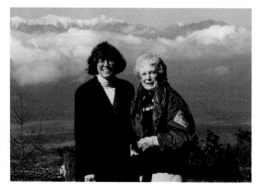

FIGURE 8.20: Esther and Charlotte Wyche, Mount Fuji, Japan, 1995.

Esther enjoyed attending the international symposium, in several of which she was accompanied by good friend, Pat Cohen, and she was particularly fond of the 1989 Symposium in Ottawa, Canada. She said that *Dale Scanlan had the program organized down to the last detail; opening ceremonies were great, and it included lots of dancing.* As Esther said, *the best one yet! Very beautiful.* Lynda McKeown attended the Ottowa Symposium, which is where she noticed a "person dancing up a storm which, of course, was our own Esther."

Along with six other US dental professionals, Esther visited the Cleland Wildlife Park in Adelaide Hills, South Australia, hosted by the Australian Personnel Placement Services.

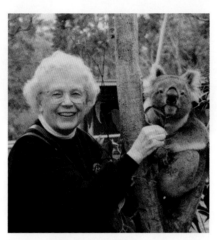

FIGURE 8.21: Esther with koala bear, Australia, 2001.

Lynn Hunt Nunn met Esther, whom she described as

" a delightful lady with a good sense of humor and a beautiful smile" at the IFDH Symposium held in Stockholm, Sweden. "I remember in particular that we stopped to tour Marbacka, the home of Nobel Prize novelist, Selma Lagerlof. On the way, Esther led us all in singing 'America' as it was the fourth of July. It was a beautiful sunny day and all of us Americans grew much closer as we belted out the words to the song." Lynn and Esther's adventures included a tour of the Karlstadt School of Dental Hygiene, conducted by Per Axelsson (who conducted research on fluoride and dental enamel), "gliding down the canals of Amsterdam, tasting international cuisine in many different countries, visiting some of the most beautiful areas of the world, and meeting dental hygienists and dentists from leading dental programs around the world." Lynn highlighted Esther's incredible sense of humor when she described their trip to North Carolina: "She and I went to the North Carolina mountains to spend a day touring Biltmore House at Asheville. It was raining throughout the day, but Esther was a terrific trouper as we left the warmth of the dry house to walk through the gardens in the rain. Of course, we used umbrellas, but our feet got wet. What did Esther do? She beamed her trademark smile and began a chorus of 'Singing in the Rain!'"

There were many stories from Esther's friends on the adventures they shared with Esther around the world during many of these symposiums and other international trips. Mary Rose Boglione said,

❝ to just relate one episode of my friendship with Esther is not possible. All our encounters were unique. One special one for me and for Esther was our visit to La Scala, the opera house in Milan, Italy. We went there the morning of her arrival in Milan, after traveling all night (a 9-hour flight)! That day had a very full agenda, but knowing that she wanted to go there.”

Mary Rose continued,

❝ the experience was gratifying; it was 'like bringing a child to a toy store' she was so excited. That morning there were orchestra rehearsals so we were able to sit, watch, and listen, which made her very happy. Then, later in the afternoon, after we worked to prepare for the course she was offering, we had reservations to see the 'The Last Supper' by Leonardo DaVinci at the Cenacolo. However, due to traffic, we missed our slot!! To say the least, Esther was upset. But Esther did not give in, with her determination she wanted to see it, and with her persistence wanted to get another time slot, and we DID! We saw it, and it was worth the waiting.”

The IFDH meeting in Florence, Italy, brought many of Esther's friends together once again. Anyone who knew Esther well is aware of her love for coffee (which doesn't even keep her up at night after having her high-test brew late at night). Marie Cole, after attending various presentations at the convention, commented with Esther about how much they missed American coffee. “We discovered a McDonald's near our hotel—and off we went together for a cup of American java!”

At the same IFDH meeting in Florence, Marie recounted that Wilma Motley had been presented with a magnificent bouquet of flowers. “When Wilma left the meeting she gave them to Esther to adorn her hotel room. I was the last to leave Florence, so when Esther left I inherited the flowers.” What Marie didn't mention but that Esther clarified,

Wilma and her daughter had placed the flowers in the bidet to keep them watered, most likely extending their life so they could be passed on to each friend as the others departed.

In 2001, the IFDH met in Sydney Australia. Barbara Dawidjan said,

❝ We were on the same plane. When we finally arrived, I was exhausted and had severe jet lag. I attended the opening ceremonies that night very tired and basically a mess from many hours of travel. At a later reception I see our good friend, Esther, dancing the night away and looking wonderful. I could not believe that she looked so well after the traveling we had done. I commented to her and she said it was because she went first class. I don't think it was that, because where there is music, there is Esther on the dance floor. Her energy is to be admired and even after traveling around the globe, she looked awesome and was enjoying herself right away.”

Esther delighted in remembering all the side trips she and her friends and colleagues took around the world when attending the IFDH symposiums, which offered to attendees choices of the various sightseeing tours of the areas they were visiting. Esther said her most memorable adventure was in London in the 1980s, where the convention was held in Seaside, South of London. After the symposium, 12 or so of the attendees, including Esther, Barbara Wilson, and several of her colleagues began a 10-day European holiday. Esther had only been in Europe once, so she really looked forward to her upcoming experience.

The trip began with a bus ride to the Waterfront, then a ferry across which, according to Esther, they were supposed to sleep upon, *but it was so crowded you couldn't move!* The first country was The Netherlands where they experienced the local culture and tourist spots, then on to Belgium where they enjoyed the museums. Germany was next, with a boat ride down the Rhine and a bus trip to the Castle on the Hill. Austria was next, then Switzerland. Esther said they were *always changing money!* The Alps were next, then on to Italy and Venice. She loved Venice, road the boat, enjoyed Italian restaurants, and the *wonderful culture.* They were in Florence a couple of days and went to museums. They spent a few days in Rome next. They saw the Vatican, then drove up the coast to France and saw the leaning Tower of Pisa. Then on they went to Sweden and saw the crown jewels, then looked down at Monaco. The tour ended on their ferry ride back to London, directly to the hotel at the airport for departure the next day. Esther remembered vividly and enthusiastically each of the segments of her European adventure with her friend, Barbara Wilson.

When Esther returned from her trips abroad, she often wrote to those responsible for making arrangements for her, including accommodations and travel to and from the airport, and the excursions in and around the places she visited. She reflected on her trip to New Zealand in 1996:

So many terrific memories dance through my head when I think of the 5-6 days in New Zealand!! Thank you for the nice things we did together—dental hygiene meetings, traveling, sightseeing beautiful Wellington, visiting the Dental Nurse School, everything. The dental hygienists are real pioneers—as their numbers increase, they will be able to self-regulate and own the world!!

Another trip for the friends was to Beijing, China. Barbara was invited with Esther to come to Beijing by the government to discuss if it was cost-effective and valuable for the hospitals to begin a program in dental hygiene rather than spend time and money educating more dentists. Barbara recalled that they set up teaching clinics for demonstration purposes.

Tina Daniels, long after her flat tire trip with Esther to Worcester, Massachusetts, "shared global experiences by trading international waters" with Esther, including 2001 at the South African Dental Association Conference in Durban, South Africa and 2004 IFDH Annual Symposium in Madrid, Spain.

❝In 2001 after learning we both were traveling to South Africa approximately the same time, we coordinated or plans to meet in Durban at a dental conference. Neither Esther nor I knew we would be experiencing history at the opening session; to our amazement, we were witnessing the first integrated South African Dental Association Conference with South African dignitaries and other honored guests, all in attendance to mark the occasion. During our stay in Durban we visited the local University's Dental and Dental Hygiene Schools; we lunched with the dental hygiene faculty and later chatted with a large assembly of dental hygiene students. I will never forget the graciousness shown to Dr. Wilkins by those students. I watched their faces as she signed their text and personally daunted over each student. That afternoon she spoke at a program where she was honored by other faculty and students. These were the times in our lives where we bonded both professionally and personally."

❝ I will be forever grateful for that cold winter day in Boston that Dr. Esther Wilkins needed a ride. Meeting Esther was a 'Mountain Top' experience in my professional journey: an experience I wish every dental hygiene faculty and student could have."

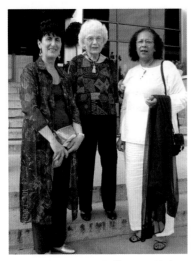

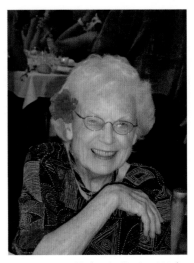

FIGURE 8.22: Mary Kellerman, Esther, and Tina Daniels, Spain 2004.

FIGURE 8.23: Esther in Spain, 2004.

Esther often remarked that her vacations all centered around her travels through ADHA or IFDH and she certainly has had lots of adventures with many different people to many different places. As she wrote in a letter to Mary Rose Boglione in 1998, *new friends from IFDH—last forever!! Just like you and me.*

Esther's propensity to be a pack-rat was pretty well known, but what is of significant note is the order in which she kept her mementos of her travels. She kept a diary of every trip she took to every single country and described with precision: the clinics, hospitals, or schools she visited, dental topics, programs and speakers, what and where she presented, curriculum, labs, instruments used, visual aids, whether a program was translated, ceremonies, deans and dignitaries she met, and awards or honors bestowed upon her, and if they used her book (or translation of her book). She noted the economy, the history, the condition of factory workers, and the availability of public transportation.

Of particular concern for Esther was the public health programs of each country, whether there was fluoridation or plans to do so, and whether dental care was available to all residents. A notation in her Australia notes: *Their program care with remote areas tends to be pain related rather than prevention.*

The excursions, boat and gondola rides, tours of museums, handcraft centers, ruins, memorials, exhibits, hot springs, beach trips, visits to villages, gardens, factories, city tours, magnificent views (especially sunsets and mountains), and friends she met were written in detail, page by page in individual booklets or notebooks. *They invited me to their Friday evening Sabbath supper—isn't that something!!* She took a tour of Fuji, visited the Peace Shrine, the Jade Buddha Temple, the Everglades, La Scala in Milan, Ayer's Rock in Australia, put her hand in the Dead Sea, Church of the Beatitudes, Sea of Galilee, the Masada, a pipeline in Saudi Arabia, the Wailing Wall, the Chagall Windows, the Great Wall of China, held a koala bear, attended an international soccer game (Italy vs. Nigeria), and drank Australian beer. Together, these comprehensive diaries could justify inclusion in yet another biography.

After each trip, a box was created (never a new one, always recycled), clearly labeled by country, preserved with care in which she carefully placed airplane and museum tickets, programs, store receipts, photographs, tour receipts, cards from admirers, postcards, and souvenirs. During one of our many interviews, I asked her why she held onto so many items. She quickly replied that everything was meaningful to her; it *kept my wonderful memories close to me forever.* She occasionally in later years looked through the folders. In a letter dated 1996, Esther wrote,

> *Such warm, purry memories of my days in Denedin, New Zealand. I loved the sightseeing. I was looking at my pictures the other day, thinking of the beautiful castle—and that rail-ride up the mountains.*

❧ THE DENTAL HYGIENE ADVOCATE ❧

Esther was the ultimate dental hygienist and her passion for the profession is unequaled. She loved the professionals who talk about it, learn about it, and practice it. Any way she could help in this regard she would do so willingly and enthusiastically. It was infectious. I asked her once why she loved the crowds, why she continued to work on yet another edition of her masterpiece well into her 90s. She thoughtfully responded that she loves dental hygiene and she would love to be remembered for a long time. I honestly don't think there is a doubt that she will ever be forgotten, and perhaps this biography will assist the profession in understanding and knowing who Dr. Wilkins truly was for generations to come. I, for one, have been endeared to this unique lady, who in 2008 prefaced an email to me with *Hello there my dear author of my biography.* She had a way about her that made you smile.

CHAPTER 9

Tufts Dental School, 1964 and Beyond

Pax et Lux (peace and light), Tufts University Seal

When Tufts College Dental School moved from Huntington Avenue to Harrison Avenue, Esther had moved to Seattle to join the faculty at the University of Washington, where she was director of the dental hygiene program. Tufts University officially became a university in 1955. According to Millstein (2008), "By 1956, Tufts Dental School had become the largest grant and contract oral research center in the country" (p. 8). Dr. Wilkins later returned to Boston in 1964 to enroll in the postdoctoral certificate program in periodontology at Tufts Dental School. Esther said that *finding Tufts in the new environment of their second home provided new experiences.*

Esther came home from Seattle, electric typewriter in one hand and her mother's sewing machine in the other, as she boarded the plane. She had just completed the second edition of her textbook, *Clinical Practice of the Dental Hygienist (CPDH)*. Esther stayed with her sister and family in Brockton until she could look for a place of her own to attend her postdoctoral studies. She located a small one-bedroom, unfurnished apartment with kitchen and bath at 8 Fayette Street in Boston, on the second floor, larger than the one she had in Seattle and close enough to Tufts to walk and arrive on time to her 8:00 AM class. She brought back most of her belongings from Seattle, including the ironing board that she used until 2016. She had to buy a bed but *had a bedroom this time.* Her friend Barbara Jasper (Simmons, Class of 1938) contributed a studio couch, which helped when Barbara wanted to visit to see Boston stage performances and would then sleep on the couch. *It slumped, so Barbara's husband made a board for it.* Esther exchanged holiday cards with Barbara up until a few years before Barbara's death. The last time Esther saw her long-time friend was at Simmons' 50th reunion in 1988.

When Esther attended graduate school, she had saved enough money and did not have to work so she could concentrate on her studies. She walked to class every day, which was in the next building over from the current Tufts Dental School. *They were building the "T" orange line then, changing it from overhead to underground.*

Esther was working on the edits to the second edition of *Clinical Practice of the Dental Hygienist* while she attended Tufts. Esther Wilkins and James Gallagher graduated in 1966, both with postgraduate certificates from Tufts University. They were married the same year (see Chapter 10).

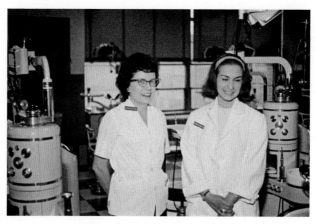

Figure 9.1: Esther and Judith Mejias, Tufts, 1965.

"Her days were occupied with teaching and administrative duties for the dental hygiene department" (DePalma, 2002, p. 2) at the University of Washington, teaching in the Periodontology Department at Tufts, working on the various editions of her book, and a very full continuing education schedule. As Esther related,

> *After two busy years as a student and receiving my certificate as a periodontal graduate, I joined the Department of Periodontology to assist in teaching the pre-doctoral students.*

✣ Tufts University School of ✣ Dental Medicine Teaching

Esther Mae Wilkins, RDH, DMD, began teaching at Tufts University School of Dental Medicine (TUSDM) as an assistant clinical professor of periodontology in 1966 through 1971; associate clinical professor, 1971–2003; was promoted to professor from 2003 to 2011; and clinical professor of periodontology emeritus in 2011. In seeking recommendations for advancement to professor, Esther reflected,

> *The letters of recommendation that I wrote to people for and collected copies (when they sent me one) are all dated in November 1999. I never did get an official letter from the committee!! I was told by a couple of the committee members (word of mouth) and then it appeared that summer in the Tufts Dental Magazine with the News of the Department or something.*

Probably of note to at least Red Sox fans, one of Esther's students in the late 1970s was Jim Lonborg, ace pitcher for the Sox for seven seasons, including the magical and Impossible Dream 1967 team, and Cy Young recipient. He was enrolled in Esther's clinical class and in Jim Gallagher's didactic classes. Dr. Lonborg became a dentist and practiced on the South Shore in Massachusetts.

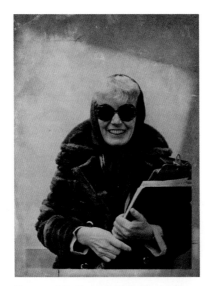

FIGURE 9.2: Esther's Tufts Yearbook, 1970s.

Tufts University completed an addition to its new building, which, according to Esther, *went skyward 5 more stories*. Esther was invited to tour the new addition before it was officially opened, donning a hard hat and looking out at her treasured city. *Tufts added five stories to the top of the building so our Perio Dept moved to the tower. I have a corner with view out over the city!!* (Christmas Letter, 2009). Her new office was housed in the new building until her retirement.

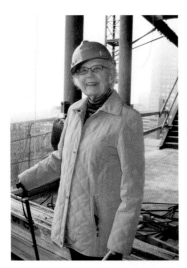

FIGURE 9.3: Esther in hard hat at Tufts topping off.

Esther was on the faculty at TUSDM for over 45 years. "During her long tenure, Wilkins became an advocate for infection control measures in the clinic. In fact, the school's first infection control handbook, published in 1990, was dedicated to her" (Wolff, 1999, p. 18).

"This manual is dedicated with sincere appreciation to Dr. Esther Wilkins for her enthusiastic efforts for better Infection Control Procedures at TUSDM by the other contributors—Infection Control Subcommittee Members 1989-1990" (Tufts University School of Dental Medicine, 1990). When she was a faculty member at Tufts, Esther scolded those who had pulled their masks down to their chins and said that they were not following protocol.

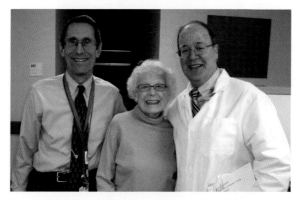

FIGURE 9.4: Drs. Wilkins, Levi, and Vankevich, 2004.

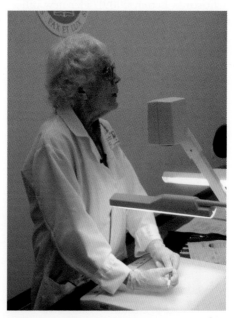

FIGURE 9.5: Esther, Tufts, Perio Lab, 2005.

Esther also taught at Northeastern University in Boston for five or six classes from 1975 to 1985. Classes were once a week for one semester—repeated once a year. The dental hygienists were completing a bachelor's degree after a 1- or 2-year dental hygiene program. Many were from Forsyth. "In addition to her teaching duties at Tufts and Middlesex Community College, she has undertaken a course called 'Advanced Periodontics' for practicing dental hygienists studying at Northeastern University" (Jim Gallagher, Christmas Letter, 1975). She was also working on the fourth edition of *CPDH*.

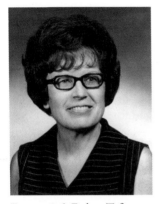

FIGURE 9.6: Esther, Tufts Yearbook, 1975.

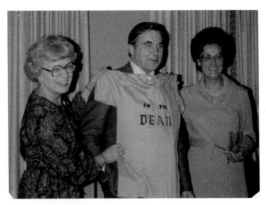

FIGURE 9.7: Esther, Dean Erling Johansen, and Inger Johansen, 1979.

Esther also continued to teach at TUSDM. Her philosophy was like that of the United States Postal Service: The mail must get through. In Jim and Esther's 1969 Christmas Letter, she said,

> *The disadvantage of living close to Tufts: we never have a cozy at-home snowbound day off as do our country faculty colleagues. With only a 10 minute walk to school, they know Esther and Jim can always make it.*

If Esther made a commitment, especially a course, she would meet her promise. Pat Cohen related one story about such a pledge: "One day Esther arrived for teaching our workshop and had a huge bandage on her left hand, so I thought she would need to sit this one out regarding the hands-on portion of the workshop, but I was wrong. She simply said, while tugging on a glove: '*If I can just get this glove over my bandage,*' and she struggled to pull the glove over her injured hand. As always, she did a great workshop with the students. Her mantra, as always, was: '*The show must go on!! Why not!!*'"

It is difficult to conceive how one woman, so small in stature, could break as many barriers as she did as a trailblazer who made significant contributions to two professions: dentistry and dental hygiene. Sometimes those two worlds would meet. In the late 1960s, Esther presented a 2-day periodontology course for dental hygienists at Tufts. As Forsyth alumnus, Beverly Whitford (who practiced dental hygiene in Connecticut) related:

❝ One day was didactic and the other day clinical. I was in awe of this tiny lady who was a dynamo in the classroom. There were other instructors involved with this program, but I can't tell you who. I only remember Esther. I was mesmerized by her energy and 'down-to-earth' demeanor. She opened my eyes to the use of curettes and inspired me to constantly research the most current standards of care."

Reflections, Dr. Ted L. Quong

Remembering fondly those days under Esther's tutelage, Ted L. Quong, DDS, who practiced dentistry in Hawaii, wrote with much enthusiasm and fondness of his mentor and teacher:

❝ I will start by saying up front that I love the woman!! She came into my life at a time when I had few academic friends and a multitude of perceived and real antagonists. It was in the Fall of the academic year 1969, during my first days in Dr. Irving Glickman's arduous Post Graduate Program in Periodontology at Tufts University. Truly anyone who was not there at that time cannot understand or appreciate what it was like back then. The tension and fear of failing that hung palpably in the air 24/7 was real and not imagined—and not unlike walking through an uncharted mine field on a daily basis. I had previously been a grad student in microbiology, U.S. Navy office, and an intern at the oldest and largest hospital in Honolulu, but never experienced anything as intense as that before."

Ted related a story:

❝ One day early in my training, in PG Perio, after an especially disheartening day, I was putting my equipment away when this beautiful, elegant, smiling lady in a white lab coat opened her locker near mine. She said to me, 'Are you the new 1st year PG student from Hawaii?' It was like a window to the normal world had been flung open and beam of humanity had burst in. It was, of course, Esther. A lasting friendship had begun. There are tipping points in everyone's life, and this was one of those for me. I don't think Esther realized that she had just thrown a life preserver to a drowning man."

Ted continued:

❝ Over the next 2 years through the *Journal of Periodontology Abstracts* Program that Esther was editor of, she became a compassionate mentor to me. She is a very knowledgeable and giving person; and I gained immeasurably from her friendship. She was a demanding teacher, but always fair—presenting fresh new perspectives on seemingly insurmountable situations. When I did graduate in April 1971, she presented me with the finest graduation gift that I received or ever would receive: an inscribed copy of her latest book, the 3rd edition of *Clinical Practice of the Dental Hygienist*." Ted enclosed a copy of the inscription and the cover of his "prized possession" to show Esther to see if she remembered that moment and thought she'd "get a kick out of it. It speaks volumes as to her humanity and character; that kind gesture is Esther."

❝ I have always felt that Esther and her contributions to dentistry were grossly undervalued and underappreciated at Tufts," wrote Dr. Quong. "It was not easy for her in a male dominated academia, where women were not taken all that seriously. Her courage was exemplary and a great debt is owed by those who followed in her footsteps. She was/is a pioneer in the truest sense of the word. One has only to go out into the rest of the country and the world to see her enormous impact in dental health education and practice."

Ted returned to Hawaii as an assistant professor and dental hygiene clinic supervising dentist in the dental hygiene program. At the beginning of each new class of entering students he taught, he held up his autographed copy of the dental hygienists' "bible," with "the admonition to memorize the book cover to cover." Ted said the response was always the same:

❝ You know Dr. Wilkins?" Ted knew he was then "in solid with them and they were more receptive to learning from me from that point on: a tremendous advantage in an age when the students challenged everything the professor said. After I retired from active practice and teaching, four of my previous students became faculty members in the UH Dental Hygiene Program: a living perpetuating legacy of Esther's philosophy, teaching, and expertise."

Ted was happy to have been on Esther's Christmas card "A" list and receiving a

❝ personal hand written note each year. Esther must have had a zillion cards to send and it was a delight to hear from her each year. She had a terrific sense of humor as you well know. I do miss her easy, uplifting, and infectious laugh."

Reflections, Dr. Joseph Kenneally and Dr. Josh Hammer

Esther's impact on students is legendary, insisting on rigor, posture, and professionalism. Former student, Dr. Joseph Kenneally, remembered:

❝ Esther was a true educator, but she was not one to put up with much nonsense from her students. To be honest, most of us were a bit intimidated by her."

❝ One of my memories of her occurred while I was treating a patient in the third floor student clinic on Kneeland Street. I was attempting to restore decay on the distal part of an upper second molar, without an assistant, so I was bent over, with my young back and neck twisted in such a way as to be able to directly see the area in question. The next thing I knew, I felt a strong hand grab me by the back of my clinic jacket and pull me into an upright position. It was Esther, who said *'Young man, if you don't learn to treat your patients with proper posture, you will not last ten years in this profession.'* Keep in mind, this was an operative dental procedure, and Esther was a professor of periodontics, whose treatment bays were on a different floor. She was just passing through. I said 'Thank you, Dr. Wilkins,' waited for her to leave the area, and finished the procedure in the same position that earned Esther's rebuke. The patient found this to be pretty funny. After that day, I tried to get an assistant, so I could sit straighter while being able to see what I was doing. I have practiced for 36 years and counting," Dr. Kenneally recalled.

Another former student, Dr. Josh Hammer, remembered an instrument-sharpening class Dr. Wilkins taught.

❝ She had an eagle eye on each of us and passionately corrected us if we were sharpening our instruments at the wrong angle. She wanted everything perfect" (Hammer, as cited in Demers, 2013, p. 7).

Reflections, Dr. Paul A. Levi

During her later years, Dr. Esther M. Wilkins taught 1 day per week in the Fall/Winter at Tufts Dental School, walking the short distance from her home, as dedicated as she was when she began her career many years ago. She taught predoctoral students at Tufts periodontal instrumentation and instrument sharpening with Pat Cohen and Dr. Paul Levi. Paul Levi, Tufts colleague and friend, related that Esther Wilkins had

❝ a total dedication to precise basics in non-surgical periodontal instrumentation. She was wholly dedicated to teaching and gave all of her students including all of her co-teachers, sound advice, and she never minced words! Her tenets were the basics, and she emphasized what she believed and believed that a healthy dentition was at the center of dental therapy. These are some of the hallmarks of this outstanding teacher and friend."

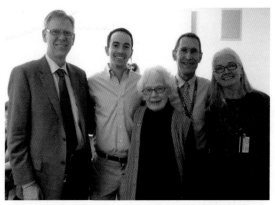

FIGURE 9.8: Esther, Pat Cohen, and Drs. Levi, Coleman, and Steffensen.

❝ I was fortunate to interact with Esther throughout my periodontal career, which began in 1964," Dr. Levi related. "Esther taught me periodontal non-surgical instrumentation when I was an undergraduate student at Tufts when she was a postdoctoral periodontal student. Previously being an accomplished hygienist, Esther was a stickler for detail and insisted on absolute perfection from me and my fellow students. As a student of Dr. Irving Glickman, my mentor also, Esther insisted that we all pay close attention when she taught. After graduating from Tufts, I entered the military and three years later I returned to Tufts to begin my training as a periodontist under the guidance of Dr. Irving Glickman, Dr. Esther Wilkins, Dr. Max Perlitsh, and many other outstanding teachers."

❝ As a postdoctoral periodontal resident, Esther and I taught the predoctoral dental students nonsurgical periodontal instrumentation and instrument sharpening, much as I had been taught five years previously. True to Esther's character, while I was working with a student, Esther would critique my teaching and advise us all to *be quiet and pay close attention when she spoke*. She would say, *Dr. Levi, when I am talking you need to pay attention*. Often this would happen after a student asked a question of me while she was speaking, and I quickly learned to say to the student, 'later, we both need to listen to this amazing lady.' After I graduated from my periodontal training, I practiced in Vermont, and I taught part-time for 27 years in the Department of Dental Hygiene with Dr. H. Charles Hill, a former Tufts periodontal resident and disciple of Esther Wilkins. We both preached the Gospel of Esther Wilkins and emphasized following exact principles of instrumentation, from diagnosis, using the TU-17 Esther Wilkins explorer, to all of the curettes and scalers that she advocated. Additionally, we insisted that the instruments be sharpened to perfection before every use, just as Esther had taught us."

❝ When I returned to Boston to teach at Tufts in 2003, I again had the fortune to work with Esther teaching the second-year dental students just as I had been taught in 1964 and as I had taught them with Esther in 1969-1971. What goes around, comes around and again Esther would chide me if I was answering a student's question while she was speaking. Would I never learn?!"

❝ Perhaps one of my greatest thrills in teaching and lecturing was about 10 years ago, giving a full-day course with Esther Wilkins. Here I was her student working with someone whom I admired greatly and giving a course to the hygienists in the State of Vermont. Because of Esther's paying attention to detail and her training that she had provided me, the course was flawless. When periodontology has to define itself, Esther Wilkins expresses the essence of our profession. I feel so very fortunate to have had the good fortune to have her as a mentor."

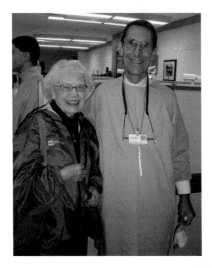

FIGURE 9.9: Dr. Levi and Dr. Wilkins.

Reflections, Dr. Kathleen O'Loughlin and Dr. Andrea Richman

Kathleen O'Loughlin, DMD, MPH, who was appointed executive director and chief operating officer at American Dental Association, was both a student of Esther's at Tufts Dental School as well as her director from 1979 to 2002. Kathy described that as a new student in the clinic,

❝ Dr. Wilkins supervised my periodontal instrumentation—preclinical and clinical. She thought I was moving too fast for my own good, and at one point thought I should stick with nursing or research, my previous profession." Kathy indicated that Esther expected the best of her students and when they failed to deliver, "we would occasionally get a little tap on the head or hand! She taught me not to expect anything less of myself. She is a trailblazer and prepared the road for my own professional success."

When Esther became one of Kathy's faculty members at Tufts, Esther's skills as an instructor became evident:

❝ Her dedication to perfectionism when it came to patient care drove me crazy as a student, but as a clinician—I valued her rigid adherence to top, superb, excellent clinical performance as a 'gold standard.' I depended on faculty from many departments to teach in my course, *Introduction to Clinical Experience*—year long and 165 students. Dr. Wilkins NEVER let me down. She was always ready, prepared, organized to teach her section effectively. I had confidence in her and the students she taught. Periodontology was one of the most effectively taught pre-doctoral programs at Tufts. My nickname for Dr. W. is the 'Ever-ready battery bunny periodontist,' always ready to go to work!"

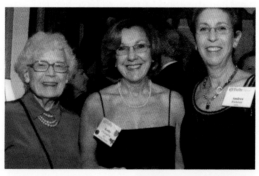

FIGURE 9.10: Kathleen O'Loughlin, Esther, and Andrea Richman.

Although she was not in her department, as a dental student Andrea Richman remembered Esther as

❝ one not to be trifled with! She could be very intense, but had a great sense of humor. She once stated in a lecture that her patients were known to quit their jobs and devote themselves to plaque control." Andrea "crossed paths with Esther quite often when they attended meetings or functions. If there was a party, she was on the dance floor in her jogging suit and sneakers—cutting a rug with her graduate students! I once testified in the Massachusetts State House on an issue, and she was testifying on the opposite side. As I walked back to my seat, she chastised me and asked when I went over with the Big Boys. Actually, I was President of the Dental Society at the time and it was my issue. Of course, this didn't carry over to our chit-chat after that."

Reflection, Dr. Tim Hempton

In remembering Esther, Dr. Timothy Hempton shared his admiration for his mentor and Tufts office mate.

    " Dr. Wilkins introduced herself to me in 1990. She was just finishing reviewing infection control protocol with a third-year dental student in the clinic at Tufts University School of Dental Medicine. I introduced myself to her as a new member of the Periodontics Department and told her that we would be working together on the clinic floor. She was very welcoming and very enthusiastic about a new periodontist joining the faculty at Tufts."

    " Through the years, Esther mentored me as to how to be a good clinical instructor. It was surprising to meet a woman well into her 70s who had so much energy and enthusiasm. In 1994, I asked if she could help me on a different level, writing review papers for dental hygiene journals. She said *yes* and proceeded to help me construct four review papers for RDH magazine. The first paper covered diagnosing mucogingival problems and the benefits of graft therapy; the second and third papers covered periodontal regeneration; and the fourth paper was a review of Juvenile periodontitis now known as Aggressive periodontitis. She was extremely helpful. It became very apparent, however, that she not only was well versed in Periodontology, but also in crafting scientific subject matter in a clear and compelling format."

Of note is Esther completed the seventh edition of *CPDH* in this same year.

    " From 2000 to 2010, we shared an office at Tufts," Dr. Hempton remembered. "During that time she provided guidance to me as I constructed continuing education lectures for dental hygienists on the topic of Periodontology and Implantology. She made it clear to me that the RDH very much wants to help patients understand risks treatment options and prognosis. To Esther it was always about helping people learn how to maintain good oral health."

During this same period, Esther also completed both the 9th and 10th editions of her textbook.

    " From Boston to Seattle, from Chicago to Miami, dental professionals everywhere are inspired by her. What she perhaps doesn't realize is truly how much she inspired and continued to inspire others" (Hempton, as cited in Camire, 2006, p. 1).

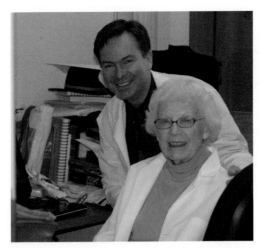

FIGURE 9.11: Dr. Tim Hempton and Esther, 2007.

Reflections, Dr. Robert J. Rudy

With deepest respect, Dr. Robert J. Rudy reflected on his 36 years of association with Esther, as her student, as her colleague, and as her friend. According to Dr. Rudy, when Esther was admitted to Tufts in 1945, she came under the influence of Dr. Glickman,

" an energetic and apparently tireless researcher" (Tufts-New England Medical Center, 1967, p. 3) who advanced preventive dentistry. He is recognized as "one of the world's leading investigators in the field of periodontology" (p. 3).

According to Dr. Rudy, Esther embraced Dr. Glickman's philosophy of a public health vision for dentistry and "became one of his many disciples." When she became a teacher herself, she became an authority in her own right. As a dentist and dental hygienist, she was passionately concerned about public health and prevention, and this passion informed all her lectures inside and outside the walls of Tufts.

" Dr. Esther M. Wilkins joined the teaching ranks of the Department of Periodontology in 1966, after successfully completing her post graduate training under Dr. Irving Glickman. Esther chose to focus her attention on the didactic and clinical training needs of the expanding pre-doctoral student body." Innovations with the teaching program at Tufts began in 1968, when new professor of Restorative Dentistry, Dr. George Mumford, "was given the responsibility of combining the areas of operative dentistry, crown and bridge, partial denture prosthesis, preclinical technic and materials science" (American Academy of the History of Dentistry, 1970, p. 26).

According to Dr. Rudy, other departments also sought to strengthen the new curriculum, including the Department of Periodontology, which made improvements, including strengthening the pre-clinical component. "Esther made that happen!" Esther was a driving force for change.

Dr. Glickman passed away in 1972, and Dr. Perlitsh was appointed acting chair. At that time, Esther was teaching in clinical, working with the didactic program. She advocated for change to strengthen training to a real clinic. With an utmost respect for Esther, Dr. Rudy said,

❝ Esther was ahead of the game; she was passionate, she was a perfectionist, and she was a terrific professional role model. She made clinical skills a reality for her students and advanced their professional lives and practice." Dr. Rudy felt Esther made him more detail-oriented and a stronger teacher.

Dr. Rudy continued,

❝ In 1973-1974, following the sudden passing of Dr. Glickman, Esther working closely alongside interim department chairman, Dr. Max J. Perlitsh, and teaching colleague, Anna Pattison, proposed a new addition to the curriculum: the Periodontics I course. Esther's carefully-outlined proposal, which strengthened and expanded the department's commitment to the periodontal education of the pre-doctoral students, was accepted by the school's curriculum committee. The new course was established in 1975 under Esther's guidance. The text assigned was Glickman's 1972 edition of *Clinical Periodontology*. "The course will offer an orientation to periodontal instrumentation. Lectures, video tapes, group demonstrations, and practice on Dentoforms and on fellow student patients will introduce the student to principles of instrumentation, periodontal examination, scaling, root planning and gingival curettage procedures. In addition, sharpening, sterilization and care of instruments will be presented" (Course Proposal, Periodontics I, 1972, Dr. Esther Wilkins and Mrs. Anna Pattison).

❝ Esther remained an active and enthusiastic participant in this course until the year 2013, when, at the age of 94, she reluctantly took a leave of absence for health related issues. Esther outlined the objectives of the program. She should be given credit for redirecting the program in Periodontology at Tufts; she set the bar."

❝ The goals of the Periodontics I course were essentially two-fold: (a) Ensure the integration of the department's didactic lecture courses and clinical training; (b) Ensure that the pre-doctoral students were competent in the following skills, each considered by Esther, indispensable to proper patient care.

    a. diagnostic and charting skills
    b. probing and calculus detection skills
    c. radiographic interpretation skills
    d. ability to formulate the correct diagnosis
    e. ability to summarize the patient's essential problems and needs
    f. preventive dentistry counseling skills
    g. manual instrumentation skills
    h. ultra-sonic instrumentation skills
    i. instrument sharpening skills
    j. phase I therapy evaluation skills"

Dr. Rudy explained,

❝ To help highlight and codify exactly what she expected from the students, Esther took on the responsibility of creating the teaching handbook known as the *Clinical Periodontics Handbook*. The handbook first appeared in 1978 and went through 35 separate editions. Esther was concerned with every possible detail and took great pride in the appearance, the organization, and the contents of each succeeding edition. *the Clinical Periodontics Handbook* served as the 'clinical Bible' for thousands and thousands of Tufts pre-doctoral students and helped to establish the 'standard of care' in the main patient care clinics of the dental school." According to Dr. Rudy, the students were to learn the material, like it or not, and she demanded they follow her guidance. "She learned from Dr. Glickman, championed Glickman, crystallized his ideas, shared his passion, and passed it on to her students." It didn't matter which audience she preached to; she championed Dr. Glickman's ideas for the need to care about public health as well as the early diagnosis and early treatment of periodontal disease.

❝ She was the lead editor of the *Clinical Handbook* from 1978 to 1994." During this time period, Esther also completed the fifth, sixth, and seventh editions of her textbook. Dr. Rudy continued: "In 1995, I became the first Director of Pre-doctoral periodontology and became lead editor of the handbook and remained so until 2013. I always did my best, however, to defer to Esther's keen judgment on the appearance and contents of this training guide. She remained enthusiastic that each year's handbook would 'out do' the previous edition. There was never an edition where she was complacent; rather, each year, she challenged herself to comb through the manuscript with painstaking attention to detail, searching for every misplaced comma, every potential spelling error, every important concept that was missing or out of place, every color of every page. Esther even insisted on having a certain number of handbooks printed just for 'left handed' students. These students were always shocked and amazed that someone had prepared for their special instructional needs."

❝ In her own right, Esther was a formidable teacher for any student to encounter. She challenged and inspired her students by demonstrating a penetrating mind, an indefatigable work ethic, and a no nonsense, non-negotiable advocacy of the highest possible standards of technical skill. Throughout her long career, Esther made a magnificent contribution to formulating the 'standard of care' in the field of non-surgical periodontal therapy as well as to enhancing the role the subject of periodontology must play in the day to day practice of general dentistry."

❝ It should be remembered that during her 45 year long tenure on the faculty of the Department of Periodontology, all of the seven department chairpersons under which she served, namely Drs. Glickman, Perlitsh, Stern, Smulow, Leone, Griffin, and Hanley, recognized and appreciated Esther's special concern for the periodontal education of the pre-doctoral student body and fully supported all of her teaching initiatives." Dr. Rudy said she was a force to be reckoned with. She was passionate about high standards and fought some battles in achieving her goals, "fighting the good fight! She scared some people, but I learned a lot from her."

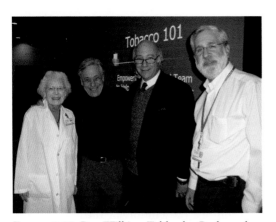

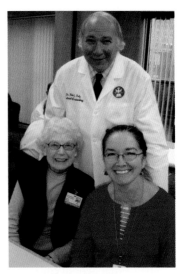

FIGURE 9.12: Drs. Wilkins, Zablotsky, Rudy, and Rosenberg.

FIGURE 9.13: Dr. Wilkins, Dr. Rudy, and Pat Cohen, 2005.

Rudy continued:

❝ In addition to her unwavering commitment to the educational mission and programs offered by her department, and perhaps more importantly, Esther herself exemplified many of the characteristics most admired by members of her chosen profession: (a) honesty and integrity in all patient care matters; (b) a desire to serve patients in such a manner that the highest standards of technical care were never compromised; (c) a desire to empower patients with the practical knowledge of preventive dentistry so they could achieve and sustain oral health for themselves; and (d) a desire to fulfill a deep sense of social responsibility by sharing her enduring passion for the field of periodontology with thousands and thousands of dental students, dental hygienists, dentists and periodontists across our nation and around the world."

Esther's Reminiscences of Tufts

Esther was asked to provide her reminiscences of her days at Tufts before they moved from Harrison Avenue to Washington/Kneeland Streets:

History of Tufts University School of Dental Medicine

Reminiscences of the history can best be told in four parts, each to describe aspects related to the four locations in Boston.

Tufts at Harrison Avenue: When Tufts moved, I had moved to Seattle to join the faculty at the University of Washington, where I was the Director of Dental Hygiene. I returned to Boston in 1964 to enter the post-doctoral program in Periodontics at Tufts. Finding Tufts in the new environment of their second home, providing new experiences. After two busy years as a student, and receiving my certificate as a periodontal graduate, I joined the Department of Periodontology to assist in teaching the pre-doctoral students.

165

Remembering experiences in that big clinic which covered nearly the whole second floor, include a snow day when nearly all the patients, especially the older ones, showed up, and many students, but a shortage of faculty. As the only periodontal faculty member present, I hurried from one patient to another, always with a long list. One of the prosthetic professors said that he checked mostly restorative cases all morning!

Plans were beginning for another move as Dean Louis Calisti saw the need for more space for research and postdoctoral clinics. The new building was being designed and built on the corner of Washington and Kneeland Streets, literally "around the corner." We moved in 1972. Now when we spoke of Huntington Avenue, it was the "old old" school for those of us who had been there. Harrison Avenue became the "old" school.

Now into another century, dental education is expanding at all levels. The new research and the need for the expansion of education for pre-doctoral students makes a great need for more space to accommodate for the needs of general practitioners to help with the problems of access to care. The new picture of the dental school going skyward five more stories will tell its own story for the future.

Tufts Dental School enjoys an impressive history. For a history of Tufts, as well as pictures of the Huntington Avenue, Kneeland Avenue, and Washington Street Tufts Dental School buildings, as well as its expansion, see two comprehensive articles by yet another friend of Esther's, Charles Millstein (1999 and 2008) and American Academy of the History of Dentistry (1970).

Esther thoroughly enjoyed teaching, although the walk to Tufts was sometimes treacherous in poor weather or as sidewalks deteriorated. In an interview conducted by Tonya Smith Ray in 1996, she asked Esther as a professor at Tufts University Dental School in Boston if she could teach her students one thing, what would it be? Esther responded, *How to have a productive, team-oriented practice with dental hygienists as colleagues, contributing to the best of their knowledge and capabilities.* Herein, perhaps, lies one of the most important contributions Esther M. Wilkins, RDH, DMD, has made to dental science: understanding and educating all professions, especially in health care, the essential value of both dentist and dental hygienist to the health care team. Because she was both a dental hygienist and a dentist, she had credibility, knowledge, and communication savvy to get that crucial message across. Many listened to what she had to say. As she stated, *I can't imagine life without dentistry and dental hygiene,* which is the reason she never considered retirement.

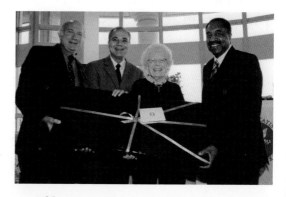

Figure 9.14: 40th Anniversary Award for Teaching, Tufts University School of Dental Medicine.

Teaching and advocating for Tufts was important to Esther, to Tufts colleagues, and to her students. In 1974, Esther represented Tufts at the Massachusetts Governor's Commission on the Status of Women held in Boston in January, which drew thousands of attendees. "The purpose of the event was to bring together women of various professional backgrounds" (Tufts University School of Dental Medicine, 1974, p. 7). Drs. Rothenberg, Wilkins Gallagher, Santis, and Fogels represented the University in sharing that "the dental profession is open to women" (p. 7).

Through the years, Esther was recognized by Tufts Dental School for her many contributions to the college (see Chapter 13) and has also had a major impact on the students she has taught through the years. Karen Neiner retold a story of her husband, whom she said she married partly because he had been a student of Esther's at Tufts back in the '80s. When she met her husband, Rick, who had said he was in dental school, she grilled him as to whether he knew of the TU-17 explorer and Dr. Wilkins. He said "yes" and that he actually would walk Esther home sometimes, as she didn't live far from him. He added that she was the toughest instructor when it came to checking out patients in the clinic, as according to Esther, *a Class I patient could even take you up to four appointments.* Karen added that she didn't realize at the time that 4 years after her conversation with Rick about Esther that she would begin work at Hu-Friedy Mfg. Co., "the company who made the TU-17 explorer per Dr. Wilkins' requirements since her collaboration and development in the 1970's."

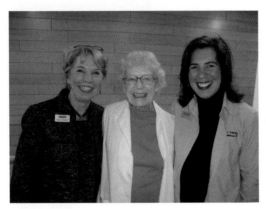

FIGURE 9.15: Dr. Wilkins, Mary Littleton, and Karen Raposa (Hu-Friedy), Tufts University School of Dental Medicine, 2012).

Esther made lifelong commitments to the educational institutions from which she graduated, acknowledging the tremendous value and impact on her professional life that her education provided. As such, she remained affiliated with Simmons, Forsyth (Massachusetts College of Pharmacy and Health Sciences [MCPHS]), and Tufts throughout her whole life. She attended alumni reunions with great enthusiasm, kept in touch with classmates for over 70 years (with Christmas cards, wedding gifts, and entrances into nursing homes), and was generous in her gifts to the three colleges.

Esther and Jim attended as many Tufts Class of 1949 reunions as possible. In 1969, they traveled *but not far: a 20th dental class reunion in New Hampshire.* Maria Tringale, former director of Development and Alumni Relations at Tufts, recalled the planning of the 40th reunion of the Class of 1949. "It was in 1989 when Esther was involved in her class' 40th reunion. This was a serious class, with the likes of Dean Erling Johansen who I revered and was a little afraid of at the time. I expected a level of seriousness in the first class meeting—but that all changed when Esther arrived—a little late. Everyone relaxed and got down to the fun of planning a first-rate party! Anyone who knows Esther knows that a good party must have dancing!! To this day, Esther is one to show the rest of the room how to ballroom dance." In 1999, the Class of D49 Tufts held its 50th reunion. Class members were asked to describe, for inclusion in a class booklet, their most memorable experiences at Tufts. Esther stated that what came to mind about her Tufts days were

Dr. Joseph Volker's super lectures and the spiral staircase between 1st and 2nd floor clinics and carrying the big old black instrument kits around. It's amazing how fast 50 years can go.

Tringale described the reunions of classes that graduated in years Esther had been teaching: "During reunion class meetings of her students, I listened to tales about Esther's persnickety demands in the clinic . . . something alumni would say that they came to appreciate and understand once they were in a PG Program or out in practice."

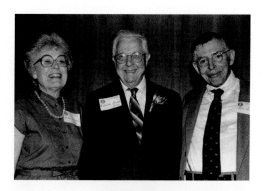

FIGURE 9.16: Tufts reunion, 1987, Esther Wilkins '49, Walter Brown '24, and Jim Gallagher '49.

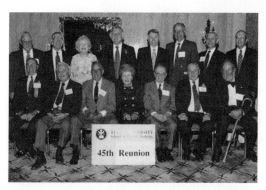

FIGURE 9.17: Tufts 45th reunion, Class of 1949 in 1994.

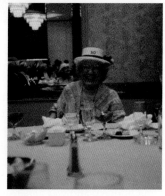

FIGURE 9.18: Tufts 50th reunion, Class of 1949 in 2009.

One student from the Class of 1979, Amerian Sones, shared, "Esther was always ahead of her time. Before ergonomics was ever discussed as an occupational concern—she was on it! It was 1976, in our first year. We were learning about root planing and scaling in small groups. When my turn came to demonstrate chair and hand position, Dr. Wilkins came over to me quickly and firmly straightened up my back and neck, pulling my shoulders back to correct the poor posture I had. *You'll never make it through a dental career with posture like that*, she quipped."

Reflections, Dr. Sheldon Duchin

Former student, Sheldon Duchin, D74, who is an assistant professor of periodontology at Tufts, described his favorite instructor: Dr. Wilkins. Duchin (as cited in Flaherty, 2012) said,

    "You had to spend a long time with her doing your periodontal diagnosis. If you did scaling with her, she would detect every small particle of calculus on a patient's tooth. And she would go through brushing and flossing with a patient endlessly, until the gums were in perfect condition" (p. 3)

Dr. Duchin suggested that Esther's influence was a big part of his choosing periodontology as a specialty. As Flaherty (2012) related,

    "Wilkins' students at Tufts knew little of her celebrity in the dental hygiene world. Duchin happened to come upon *Clinical Practice of the Dental Hygienist* with Wilkins' name on it in the library. When he asked her about it, she said, 'Yeah, I actually wrote the dental hygiene bible.' His helpful instructor, he discovered, was 'really quite a famous person" (p. 29).

    "You often decide to do things based on how enthusiastic your instructors are, the excellence they exhibit, and I think that's what happened to me. Somehow the message went across that periodontics was the way to save patients' teeth, that this was a very important part of dentistry. And that's what I decided I wanted to do" (Duchin, as cited in Flaherty, 2012, p. 3). According to Flaherty (2012), "When Duchin was accepted to Harvard's graduate program in periodontology, the first person he told after his parents was Wilkins" (p. 3).

Reflections, Dr. Ed Cataldo

Esther had an office at Tufts until she was well into her 90s. Tufts Professor Emeritus Ed Cataldo wrote

    "As a colleague of Esther's at Tufts, whenever I made a presentation to hygienists, I would always mention that my claim to fame was that my office was directly across the hall from Esther's office. Just this would give me instant celebrity status and usually, in the post presentation question time, most of the interest expressed revolved around Esther, rather than the subject material" (personal communication, May 25, 2012).

Reflections, Pat Cohen

Pat Cohen saw Esther as a powerful role model.

❝ Her usual approach to new ideas and projects is 'Why not?' And that's not a
question. It's her way of saying, 'Let's do it, and let's do it now!" (Cohen, as
cited in Flaherty, 2012, p. 4). Pat related a story of Esther's determination:

❝ Esther's office was relocated to the newly-built tower, where she quickly chose
the desk by the window, to look out at her city. After a 2-hour lesson in the sim-
ulation learning center, we returned to Esther's brand new office on the 12th floor.
The outside wall has half/wall windows with a beautiful view, the sidewalls have a
few shelves over desks and the fourth wall is the perfect spot for a bulletin board.
Esther spoke with Coletta from the perio department and Coletta told her that she
could order a bulletin board but it would take a few months and at this time the
rule is 'nothing should be hung on the walls.'"

❝ But Esther had an idea . . . she thought out loud 'I'll just get my old bulletin
board from my old office downstairs on the second floor.' Coletta's quick reply,
'There's nothing left down there in your old office; everything has been cleared
out.' But Esther had another idea . . . *I still have a key, Pat. We can go see what's there.*
I said 'Let's go!' *'Now?'* Esther asked. 'Sure!'"

❝ We quickly went down to the second floor and snuck into the old office where
there was a bulletin board still on the wall, attached very securely with four
big screws. We pulled out our screwdriver, got up on a chair, and started turning
the first screw. It must have been six inches long, but finally it came out. Repeat
the effort three more times, and finally the board drops to the floor. It was heavy,
maybe 40 pounds or more."

❝ Due to a little dumb luck on our part, I had my wheelie suitcase with me
and so we perched the giant sized board on my suitcase and against my head,
balancing and pulling it along carefully. The board hardly fit through the doorway.
We moved the board down the hall, laughing and feeling very naughty."

❝ When we got to the elevator, the doors opened and the elevator looked a little
full, but onto the elevator we squeezed. I think the other folks on the elevator
thought they were on 'Candid Camera.' I had a big board perched on my head and
Esther was navigating, because it was not easy for me to move my head around to
see where I was going. In hindsight, why didn't anyone offer to help us? We were
certainly struggling. No one was around to see us sneak the huge bulletin board
into Esther's office. We tucked it behind a desk against the wall. A phone call to the
facilities department and a request for someone to come up with an electric drill,
we will have that bulletin board up on the wall in no time at all."

❝ And the rest of the perio department will wonder: How the heck did Esther get
that big heavy thing up here? And how did she manage to hang it?" *Let them
wonder, it's fun,* she replied. "When Esther has an idea, nothing can stop her. She's a
moving target and a laugh a minute; an inspiration and an amazing wonder to us all."

Commitment to Tufts

Regardless of whom you speak with at Tufts who knew Esther, you will hear words, such
as trailblazer, pioneer, ambitious, rock star, teacher, mentor, force of nature, tough, educator,

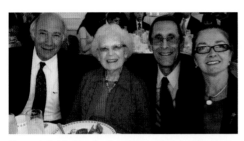 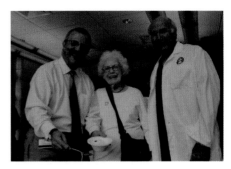

FIGURE 9.19: Faculty luncheon, Esther, Dr. Rudy, Dr. Levi, and Pat Cohen.

FIGURE 9.20: Esther, Dr. Rudy, and Dr. Huw Thomas.

professor, enthusiastic, perfectionist, lifelong learner, and to her, above all else, friend: As Dr. Robert A. Faiella, past President of the American Dental Association, reflected,

❝ Esther was a great friend and iconic figure in dentistry!"

Esther was quite excited when for the first time in Tufts Dental School history, two women were serving as class presidents (see Flaherty, 2012). Tufts honored Esther and Hilde Tillman (both also graduates of Simmons College) with special lifetime achievement awards, during their 60th reunion at Tufts University School of Dental Medicine, in June 2009.

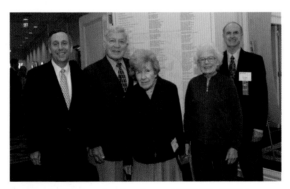

FIGURE 9.21: Reunion luncheon, 2009, Dr. Wilkins, Dr. Tillman, and colleagues.

The two women class presidents, Meghan Dombrowski and Inga Keithly, presented the awards to these pioneers in dentistry. These two women were the first female presidents of two classes at Tufts, which made Esther smile.

Considering that 70 years ago, Esther enrolled in a Tufts dental program where women were a small minority and Harvard Dental School could not consider admitting her due to her gender, she trailblazed through the evolution of dental history.

Tufts University remained a very important part of Esther's life. She perpetuated her support of the university in her establishment of the Dr. James B. Gallagher Jr., A47, D49,

DG68, and Dr. Esther M. Wilkins, D49, DG66, Scholarship Fund. Lawrence S. Bascow, President of Tufts University, acknowledged Esther's contributions:

    ❝ Your philanthropy and your own outstanding accomplishments as a leader in dental medicine both provide tremendous encouragement to others" (personal communication, April 2, 2010).

In 2011, Dr. Wilkins was bestowed with the title "Clinical Professor of Periodontology Emeritus" by Tufts University School of Dental Medicine.

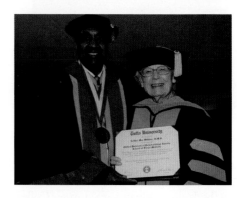

FIGURE 9.22: Emerita, Tufts, 2011, commencement.

Esther was posthumously awarded the Dean's Medal, the highest honor a dean can bestow, shortly after her death. Esther's niece, Betsy Tyrol, accepted the award on behalf of her family.

Esther stored her dental degree and graduate certificate from Tufts tucked away in her closet, still rolled up in their original tubes. Dr. Bjorn Steffensen, chair of the Department of Periodontology at TUSDM since 2013, accepted these documents on behalf of the college and department. Thanks to the generosity of Dr. Robert Rudy who had them framed, they are now displayed in the Glickman Library at TUSDM.

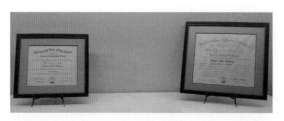

FIGURE 9.23: Esther's framed degrees.

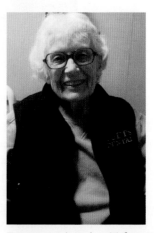

FIGURE 9.24: Esther, Tufts, 2013.

CHAPTER 10

Esther and Jim

His dedication to dental education was a true inspiration for me.

Born on March 26, 1926, in Brockton, Massachusetts, James B. Gallagher, son of Dr. James Bernard Gallagher, Sr., a practicing dentist, and Katherine Francis Keough, grew up in Rockland and graduated from Rockland Public High School in 1943, followed by service in the Army during the Korean War, stationed in Germany.

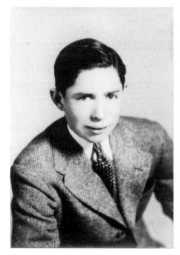

FIGURE 10.1: James B. Gallagher, Jr., Rockland High School, 1943.

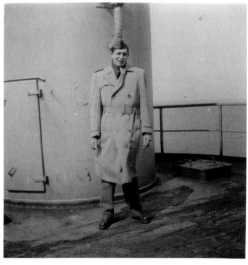

FIGURE 10.2: James Gallagher on boat to Germany.

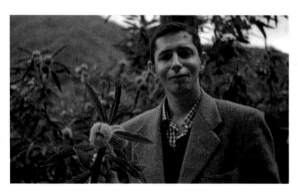

FIGURE 10.3: Jim Gallagher.

After the war, in 1946, at the same time as Esther Mae Wilkins, RDH, Jim enrolled in Tufts Dental School in Boston, both in the Class of 1949. They were classmates, although they were just friends back then. As the circulation manager of *Tufts Dental Outlook*, treasurer of the 1949 Class, a member of the Louis Pasteur Society, and treasurer of Delta Sigma Delta, Mu Chapter fraternity, the first Greek letter, Jim was, like Esther, actively involved in Tufts activities.

After Jim graduated from Tufts Dental College in 1949, he practiced dentistry with his father for 12 years in Rockland, Massachusetts. He was also the school dentist in Halifax for a short time and a dental officer for the Army from 1952 to 1954. While in private practice, he was also a visiting dentist at the Plymouth County Hospital. Jim was married to Cecelia M. Lauricella, a registered nurse, in Lynn, Massachusetts.

Jim returned to Tufts Dental College in 1961 as a part-time instructor in the Department of Complete Denture Prosthetics. In 1962, he became a full-time instructor and then assistant professor in 1964. Jim's wife passed away at 43 years old in 1964, shortly after she and Jim purchased the Brant Rock cottage.

❧ ESTHER AND JIM RECONNECT ❧

During his two postdoctoral years at Tufts from 1964 to 1966, enrolled in a graduate certificate program in periodontology, Esther reconnected with her former Tufts classmate:

> *We met at Tufts in September of 1964 when I was there from Seattle to register for the periodontal graduate program. He was coming down the hall on crutches, having broken his leg in April of that year. He was in his office and the light bulb blew overhead. He climbed up on a stool to change the light bulb and fell. It was April 15, 1963.*

Jim's disability from this accident lasted the rest of his life.

They began spending time together while at Tufts, the romance kindled, and Esther and Jim's friendship evolved into love. Jim asked several times for her to marry him, but she said she tried to explain how "The Book" was *such a big part of my life and a full-time job and I couldn't give it up.* Esther was working on the third edition of *Clinical Practice of the Dental Hygienist* (CPDH). She finally agreed when Jim said he *didn't think he would suffer much and could put up with it.* Shortly before they both were scheduled to graduate in 1966, they talked it over with a priest and Esther agreed to get married in the Catholic Church.

Esther did say, in retrospect, that she thought her dedication to the book did become a burden on him, as much of her time was spent on subsequent editions.

❧ THE WEDDING OF JAMES GALLAGHER ❧ AND ESTHER MAE WILKINS

James Gallagher and Esther Mae Wilkins were married in a small ceremony at St. James Church on Harrison Avenue in Boston, by a Catholic priest (Jim was Catholic) near Tufts Dental School, on August 5, 1966.

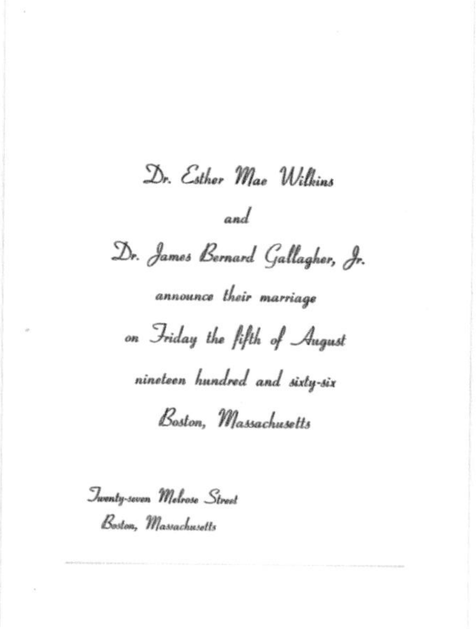

Dr. Esther Mae Wilkins

and

Dr. James Bernard Gallagher, Jr.

announce their marriage

on Friday the fifth of August

nineteen hundred and sixty-six

Boston, Massachusetts

Twenty-seven Melrose Street
Boston, Massachusetts

FIGURE 10.4: Esther and Jim's wedding invitation.

Jim's colleague and friend from Tufts, Dr. Albert Yurkstas, stood up for Jim. Esther's sister, Ruth, was Maid of Honor, accompanied by Ruth's husband, Rev. Richard Colby and Esther's niece, Betsy; Jim's brother, his wife, and their two daughters; Yurkstas's family; and long-time friend, Mary Dole, were invited guests.

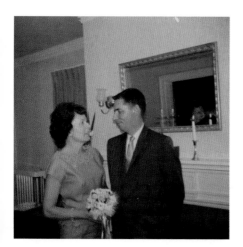

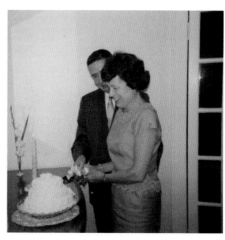

FIGURE 10.5: Esther and Jim's wedding day, Boston, August 5, 1966.

FIGURE 10.6: The wedding cake.

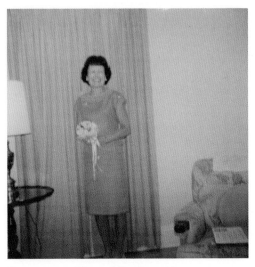

FIGURE 10.7: The wedding bouquet.

Esther's sister, Ruth, gave them a celebration dinner later in the fall, which Mary Dole described as a lovely reception.

❝ Esther and Jim were a happy couple, and they loved to dance, probably what attracted them to each other."

Spending just two nights on the Cape, Jim and Esther returned home. As Jim related in their 1966 Christmas Letter: "It was a weekend on Cape Cod before settling into

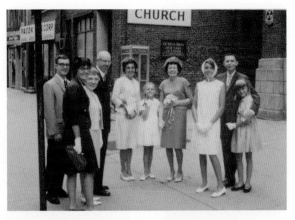

FIGURE 10.8: Wedding party and guests, 1966.

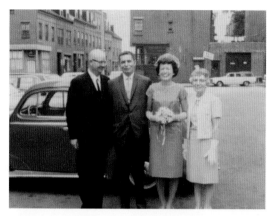

FIGURE 10.9: Ruth and Dick Colby, Esther and Jim, wedding day, 1966.

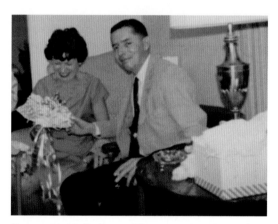

FIGURE 10.10: Esther and Jim, reception, September 1966, Brockton, MA.

our cottage at Bluefish Cove in Brant Rock (Marshfield, Massachusetts), for August (and about every weekend since)." During Christmas week, Esther and Jim vacationed for a week in San Juan, Puerto Rico, for their honeymoon:

> *What a wonderful belated honeymoon it was in that tropical land. We shared a room in a guest house with a little chameleon who lived on our window sill and watched our comings and goings. There was plenty of sightseeing around old and new San Juan, and we flew to St. Thomas for a typical shopping spree for tax-free goodies. For New Englanders to lie on the beach and swim in such warm water, especially on Christmas Day, was as unusual as the Christmas Eve celebration hosted by our landlord*

with roast pig in an air-conditioned house. We boarded our plane in summery weather with our packed wet bathing suits, mildewed shoes, and our bag of 'smuggled' pineapples, we were scarcely in the mood for the cold wintry Boston that greeted us" (Jim and Esther's Christmas Letter, 1967).

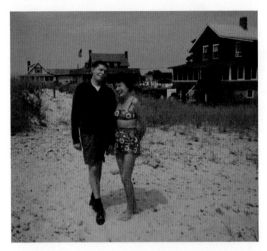

FIGURE 10.11: Esther and Jim in Brant Rock, 1967.

Esther moved out of Fayette Street where she had been living and into Jim's Apartment in Bay Village in Boston, which Jim described as "cozy," where they could look out at the brick fronted houses of this old section of Boston.

We are just 5, 10, or at the most 15 minutes' walk from everything in downtown Boston, especially Tufts Dental School [where Jim teaches full time in the Complete Dentures Department and Esther half-time in Periodontics].

When Esther and Jim lived in Bay Village, in a wonderful apartment, according to Judy Harvey (Forsyth Institute), "Edna Bradbury and a few of us did some partying in those days!"

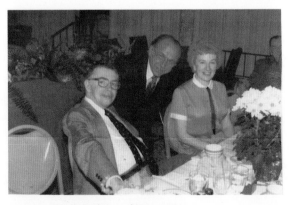

FIGURE 10.12: Esther and Jim, 1971.

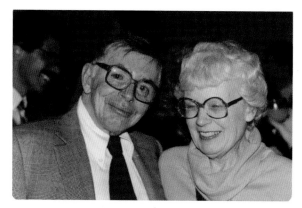

FIGURE 10.13: Esther and Jim, 1972.

Esther and Jim moved to 22 St. Paul Street #2, in Brookline, Massachusetts, from 1972 to 1979, before moving to Tremont Street in Boston in 1979. Esther didn't like the commute from Brookline to Tufts, as she was *used to just walking close by.*

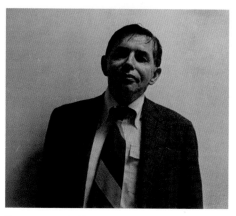

FIGURE 10.14: Jim, 1975.

❧ JIM AS EDUCATOR AND SCHOLAR ❧

Jim was as passionate as Esther about education and students, and he truly enjoyed teaching. Jim became an associate professor in 1968 after completing a masters in science (MS) in prosthodontics, and over the years, he advanced to become professor in prosthodontics. Jim published numerous articles in professional dental journals, in addition to "An Evaluation of the Transfer of Information by Printed Materials Without a Formal Lecture" in 1970, which was a part of his thesis submitted as a requirement for this MS degree, and which he dedicated, "With Love to Esther, My Inspiration."

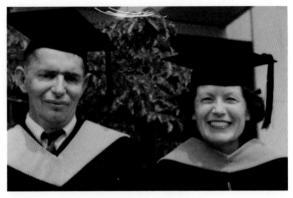

FIGURE 10.15: Esther and Jim, Tufts Commencement, 1968.

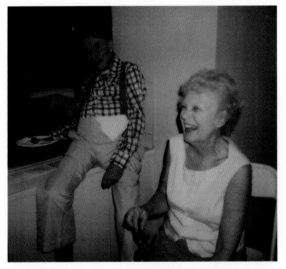

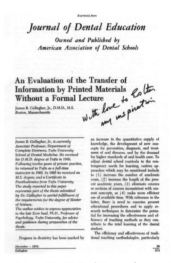

FIGURE 10.16: Esther and Jim in Boston, 1970.

FIGURE 10.17: Jim's journal article, dedicated to Esther, 1970.

The graduate degree journey was documented in their 1968 Christmas Letter:

1967 had originally been called the "Year of the Thesis," but by the end of April 1968, a better name for that period of time was the "Year and 1/3 of Thesis." The climax came June 9, which dawned a bright (and hot, of course, because Tufts' Commencement is always hot) day over the main campus in Medford where Jim received his M.S.

A later comment by Esther on that journey was that she *nagged and edited his references.*

Jim served from 1976 to 1987 as associate editor of the *Journal of Prosthetic Dentistry*, as well as an editorial consultant for the *Journal of the American Dental Association* during those same years. Recognized for his expertise in prosthetics, he served as a consultant in full denture prosthetics at the U.S. Public Health Service Hospital in Brighton, Massachusetts, as well as a consultant in dental medicine at the Chelsea Soldier's Home in Chelsea, Massachusetts, both from 1972 through 1987. From 1980 to 1982, he served as chairman of the Removable Prosthodontic Section of the American Association of Dental Schools in Chicago.

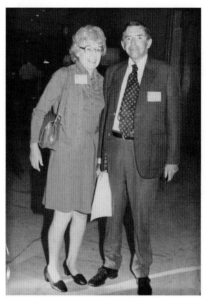

FIGURE 10.18: Esther and Jim, American Association of Dental Schools meeting, Miami, 1976.

Jim also attended postgraduate dentistry courses at Chicago State University and the University of Michigan.

Jim, like Esther, enjoyed presenting at many dental conferences. In 1968, he was *on the American Prosthodontics Society Program* (Christmas Letter, 1968). His memberships in professional organizations included Massachusetts Dental Society (he was appointed chairman of the Council on Dental Education in 1974), Northeastern Prosthodontic Society (where he held several positions), American Dental Association, Metropolitan District Society, Tufts Dental Alumni Association, and Delta Sigma Delta (the oldest and largest international professional dental fraternity). Jim was honored as a fellow of the American Academy of Dental Science in 1968 and a fellow in the International College of Dentists in 1972. Tufts University School of Dental Medicine (TUSDM) presented Jim with the Alumni Award in 1986.

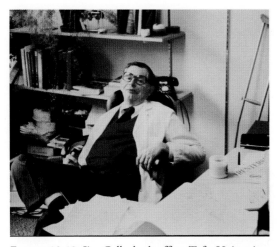

FIGURE 10.19: Jim Gallagher's office, Tufts University School of Dental Medicine.

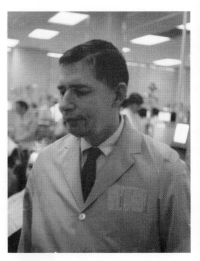

FIGURE 10.20: Jim in lab coat, Tufts University School of Dental Medicine.

Extremely well-liked by his students, they described him as a "gentle gentleman," which Esther thought was an appropriate description. Esther often spoke affectionately of

Jimmy. His dedication to dental education was a true inspiration for me. He had a great sense of humor, and he cared deeply about his students and they respected him.

Later in life, Esther would meet his former students, especially at Yankee Dental Conference in Boston, who *remembered him with great fondness, one of their favorite teachers.*

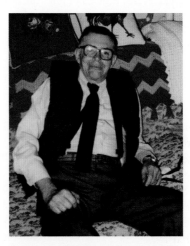

FIGURE 10.21: Jim, 1983.

❧ ESTHER AND JIM ❧

Esther and Jim shared many things, from a passion for dentistry, a love for dancing, and the time they spent at Brant Rock, enjoying the friends they met there, as well as those in Boston and beyond. "More than anything we look forward to seeing more of our friends in 1976" (Christmas Letter, 1975).

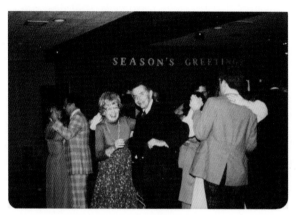

FIGURE 10.22: Esther and Jim dancing, 1976.

When not teaching or traveling, Esther and Jim spent as much time together as possible, primarily at the dance halls, museums, and theaters, all within walking distance of their home.

Jimmie, as Esther fondly called him, *was a very kind and gentle man.* He needed a lot of help due to his health. Esther laughed in remembering when she *did something dumb* when driving the car (or any time), he would say "glad I didn't do that!"

He never minded what I cooked for him; he was glad to have someone home and company. He had been alone for almost 2 years by himself, so he had eaten out a lot.

The couple's love of jazz, music, and dancing lasted all their lives. "Here in Boston we dance nearly every week" (Christmas Letter, 1966). They enrolled in dance classes, took art lessons, and became subscribers to the Huntington Theater. Both Esther and Jim had little extra time outside of teaching obligations and work on CPDH. In their first Christmas Letter, 1966, Jim wrote, "there isn't too much goofing off time." Travels for continuing education, dental hygiene and dental meetings, white coat ceremonies, dedications, and alumni meetings took Esther away quite frequently from Boston and Brant Rock.

Yet, the hidden gems of their relationship found in carefully tucked away letters, telegrams, and postcards revealed they remained connected. Sometimes, sent each day of a longer journey, Esther shared the dental programs in which she presented or attended, the area or country, the wonders of the world she had seen, the food she had sampled and the joys and tribulations of hotel stays and airplane transportation. Quite often, Esther described food or places and wrote to Jim *like you would love*, followed by *love, Esta*.

Today we toured the Colosseum, Pantheon, St. Peter's, the Sistine, the Catacombs as well as seeing points in between. We start really early tomorrow, 450-500 mile ride to Nice. Love Esther (postcard from Rome, August 8, 1981). Toward the end of a journey, the postcard reflected her eagerness to come home. *Hope to see Westminster Abbey tomorrow. Wish I was home with you. I love you, Esta* (postcard from London, 1981) and from Heidelberg Castle in 1969, *wish I was home with you. This trip is too long. Lots of Love, Esta*.

It seems she enjoyed sharing each adventure with Jim, filling the postcard message space completely, with the detail of a daily diary.

The wedding was today, which we watched on the big screen in our lecture room. Harvey Company donated Harvey's Bristol Crème for us to toast the happy couple (From London, July 29, 1981, Princess Diana and Prince Charles Wedding Day). The next day, July 30, she bought a postcard with a stamp of the couple: *Hi Dear: Thought you'd like one of these and the special stamp for a souvenir. Love, Esta*.

Jim was somewhat of a sentimentalist and, according to Esther, *very thoughtful*. When Esther was in Venice on August 4, 1981, Jim sent a Western Union Mailgram with a simple message: "HAPPY ANNIVERSARY ANTICIPATING A CELEBRATION ON YOUR RETURN, LOVE JIM." The next day, August 5, 1981, would be their 15th anniversary.

On August 5, 1981, Jim received a postcard:

Arrived in Venice and here was your telegram waiting for me! Thank you, Jim, you are thoughtful and kind. I love you and miss you very much. Lots of Love, Esta. Jim received yet another telegram from Esther dated August 6, 1981, in which she described her tour of Venice and acknowledging his postcard yet again: *We toasted to you last night for the anniversary! Thank you again for the beautiful telegram. Love, Esta*.

Sometimes, Jim received letters from Esther with restaurant menus enclosed:

It was a very lovely day in S. F. and we walked back. It reminded me of when you were here with me! Love to you—next letter from Beijing. Love Esther. She worried about him, especially when she was on a particularly long trip. *Hope Ailsa gave you a nice meal, and that you'll eat out some so it won't take up all your time cooking and making lunches*.

Esther and Jim shared many things, from a passion for dentistry, a love for dancing, and the time they spent not only together whenever they could at Brant Rock, but with their enjoyment of their mutual friends. Jim liked to do most of the driving. While driving to a dental meeting in Washington, DC, Esther *got to drive only while he ate the lunch she had packed*. They took turns eating lunch while the other drove! It was a 9- to 10-hour drive. Jim was a smoker, which displeased Esther, but she was the first to celebrate Jim's

CHAPTER 10 ~ ESTHER AND JIM

New Year's resolution for 1970: *After over 30 years of heavy smoking, he smoked his last on Friday, January 2, 1970, at 12:15 PM.*

~ IRELAND, FEBRUARY 1978 ~

Esther and Jim were scheduled to speak as guest lecturers at a dental program in Sligo, Ireland: she on periodontology and Jim on dentures. A dentist friend of theirs went every year and often invited guest speakers from United States. They were scheduled to fly out the morning of the Blizzard of 1978, but Logan Airport was closed and traveling was perilous at best. They received a call (Esther said the phones were working so electricity must not have been out in the Boston area) by their friend who said plans changed, they would go by train to New York and fly out from there that day.

Jim resisted and pointed out that what streets were plowed out were policed, and cars were not permitted. *But we were to go anyway*, Esther said. A friend and his son arrived to pick them up. They all left Brookline in a station wagon (the son hopped in the way back and hid, saying that if the cops stopped them, he wasn't going to be involved). Esther was concerned for them, because he was going to have to take the car home after he left them at the train.

South Station was crowded, suitcases were in the aisles on the train, but it hadn't snowed quite as much in New York. Esther recalled,

our plane "got out okay," and we were finally off on our much anticipated trip to Ireland.

Esther and Jim had their trip all mapped out: first, the dental meeting in Sligo, then renting a car for touring around Ireland sightseeing. The couple arrived in time

to reach the dental meeting in Sligo after an all-day drive, just in time for our presentations. In addition to being welcomed by their wonderful Irish hospitality, we were also welcomed by their worst snowstorm in 50 years.

Esther said she was cold the whole trip. When the program ended, the next day, they were to travel to Dublin, but once again, it snowed so they took the train. *We took trains to Dublin for sightseeing, then on to Killarney.*

Although cold and rainy in Dublin, they did visit the Olympia Theatre, which, according to Esther *was unheated!* Esther visited the old Dublin dental school, but only briefly, while Jim waited downstairs. As Esther remembered, at the world famous National Museum of Ireland,

the notorious Book of Kells was touring America. Overall our plans had to change due to weather. We then took a train to Cork, where they had no snow, but it was still colder weather than normal for that area.

Finally, they were able to pick up a car. *Jim drove on the way to the motel where we had a reservation.* They went to a mansion, where the gardens were featured during spring and summer, but they could only tour the inside, which proved quite challenging for Jim, *with all its stairs to go up and down.* Then, an incident happened (not unlike Esther's later fall in South Carolina in 2006). Esther recalled,

> *in coming down one set of stairs, Jim fell and broke his leg. I got help to call an ambulance. Everywhere we went, everyone was always warm and friendly. The sweet Irish museum manager came up the stairs where Jim was lying waiting, and said "Dr. Gallagher, want a cup of tea?" And she bustled off.*
>
> *The ambulance came and Jim was taken to County Hospital, a Catholic hospital. I followed the ambulance with a first-time try at driving on the "wrong side" of the road in a strange country. At the hospital, everyone was very gracious and kind. The physicians and nurses attended to Jim's x-ray and decision about splinting. Patients were all in one ward together, but Jim was given a nice quiet corner of the ward so he wouldn't be disturbed.*

The hospital staff located a nearby motel for Esther, so after Jim was settled in, she had *to drive and find the motel myself.* There was no restaurant, no food, and no heat, although the motel manager made her some sandwiches and hot tea. He also provided a space heater, challenging in and of itself with its frayed cord and all, but at that point Esther was grateful for a bed with an extra blanket or two.

> *The accident was on a Wednesday, and our tickets for going home were the following Monday, so the next few days were busy planning for the plane ride that depended on the physicians' decision that Jim would be able to take the long flight. Calls were also made to Boston, and Dr. Al Yurkstas arranged for the arrival at the Tufts New England Medical Center. My sister, Ruth, was contacted and she and her husband, Rev. Colby, also planned to meet the plane at Logan.*
>
> Each afternoon, Esther went to the hospital to spend time with Jim. *Every day at 6:00 the lights would dim in the ward and suddenly everyone was still and quiet for the Rosary. That was a very special time of our visit.*
>
> *When the physicians gave permission for travel, the final arrangements were made. To accommodate the leg-length splints, a chair had to be removed in the airplane, which meant paying for two tickets. From the hospital, the ambulance had two big husky, handsome Irishmen, who picked Jim in his stretcher up like a toy, and settled him into his place on the airplane. The physician at the hospital had given me a bottle of "sleepy" pills and told me to give him two to start when we were on the plane. Jim went to sleep and slept the whole trip.* When the steak dinners were served, there were two, both for Esther, because Dr. Gallagher was sound asleep.
>
> *We were met as planned at Logan, and after Jim's settling in at Tufts Medical Center, Ruth and Dick drove me to our Brookline home. There we found the condo had been broken into and several things taken. The entrance through a front window seemed apparent. The back door had been left unlocked where the robbers exited. Welcome home!!*
>
> *Ruth had brought supper with her—a delicious beef stew—so that made a slightly happy ending for the long tiring day.*

Jim was in the hospital and rehabilitation at New England Medical Center Hospital (NEMCH) for most of the spring. He spent his birthday in the hospital. Esther commuted back and forth as usual from Brookline, and spent the evenings with him.

Jim was able in May to teach his preclinical curse when it started, by being lifted to the platform in his wheelchair. While Jim was in the hospital he set two goals: to dance at the "Hardy" prosthetic conference in September, and to fulfill a commitment to the A.D.A program in Anaheim. Now, with both of those goals achieved he is walking to work daily and all is progressing well. The Anaheim trip included some sightseeing, notably to Tijuana, Jim's first trip to Mexico, where most of the short trip was spent in line at Customs to get back into the USA!! Another special was watching the dress rehearsal and final taping of a Lawrence Welk Show
(Christmas Letter, 1978).

After Jim and Esther's memorable adventure in Ireland in 1978, she began looking for a different place to live. Jim had been in the hospital and rehabilitation for most of the spring after his accident. In May, she began thinking about moving and visited the Tremont on the Common with a postdoctoral dental student who lived there. She brought Jim up in his wheelchair (still recuperating from his accident) to *see the place.* One of Esther's favorite photos and one she insisted be included in her biography, is one of Jim in the wheelchair, being wheeled up Washington Street in front of the Two O'clock Lounge through the Combat Zone (a former shady part of town, since revitalized) by Jim's friend, Paul Parise, the laboratory technician in Tuft's Denture Department. It was a nice spring day, and they wheeled up to Tremont on the Common at 151 Tremont Street.

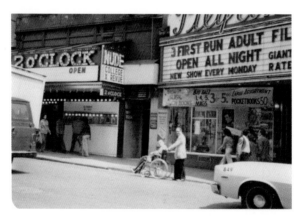

FIGURE 10.23: Jim's wheelchair being pushed through the Combat Zone, Boston, 1978.

Esther immediately put their name on the waiting list for a two-bedroom apartment. Sooner than they had hoped, an apartment became available and *it was promptly held for me.*

It was perfect: 12th floor (now condominium) facing Boston Common, parking spot in the garage below, elevators, and staffed security system. The skating rink on Boston Common is located in front of the building, the gazebo is to the left, Prudential on the left, the State House is up front on the top of the hill. It had a balcony, high enough not to hear the traffic but close enough to see all the activity as well as the fog that sometimes sits over the Common: Esther likes fog!

It was 1978 that Esther and her husband, Jim, came to live at 151 Tremont Street in Boston.

Jim nurtured a garden on our balcony, 12 stories above the teeming traffic of Tremont Street . . . pots of the healthiest, handsomest tomato and lettuce plants ever. We are still enjoying tomatoes from our abundant harvest even now, after Thanksgiving
(Esther and Jim's Christmas Letter, 1980).

When the apartments turned condominium in 1984, Esther and Jim wrestled with whether to buy it or not; it seemed like so much money back then. They weighed the advantages: two full baths and bedrooms, the magnificent view, location in the heart of the city, full elevator access, a parking space in the garage, exercise room, outdoor pool on the sixth floor, and handicapped key access to the building, no stairs at all, which accommodated Jim's disability: *so we made the buy!* In their 1981/1982 Christmas Letter, they wrote about their decision: *The black cloud that was hovering over Tremont-on-the-Common (TOC) this past 2 years has been a threat of "going condo." Well, it is, but the cloud has turned up with a silver lining and present plans are that we will stay.* Esther said many years later that she *thanked her lucky stars* for having such a wonderful place to live and work all these years.

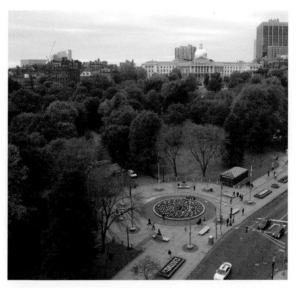

FIGURE 10.24: Boston condo view.

Jim retired on July 1, 1984,

a major event to record in our Christmas Album. That date was preceded by a series of terrific celebrations—in May the faculty, staff, and students at Tufts Dental School had a big reception. That was when he received his Tufts Chair—after 23 years it was indeed well-earned. Then in June the Dept. of Complete Dentures had a mammothly great testimonial

188

*dinner at the Park Plaza which brought out faculty, friends, relatives, everybody repre-
senting every phase of activity in Jim's career. It was a beautiful party, and the album is
filled with cards, letters, and pictures to enjoy over and over. However, he didn't leave Tufts
entirely and still goes over to school at least once a week for Admissions interviews, special
classes, department activities, etc.* (Christmas Letter, 1984).

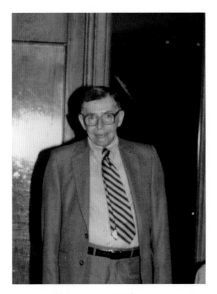

FIGURE 10.25: Jim, 1984.

Jim's retirement was documented in their Christmas Letter of 1985: *Since Jim retired
he doesn't have time to do a lot of things he planned to do when he retired. The days are full of
good things, however, and now one painting class has grown into one portrait painting class
plus one drawing class.* Showing her pride for Jim's dedication to his art, she wrote, *you'll
never guess what; he sold his first painting and so joined that elite group of "selling artists"!*

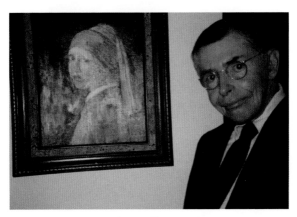

FIGURE 10.26: Jim and one of his paintings.

Jim continued to go regularly to Tufts Dental School: *No responsibilities and lunch with old friends beats working for pay, he says.* As they did since they married in 1966, they enjoyed the years in Boston and Brant Rock, enjoying their activities and the many friends they made through the years.

Jim was diagnosed with a brain tumor in December of 1987 and passed away the following year, after four days in a coma. His funeral was at St. James Church, the same church in which he and Esther were married 22 years before. Esther established an endowed scholarship at TUSDM in Jim's name in 2009. The Dr. James B. Gallagher, Jr., A47, D49, DG66 and Dr. Esther M. Wilkins, D49, DG66 Scholarship Fund at TUSDM provides aid to a third-year student who demonstrates academic achievement.

It's a memorial to my husband and his devotion to teaching, but it also reflects my own experiences as a student who struggled with finances to pay for college.

Esther remained in contact with Jim's family for a short time. Jim's brother, Robert E. Gallagher of Marshfield, passed away in 2004.

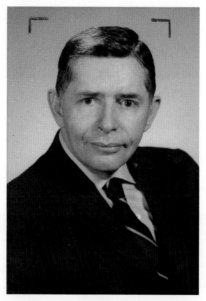

FIGURE 10.27: James B. Gallagher, Jr.

CHAPTER 11

Forsyth School for Dental Hygienists at Massachusetts College of Pharmacy and Health Sciences University

I quickly realized how lucky MCPHS, The School of Dental Hygiene, and the profession are to have Esther as an elder stateswoman for the profession (Michelle Kalis, PhD, former vice president for Academic Affairs, Massachusetts College of Pharmacy and Health Sciences).

Massachusetts College of Pharmacy and Health Sciences (MCPHS), the oldest institution of higher education in the City of Boston, was founded in 1823 and granted a charter by the State of Massachusetts on April 3, 1852. The College currently offers more than 95 degree and certificate programs across three campuses: Boston and Worcester, Massachusetts, and Manchester, New Hampshire.

❧ THE ESTHER M. WILKINS FORSYTH ❧ DENTAL HYGIENE CLINIC, BOSTON, MASSACHUSETTS

The Forsyth School for Dental Hygienists became part of the MCPHS in July 2002. During the first few years, students took didactic courses at MCPHS and travelled back and forth to the clinic at the Forsyth Institute, located just a few blocks away. But through the generous support of Dr. Wilkins, students began receiving clinical instruction in the state-of-the art Dr. Esther M. Wilkins Forsyth Dental Hygiene Clinic, which was dedicated on August 29, 2005.

As friend, Mary Dole, recalled the day: "The ceremony and dedication of the clinic was held with a large attendance of alumni and friends, as well as Boston Mayor Menino who told the many alumni, dignitaries, members of the Tufts and Simmons community, friends, and colleagues, "I'm a Forsyth kid; I grew up in Hyde Park and went to Forsyth for my dental care for many years. It was the best and most affordable. That tradition continues today" (MCPHS, 2005, p. 20). Menino concluded with the acknowledgement that Dr. Wilkins "is a living legend in dental hygiene circles" (p. 21). The evening of celebration included refreshments and a video presentation of Dr. Wilkins receiving the honorary doctorate from the College in 2004. Students gave tours of the clinic, fully dressed in their blue scrubs. At the end of the day, the clinic was officially opened in a ribbon-cutting tradition.

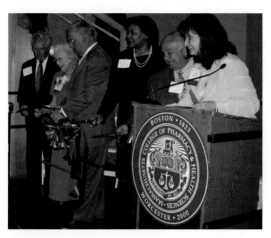

FIGURE 11.1: Ribbon-cutting, Esther M. Wilkins Dental Hygiene Clinic, 2005.

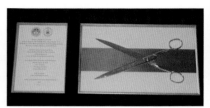

FIGURE 11.2: Ribbon-cutting scissors and plaque, Esther M. Wilkins Dental Hygiene Clinic at Massachusetts College of Pharmacy and Health Sciences.

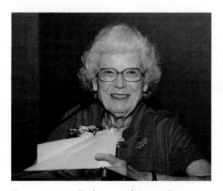

FIGURE 11.3: Esther speaking at Boston clinic dedication.

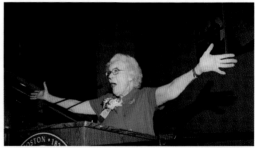

FIGURE 11.4: Esther's "Wonder of It All" speech, clinic dedication, 2005.

The 500 square-foot clinic is located at the Palace Road entrance to the College and has a formal picture of Dr. Wilkins next to the inside entrance to the clinic.

The big picture window facing the street has the clinic name etched in glass. Pat Ramsay related, "one day as I returned from lunch I noticed that a new pane of glass had been hung near the clinic. As I approached I noticed that the name of the clinic was etched in the glass. I quickly called Esther and shared my feelings about it. My words were 'Esther, it made the hair on my arms stand up.' Two days later I received a call from Esther who said, *It is quite a feeling, isn't it?* It makes me smile every time I saw Esther standing at this same pane of glass with friends that she brought over to see 'her' clinic."

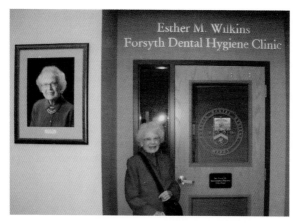

FIGURE 11.5: Esther in front of inside clinic door.

The Dr. Esther M. Wilkins Forsyth Dental Hygiene Clinic is a modern public health clinic that includes educational and clinical design concepts which allow for the delivery of preventive oral health care services within an educational setting. It has a welcoming reception area with multimedia displays of the latest guidelines on oral health care and prevention information. The Warren and Mary Dole Gallery of Forsyth class photographs was relocated from Forsyth to the Esther M. Wilkins Forsyth Dental Hygiene Clinic.

The clinic is equipped with 28 operatories, some of which are partitioned for privacy; digital radiologic imaging technology; intraoral cameras; state-of-art, ergonomic patient and operator chairs; digital panoramic technology; and computerized chairside charting. There is a spacious dental materials laboratory with magnification and flat screen monitors to enhance student learning. Several instructor stations have computers and monitors. Beyond preparation for entry-level clinical practice, Forsyth graduates will enter workforce

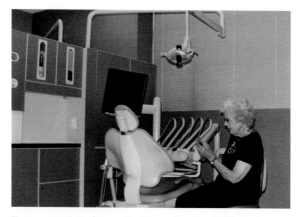

FIGURE 11.6: Esther at the Massachusetts College of Pharmacy and Health Sciences clinic lab, 2005.

193

settings that will advance oral health scholarship, education, public health, research, and industry. "The new clinic helps to advance the College's mission and enhances several innovative, proactive approaches to oral health care education that address the shortage of baccalaureate-educated dental hygiene graduates, particularly in the areas of academic, public health, and the dental industry" (MCPHS, 2005, p. 20).

The clinic has a culturally diverse patient population, which provides students with an array of outpatient experiences for professional growth and development. Handicapped-accessible, it provides dental services (oral prophylaxis, nonsurgical periodontal therapy, oral exams, dental radiographs, dental sealants, athletic mouth guards, and tooth whitening) and offers discounted rates to promote maximum utilization of services by MCPHS students, faculty, and staff, as well as those of the Colleges of the Fenway, and neighboring community residents.

According to Ann Marie Niemyski, Class of 1969,

❝ this event brought members of the Forsyth community together, sparked the interest of the local, regional and national dental communities, and attracted guests from as far away as California."

Not only were members of the MCPHS community present but also Esther's family, faculty and administrators from Simmons and Tufts School of Dental Medicine, colleagues from other dental hygiene and dental schools, and friends from around the world. Niemyski concluded,

❝ the Esther M. Wilkins Clinic is truly the talk of the town"(MCPHS, 2005, p. 22).

Esther's "Wonder of It All" speech celebrated the beginning of the next era in the story of the Forsyth Dental Hygiene Program from which she graduated in 1939, important milestones in the Forsyth history, and her pride in the opportunity to contribute to continued learning as the research continues to link oral health to overall body health (see Appendix F, accessed via the online e-book).

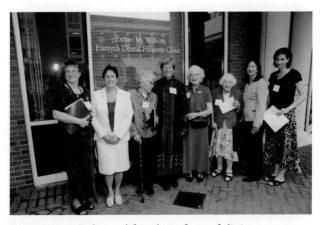

FIGURE 11.7: Esther and friends, in front of clinic.

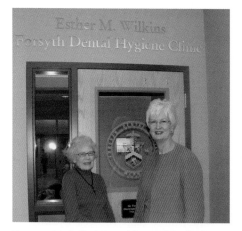

FIGURE 11.8: Esther and Lana Crawford.

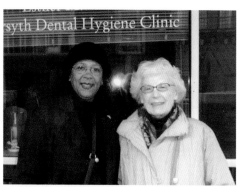

FIGURE 11.9: Esther and Tina Daniels.

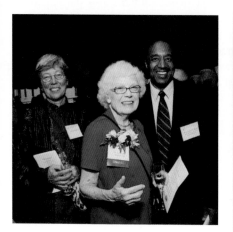

FIGURE 11.10: Charlotte Wyche, Esther, and Dean Norris (Tufts) at dedication reception.

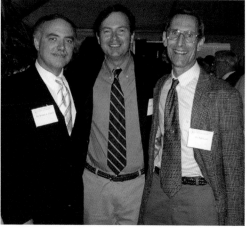

FIGURE 11.11: Drs. Faiella, Hempton, and Levi, clinic reception, 2005.

In September of the year of the clinic dedication, Esther gave a course in Harlingen, Texas:

> *No one there knew ANYTHING about the new clinic—sort of fun having a little secret inside that still made me smile privately!!!* (email to author, September 14, 2005).

In answer to the question posed to her on what she considered her proudest accomplishment, with a wide grin and large excited eyes, Esther responded, *the Clinic!* Whenever anyone came to visit Boston, they were taken on a tour of her clinic, proudly and personally conducted by Esther, who introduced guests not only to the clinic and the

College but also to its faculty, students, staff, and administration, with whom Esther kept in regular contact.

Mary Dole, Forsyth alum, Class of 1941, and recipient of the Forsyth Distinguished Alumni Award (renamed the Esther M. Wilkins Alumni Award in 1994,) commented that "the students are very fortunate to have this state-of-the-art clinic built at MCPHS. We, as alumnae, all envy the students of today to have the opportunity to train in such a high-tech clinic." Many alumni from Forsyth have vocalized the advantage dental hygiene students have by being an integral part of the College student body and part a university that is on the cutting edge for equipment, technology, and clinical excellence. They spoke positively about the opportunities for students to work with the newest equipment, a state-of the-art clinic, and a health sciences environment, as this will prepare them for the modern dental office.

The Forsyth School of Dental Hygiene, now at MCPHS, is the longest continuously operating dental hygiene program in the United States, more than 100 years young. In addition to lectures and seminars that provide complementary evidence-based information and knowledge that support clinical competencies, students also participate in community-based extramural clinical rotations to enhance on-campus clinical learning experiences. Program offerings have expanded in the last decade and include dental hygiene bachelor of science (BS) degree (accelerated BS track, fast track, predental track, and degree completion); masters of science (MS) degree; associate degree (AS) to MS bridge; oral health professions education certificate, and dual MS to masters in public health (MPH).

❧ Esther M. Wilkins Dental Hygiene ❧ Clinic, Worcester Campus

The Esther M. Wilkins Dental Hygiene Clinic on the Worcester Campus, located at 10 Lincoln Square, was dedicated in September 2013. Referred to by MCPHS President, Charles Monahan, as the Florence Nightingale of dental hygiene, Esther began her speech at the dedication with *Go Red Sox* as she shot her hand into the air. She proceeded to emphasize the importance of oral health and her pride at being part of the expansion of the dental hygiene program at MCPHS. "Since we picked her up we can't keep up with her" (Monahan, as cited in Knothe, 2013). "It means a lot to be able to use Dr. Wilkins's name for the school's second location" (p. 1). In a story published a few days after the dedication of the Forsyth clinic in Worcester, it was clear that the new addition to the city was welcomed: "Where once was a hotel—the Crowne Plaza at 10 Lincoln Square—there is now a center for dental hygiene. We welcome MCPHS University's dental hygiene clinic to the school's downtown array of classes, labs and services. And we are glad to note that the clinic carries the name of a woman who, at the age of 96, still delights in all things dentistry" (Telegram, 2013, p. 1).

A satellite of the Boston Department of Public Health license, the state-of-the art clinic is located in the center of Worcester and provides dental services to the public.

❝ With this new clinic and its focus on oral health, the Worcester area can enjoy attention to increased overall health" (Wilkins, as cited in Knothe, 2013, p. 1).

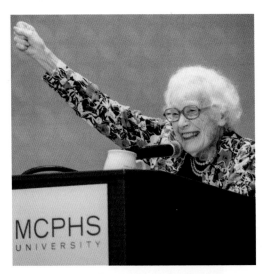

FIGURE 11.12: Esther speaking at Massachusetts College of Pharmacy and Health Sciences Worcester dedication.

❝ Students deliver high quality oral healthcare services to the public, empowering them to gain hands-on experience by working with real patients, while also giving back to our broader community (MCPHS, 2016d, p. 1).

❧ ESTHER M. WILKINS'S IMPACT AT ❧ MASSACHUSETTS COLLEGE OF PHARMACY AND HEALTH SCIENCES

Esther's dedication to the College extended beyond her generosity in establishing clinics in her name. Her impact on the program, its students, and the faculty continued, not only through her financial assistance but also in helping to assure that Forsyth students enjoy the benefits of a college that could provide more opportunities than if Forsyth stood on its own. Students take classes in specialty areas and electives taught by MCPHS faculty; they take part in the multitude of student activities and events sponsored by MCPHS and the Colleges of the Fenway; and they enjoy the facilities, equipment, and expertise of MCPHS that continued to expand. Importantly, Esther's name association with the College and the clinics has tremendous impact on others. Michelle Kalis recalled,

❝ The Forsyth/MCPHS alumni group was in the midst of a campaign to 'name' chairs within the clinic that bears Esther's name due to her generous contributions to the College. The group hosted an event on campus for alumni to come and tour the clinic and hopefully to encourage the attendees to consider a donation. These are always difficult events, because everyone has their guard up since they know they will be solicited for money. Several MCPHS staff members, including myself, said a few words and then Esther said a few words. I will never forget how adept she was at gauging the mood of the audience and finding just the right thing to say. She essentially said that she personally thought about how and when to provide a donation and decided that she wanted to make the donation while she was alive to witness the impact. She said it with just the right amount of humility and humor that it clearly had the desired impact. It was impressive."

As a graduate of Forsyth herself, Class of 1939, Esther made a commitment of time, energy, and support to her alma mater, a life-long dedication to Forsyth and to the students who sought dental hygiene as a profession. Esther was "committed to the education of dental hygiene students, and generations, of Forsyth School of Dental Hygiene students have experienced her expertise, wit, and encouragement first-hand, as she was an active presence on campus. She served as guest lecturer in countless dental hygiene classes over the years, inspiring dental hygiene students with her passion" (MCPHS, 2016c, p. 2).

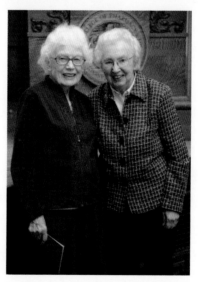

Figure 11.13: Esther and Rita Snow Keylor, Forsyth reunion.

Long-time friend Beverly Whitford added,

❝ Esther is an avid philanthropist. She continues to enhance the profession with her generosity as a major contributor to the Esther Wilkins Clinic at Forsyth/ MCPHS. It was my pleasure to work with Esther on the Steering Committee of that project and to hostess a 'House Party' for Connecticut and Rhode Island Forsyth Alumnae at my home in Connecticut. How awesome it was that day to have this internationally known treasure arranging cookies on a tray in my kitchen and later making a hospital visit to our mutual friend, Laura Fitch. Little did we know that it was to be their last personal encounter here on Earth."

Patricia (Pat) Ramsay (Forsyth Class of 1964 and past president of American Dental Hygienists' Association [ADHA]) served for a number of years as the director of Forsyth Alumni Programs and had been a friend of Esther's for over 30 years.

❝ There is some special connection between Esther and dental hygiene students. Students flock to her and she seems to gain strength as she spends time with them. How many of us have marveled at how she stops and has a special word with each student who approaches her to sign a copy of her book."

Esther M. Wilkins, RDH, DMD, received an honorary doctor of health science degree from MCPHS on May 16, 2004, at the commencement held at the Bayside Exposition Center in Boston. Charles F. Monahan, Jr., President of the College, acknowledged Dr. Wilkins's 66 years of outstanding achievement in the fields of dental science and dental hygiene, for "her unselfish mentorship of students and colleagues" (Dentistry-IQ, 2004, p. 1), which has made her "one of the most beloved figures in the profession" (MCPHS, 2016c, p.1) (see Chapter 13).

❧ MASSACHUSETTS COLLEGE OF PHARMACY ❧ AND HEALTH SCIENCES ESTHER M. WILKINS DISTINGUISHED ALUMNI AWARD

Dr. Wilkins frequently visited at MCPHS, as she was invited to many ceremonies and events involving both faculty and students of the Forsyth School for Dental Hygiene, as well as college-wide events, including alumni and continuing education. Esther was particularly fond of attending the MCPHS Formal Gala each year, where she could share the dance floor with so many partners.

Students flocked to her upon her arrival, seeking autographs and just spending time with the matriarch of the profession they were training to enter. "Dr. Wilkins was meeting weekly with small groups of dental hygiene students for lunch and conversation. The students always brought their texts for Esther to sign. She delighted to be with these students in an intimate setting and shared with them her pearls of wisdom. I believe many relish this memory of their time with her," shared faculty member Christine Dominick.

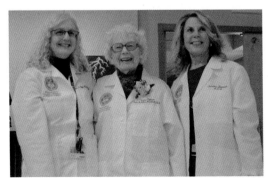

FIGURE 11.14: Esther's 95th Birthday, 2011, Linda Boyd, Esther, and Christine Dominick. (Photo courtesy of Susan Jenkins, RDH, MS.)

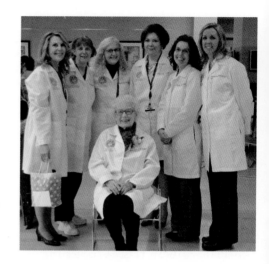

Figure 11.15: Esther's 95th birthday, 2011, Massachusetts College of Pharmacy and Health Sciences faculty. (Photo courtesy of Susan Jenkins, RDH, MS.)

The Esther M. Wilkins Distinguished Alumni Award (originally named the Forsyth Distinguished Alumni Award) is awarded each year to a dental hygiene alumnus, which Esther enjoyed presenting in person. The award encompasses the characteristics valued in the profession and embodied by Esther herself, including mentor to others, distinguished in his or her career, respected by peers and community, passionate toward the profession, loyal to Forsyth, and the epitome of one or more roles of a dental hygienist. Esther was the first recipient of the award in 1991.

Mary Dole said that "after this award was established, I had the privilege to serve with Esther on the committee that selected the candidates each year." Mary continued to practice dental hygiene until she was 90 years and was the recipient of this coveted award in 1994. When Esther presented the award to her, she told a little story about John Kenneth Galbraith, scholar, ambassador to India, and advisor to Presidents of the United States.

Mary recalled Esther's story:

❝ On his 85th birthday, a big dinner party was held for Galbraith, in the beautiful Bates Hall Reading Room of the Boston Public Library. Many famous people attended, writers, reporters, and political figures. The day after the party, the Boston Globe printed a good part of the speech he made. His concluding remarks were that he suffered from the *Still Syndrome*. He said that when he goes for a walk, he hears 'Oh, you're still getting exercise?' or gives a talk, 'Oh, you're still lecturing?' or he goes to a meeting, 'Oh, you're still interested in politics.' At that time, Esther thought that I also had the *Still Syndrome*."

Mary Dole concluded,

❝ there are very few dental hygienists at 93 years old today who are still involved in dental hygiene and dentistry. Esther has given so much to the profession."

Mary Kellerman, a 2007 recipient of this coveted award, was proud to receive it from the

❝ very person who has inspired many, many countless dental hygienists. Esther made sure I got up there and said a few words—she told me what to say—how I completed community service and volunteer work." Mary outlined what she felt was Esther's motive in that advice: "She gave me an assignment that I was to develop a course on volunteerism! That is Esther—she is always ever promoting the DH field for the future. I call her the millennium lady!"

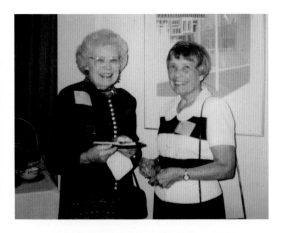

FIGURE 11.16: Esther and Mary Dole, Pre-Pops Concert, 1996.

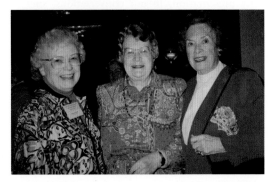

FIGURE 11.17: Esther, Barbara Wilson, and Edna Bradbury, 1993.

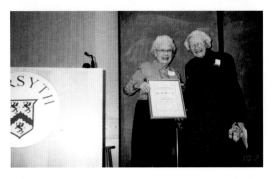

FIGURE 11.18: Esther awarding recipient, Laura Peck Fitch, past president of American Dental Hygienists' Association.

❧ ESTHER'S TEACHING AND ❧ PRESENTATIONS AT MASSACHUSETTS COLLEGE OF PHARMACY AND HEALTH SCIENCES

Esther was appointed adjunct clinical professor, Forsyth School for Dental Hygiene at MCPHS in 2004 and visiting professor in 2010. "She served as guest lecturer in countless dental hygiene classes over the years, inspiring dental hygiene students with her passion" (MCPHS, 2016c, p.1).

Esther became educator, mentor, and friend to many of the Forsyth faculty through the years. As they reflected on Esther's close ties to Forsyth and many interactions with her, they recalled her sense of humor, her subtle way to advance them in their careers, and how she provided opportunities for them to grow individually and collectively.

❝I first met Esther when I was a student at Middlesex Community College, 1976. My class was fortunate to have Esther as our periodontology professor. The course was rigorous, but we learned perio. As I reflect on this experience, the impact she had on me may be one of the reasons I currently teach perio to dental hygiene students," said Susan Jenkins, Forsyth faculty member.

Susan continued,

❝as a student, I was fortunate to be chosen to present a table clinic at ADHA's Annual Session. Esther critiqued my presentation. In our conversations, she asked if I had a pointer. In 1976 there were no laser pointers. Esther used a collapsible pointer. She offered that I take her pointer with me to Chicago. When I returned her pointer, I was excited to let her know my table clinic won 1st place. I remember she smiled and commented *that is because you had my pointer*. I did not really get to know Esther until I became a full time faculty member at Forsyth. During the past 16 years I had the pleasure of spending time with her in various places, at MCPHS, on the dance floor at ADHA, organizing student pictures with her at ADHA, and taking her grocery shopping. I was also one of her personal chauffeurs. It was during our time in the car that we had wonderful conversations and really got to know each other."

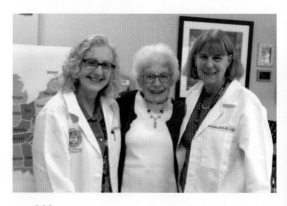

FIGURE 11.19: Linda Boyd, Esther, and Susan Jenkins. (Photo courtesy of Susan Jenkins, RDH, MS.)

Susan said,

❝ the greatest honor I had was being asked to contribute to two chapters of the 12th edition of *Clinical Practice of the Dental Hygienist*." She was forever grateful for the opportunity Esther gave her to be part of such an important work. "Over the years we always heard how respected Esther was in the dental hygiene arena. This really hit home for me when several faculty from Forsyth were included in closing her condominium when she moved to Laurel Place in 2016. She had file cabinets full of thank you notes from all over the world for presentations she had given. It was amazing to read how excited dental professionals were that she had taken time to visit with them. Esther was a great lady. She was a rock star. I am lucky to have known her. I will miss her," Susan concluded.

MCPHS faculty members were indeed fortunate to benefit from Esther's presence at the College. Lori Rainchuso, graduate program director at Forsyth reflected,

❝ Dr. Wilkins was a champion of higher education for dental hygienists. She had a unique way of making a personal connection to everyone she encountered. I had the unique opportunity of working with her on one of the chapters in the Wilkins textbook, and she was so sharp in her suggestions and attention to detail. The last time I saw her was at the Esther Wilkins Symposium. After a long day of courses and a birthday celebration, I was assisting her into her niece's car. I asked her how she felt, and she said, *I feel like going dancing*, and with that she did a little up and down bobbing movement to go with it. She was an inspiration to us all, not only in the physical and mental aspect, but aspiring us to take chances, seek out opportunities, and to live life to its fullest."

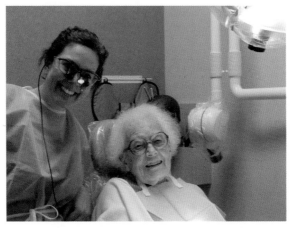

FIGURE 11.20: Lori Rainchuso and Esther in Forsyth Dental Chair. (Photo courtesy of Susan Jenkins, RDH, MS.)

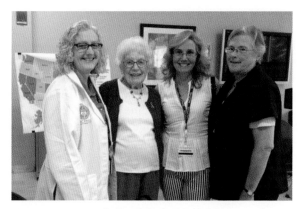

FIGURE 11.21: Linda Boyd, Esther, Julie Martin, and
Nancy Barnes at Massachusetts College of Pharmacy and
Health Sciences, 2016.

Esther also enjoyed presenting to many dental hygiene students at MCPHS and many
alumni of Forsyth through continuing education presentations, including those offered in
cooperation with the Forsyth School of Dental Hygiene Annual Esther Wilkins Symposium,
the first of which was held in 2007. Through the years, until her death in 2016, Esther offered
inspiring reflections at the symposium bearing her name on the profession of dental hygiene
and the crucial importance of oral health. According to MCPHS (2014), the symposium is
an "educational resource for the latest developments in the dental hygiene profession, but also
the perfect opportunity for MCPHS/Forsyth alumni to gather for reminiscing, re-connecting,
lively discussion, and networking, not to mention hobnobbing with Dr. Wilkins herself" (p. 1).

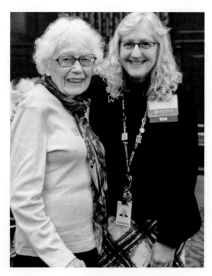

FIGURE 11.22: Wilkins symposium,
2013, Esther and Linda Boyd.

Current dean of the Forsyth School of Dental Hygiene at MCPHS, Dr. Linda Boyd, provided introductions to the many speakers who have presented on varied topics during previous symposium events. The 11th Annual Esther Wilkins Symposium was held at MCPHS in October of 2017 (MCPHS, 2017). The program included a dedication to Dr. Wilkins and speeches by Betsy Tyrol, Esther's niece; Charlotte Wyche; Tina Daniels; and Pam Bretschneider, her biographer who included milestones of Esther's long and trailblazing career in both dental hygiene and dentistry.

❧ THE COLLEGE MEDAL ❧

In June of 2012, the College awarded Esther M. Wilkins the College Medal, a prestigious recognition, at Commencement at the Seaport World Trade Center in Boston Massachusetts (see Chapter 13). The College Medal, first given in 1982, is awarded in recognition of extraordinary service to the College in teaching, fund-raising, administration, management, generosity, and multiple labors within the College community and the health professions. According to George Humphrey, then vice president for Academic Affairs, she was only the sixth person in the history of the College to receive both the College Medal and an honorary degree (see Chapter 13). In Esther's response to the vice president, she said, *thank you, George, I am indeed honored and very humbled. I will bring a cough drop to talk clearly!* (see Appendix I, accessed via the online e-book).

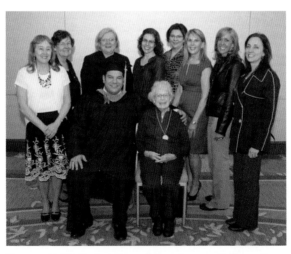

FIGURE 11.23: Esther, Betsy, Massachusetts College of Pharmacy and Health Sciences faculty and staff, and Peter DiBona, 2012 dental hygiene graduate, at the reception for her College Medal, World Trade Center, Boston, 2012.

❧ Dental Hygiene Advocate ❧

Esther's association with the College encouraged alumni participation, corporate partnerships, and gifts, such as the one generously donated in 2007 by Delta Dental of Massachusetts. This gift was a generous $3 million gift to Forsyth School for Delta Dental of Massachusetts (MCPHS, 2007). The endowment facilitated the creation of a faculty position to support expansion of community outreach. The faculty position fostered additional faculty development through creation and administration of a MS in dental hygiene degree program, with a special focus on community oral health that include tracks in public health and dental hygiene education. The faculty position continues today to integrate oral health curricular into other health science disciplines at MCPHS.

Esther was excited about the opportunity for students to advance their education, including the opportunity to provide the profession with additional quality faculty with advanced degrees. She stated,

❝ Dental hygiene is an evolving profession, and we're going to need educators and practitioners who are capable of meeting the challenges ahead. An advanced education will serve you well and the profession when you are able to impart your wisdom and experience to future dental hygiene professionals" (Wilkins, as cited in Stooksberry, 2004, p. 1).

Extending those thoughts, in an audio interview in *Dimensions*, Esther discussed the role of current dental hygiene teachers to recognize the talents of their students who show promise to become educators themselves. Esther felt that as motivational role models, teachers have a responsibility to encourage others on that path. One of her passions was her belief that a 2-year curriculum didn't provide enough time for students to learn all that is necessary for practicing in the profession, and that all of the BS and advanced degrees should require *more advanced periodontal subject matter.*

Esther strongly emphasized that *dental hygiene is going to grow, and it is important for dental hygienists to know a lot more.* She was excited about the advanced dental hygiene practitioner (ADHP) who is both teacher and clinician, as it provides an opportunity for specialized care, such as for the elderly, patients with disabilities, and those for whom access to care is limited.

❧ Esther's Legacy ❧ AT MASSACHUSETTS COLLEGE OF PHARMACY AND HEALTH SCIENCES

Forsyth School of Dental Hygiene celebrated its 100th Anniversary in 2016. Supporting her alma mater, Forsyth School of Dental Hygiene, at many events at the College or at off-site events, Esther M. Wilkins continued to inspire. Just her presence brought crowds to meet her for the first time or a repeat handshake. She felt proud to represent the College but more so to meet new Forsyth graduates just entering the career to which she was personally committed all her life.

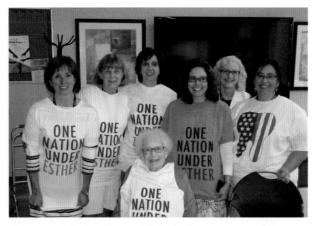

FIGURE 11.24: One Nation Under Esther, graduate orientation.

The number of outside events Esther could attend reduced in number through the years, but she made every effort to attend the events she could, especially the Forsyth Alumni Reception at the Yankee Dental Conference held each January in Boston, Massachusetts, student orientations at MCPHS, and the Esther Wilkins Symposiums.

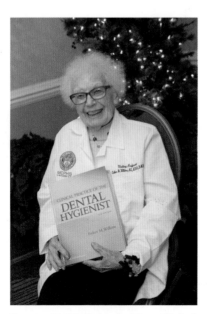

FIGURE 11.25: Esther holding *Clinical Practice of the Dental Hygienists*, Massachusetts College of Pharmacy and Health Sciences, 2015.

Chapter 12

Continuing Education

Wyoming at last!

"Here stood a diminutive woman [with] snowy white hair who commands more respect than anyone in the profession. She may be small in stature, but she is a giant of a woman! She lectured in the old-school style with an overhead projector and illustrated her points with colored markers. She also used some PowerPoint slides to highlight particular points. Her ability to connect with the audience comes from her passion for teaching and her vast knowledge of the subject matter. Nobody does it like the master" (Watterson, 2009, p. 2).

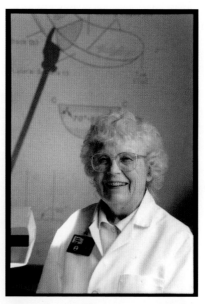

FIGURE 12.1: Esther presenting biofilm lecture.

Reaching beyond her active roles at Simmons, Forsyth, and Tufts, Esther's successful career resulted in an extensive international teaching and lecturing circuit. Her love of learning and teaching was evident in her continuing education courses, and she committed to as many presentations as possible in order to advocate for oral health and the dental hygiene profession. She was disappointed when a previous engagement or work on *Clinical Practice of the Dental Hygienist* (CPDH) prevented her from speaking to another group, and she encouraged her peers in the profession to follow her lead in maintaining strong ties to alumni organizations, always following one of her most heartfelt mottos: "Keep reaching out and influencing the oral health of all whose lives you touch" (Quinsigamond Community College, 2008, p. 4).

Esther became one of the most highly sought speakers in the United States and abroad, including the very first dental hygiene program developed in Shanghai, China. Her name was recognized across the globe, and these presentations were booked a year in advance. Announcements for her course were often prefaced with "Esther Wilkins, RDH, DMD: Internationally Renowned Speaker and Author," although once they must have run out of "D's."

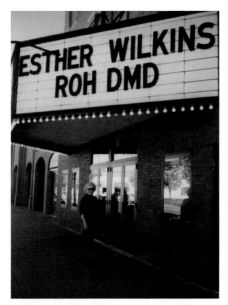

FIGURE 12.2: Marquee, Esther M. Wilkins, ROH [sic], DMD, Michigan, 1994.

Once Esther committed to a continuing education date, she wrote a letter making her specifications known, such as how the room was to be configured, the topic on which she was to speak about, brochure content, microphone availability, the plans for marketing the event, and expectations for attendance. A letter to one group dated May 5, 2000, evidenced this level of specificity:

Did I ever ask you how many people usually attend your lecture day? Of course, if it is to be 50 or under, we could hear the audience questions OK, but when it gets up higher, it is so much better to have at least one and preferably two walking mics with a couple of your committee members, or other scouts, wearing their flatties and up and down passing the hand mic around.

Esther prepared extensively for every continuing education course. She planned weeks in advance for her script, conducted research-prepared PowerPoint presentations and handouts, and made word changes just before her presentation. She shared her extensive knowledge to her audiences. It resulted in the feeling by coordinators and attendees that Esther's "presentations were always polished and comprehensive" (McKeown, 2017, p. 57). It was a lot of work, but in a 1994 letter to a colleague, she reflected on the importance of her presentations.

My courses this fall, besides Tel Aviv and Jerusalem, take me to Michigan, Maine, and Detroit. I meet so many wonderful people on these trips and although it is a lot of hard work to get ready and present, I appreciate my contacts very much. Our current emphasis is on the RISK factors—for periodontal infections. We were already pointing out the risk of diabetes, HIV infections, Down's Syndrome, and certain drugs used in therapies. All put together it makes for real meaning to a dental hygienist's career.

Esther took her commitments seriously and embraced the culture of whichever particular school or organization hosted her. In 1999, Esther was included as one of a number of speakers who gave lectures for dental hygienists, offered by AstraZeneca. Topics she offered included New Research, The Initial Periodontal Examination, Nonsurgical Periodontal Therapy, and Early Childhood Caries. In 2000, Esther and several colleagues were selected to participate on the Oral-B Advisory Board.

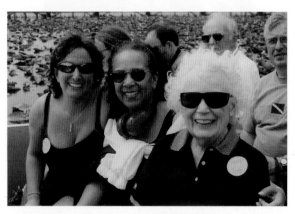

FIGURE 12.3: Esther, Tina Daniels, Joyce Turcotte, airboat ride, Oral B advisory board, Everglades, 2000.

Esther sought to better know the people, students, and faculty to more effectively reach her audience. Her events were highly anticipated and created quite an impact for the members of the communities who hosted them. When it was announced that Esther would be presenting, the response it generated was "THE Esther?" Forsyth classmate, Barbara Wilson, recalled,

❝ it was Esther Wilkins who changed dental hygiene *training* to dental hygiene *Education*. I believe Esther Wilkins is responsible for making it a *profession* we all love."

Esther reciprocated this enthusiasm from students and fellow educators. Insisting on the same level of detail for her workshops as for her editions of CPDH, she sought excellence and with a personal touch.

In a 1982 letter to the event planner at Loyola in Illinois, Esther wrote,

Please call me Esther. We have a long-term friendship developing and no doubt a file full of letters before we get it all planned! Also, for the brochure or other announcements, use Dr. Esther Wilkins, which is how the hygienists would recognize me. Theoretically, I have never been Dr. Gallagher! (Only Mrs. G). As someone said "Dr. Wilkins and Mrs. Gallagher" in the tone of "Dr. Jekyll; & Mr. Hyde!" Now to serious business. Enclosed is a CV but for Goodness sake's, don't put all that on anything!

❧ THE FIRST CONTINUING EDUCATION ❧ COURSE AND BEYOND

In May of 1967, at the annual meeting of the New York State Dental Hygienists' Association, Esther offered her first continuing education course. The topic for the course was instrumentation, and the presentation took place in a valley with resort hotels outside New York City. She presented with Roxie Spitzer, the chair of the dental hygiene program of one of the community colleges, and together, they presented a talk for each school at individual tables on periodontal, instrumentation, and forms. Members of the Dental Hygiene Association of New York attended, although it wasn't required for licensure and continuing education units (CEUs) were not yet in existence. The rest, as they say is history, as this first continuing education was followed by multiple requests for presentations.

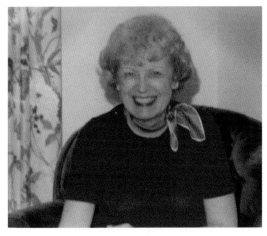

FIGURE 12.4: Esther, Columbus, Georgia, 1977.

From the 1970s to the 2000s, Esther presented at least 10 continuing education courses every spring and fall. Jim accompanied Esther on several continuing education trips and described in detail where they went, what they saw, the side trips they took, the museums and galleries they enjoyed, the people they met, as well as the challenges of traveling, often to several cities in a short amount of time.

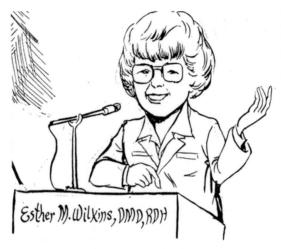

FIGURE 12.5: Jim's caricature of Esther presenting continuing education.

In their Christmas letters through the 70's and 80's, Jim chronicled every continuing education course Esther presented in each year: "In May, Esther went to China with a dental hygiene exchange program" (Christmas Letter, 1983). "There was Bismarck (where she crossed the wide Missouri and learned a lot of history about Sitting Bull); Roanoke; Cleveland; Orlando (including a trip to Epcot); Little Rock (delicious catfish); Grand Rapids (home of fluoridation); and Denver" (Christmas Letter, 1984).

In their 1985 Christmas Letter, "Esther has been skidding around on her roller skates as usual. . . . Of special note among her travels was the trip to Dhahran, Saudi Arabia, last January, to present continuing education for the nearly 30 dental hygienist of ARAMCO. *Such sights to see . . . a really terrific experience.* Another trip to China, this one with some different sights than in 1983. Special to appreciate was the visit to their first dental hygiene school in Shanghai."

The year 1993 brought Esther to Florence, Italy:

What a fabulous experience. There were side trips on the train to Genoa (to the dental and dental hygiene schools and to lunch overlooking the Mediterranean, and another trip to Bologna). Esther also gave a continuing education program in Seattle *always a sentimental journey. There are too many nice things connected to each trip to write here. In 1996, I went below the Equator!! To Australia and New Zealand!! Now I only have 3 more continents to visit. I was entertained at the Dental Hygiene and Dental Schools in Dunedin and met with RDH's in all three cities. Delightful moments of a lifetime.*

Yes, I finally got to travel through the Panama Canal, after thinking about it for years. It Really is a remarkable engineering marvel of the century. Our country really goofed when

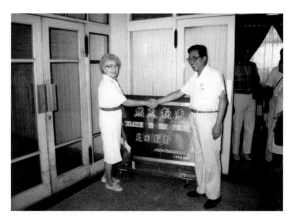

FIGURE 12.6: Esther in Beijing, China, 1985.

they "gave" it away. I'm a sightsee-er at heart. Other notable travels of the year were for presenting CE from sea to shining sea and from border to border. I presented in Idaho in September—which leaves only one more state to complete all the USA—Wyoming! Then it was over the ocean to Milan, Italy where the Italian translation of the textbook was launched (Christmas Letter, 2000).

There were initially small honorariums associated with Esther's continuing education presentations, and eventually when additional information in the field required further development, she received a fee plus expenses. As her popularity and notoriety increased through the years, she was often approached primarily by students who sought to have their CPDH textbooks signed. "Students inevitably crowd around her, clutching their textbooks, hoping to snag an autograph or snap a photo with her. She complies, of course, usually with a wide smile, *that's just what rock stars do*" (Flaherty, 2012, p. 1). Esther prided herself on the originality of her programs, and she made a point of attending continuing education courses taught by her colleagues as well *to learn more.*

As Lynda McKeown recalled,

❝ Esther [set] an example for continuing education. Not only [did] she provide continuing education for dental hygienists all over the world, she also engage[ed] in continuing education herself. Esther wanted and needed to remain current and knowledgeable in scientific evidence and societal trends as they impact upon dental hygiene. After a long day of speaking and answering questions, most presenters would be tired and ready to slow down. However, Esther attended the wine and cheese reception, and continued on to a documentary film of some intensity."

Esther's passion for collaboration was contagious, and her colleagues responded to it in a way that echoed her students. Nancy Sisty LePeau related her experiences in organizing a program with Esther,

❝ . . . when dental hygiene instructors from the State of New York traveled to Boston for an instrumentation continuing education program developed and directed by her. As members of the Dental Hygiene committee for the State of New York planned for the program under Esther's tutelage, her special and dynamic techniques as an educator began to unfold. She involved the audience by asking very interesting questions that focused on why we do things the way we do. She challenged the instructors and participants to think outside the box and to base decisions on research. Her approach differed from the way I had been taught as a dental hygiene student, and I tried to incorporate some of her techniques in my teaching at Columbia University and in subsequent years as a dental hygiene educator."

Dr. Wilkins had offered over 1,000 courses, and at that point, she stopped counting. "Wyoming at last" in 2001 celebrated her presentations that encompassed all 50 states. Internationally, she presented in several countries, along with those she toured with International Federation of Dental Hygienists (IFDH), occasionally with multiple visits: Australia, Canada, China, Israel, Ireland, England, Egypt, Panama, Costa Rica, Spain, Sweden, Switzerland, Holland, Italy, Japan, New Zealand, Saudi Arabia, and South Africa. Her presentations ranged from hour-long lectures to all-day programs and occurred in a variety of venues.

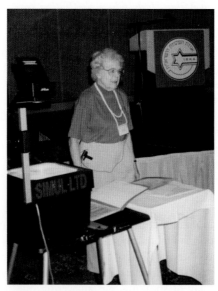

FIGURE 12.7: Esther presenting overheads in Israel, 1994.

Esther's presentations were sometimes sponsored by companies and were many times presented in association with professional organizations, including the American Dental Education Association, Yankee Dental Congress, Greater New York Dental Meetings, the Massachusetts Dental Society, Student American Dental Hygienists' Association (SADHA), and the American Dental Hygienists' Association (ADHA). Esther's Saudi Arabian trip was at the invitation of the Arabian American Oil Company.

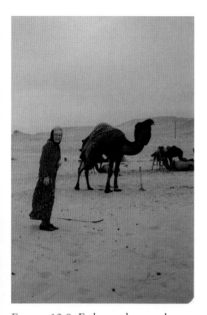

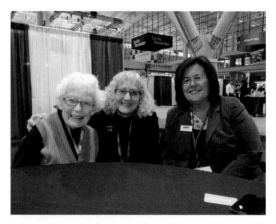

FIGURE 12.8: Esther and a camel, Saudi Arabia, 1985.

FIGURE 12.9: Yankee Dental Congress, Linda Boyd, Esther, and Patti Parker.

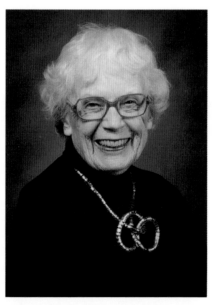

FIGURE 12.10: Esther in Boston, P & G seminar, 2007.

In 1991, Esther gave a continuing education program for the Army Dental Care System, after which she received a note and a photograph expressing gratitude:

❝ I can truly say, your dedication to the dental hygiene profession has inspired soldiers throughout the Army Dental Care System. ”

When organizing a function and determining its course of study, Esther would often ask, *what strikes your fancy?* Essentially, this wizard of dental hygiene could lecture on any subject, although admittedly her favorites were public health, dental caries (especially root caries), instrumentation, fluoridation, prevention programs, risk factors for periodontal infection, and new research in the field.

Despite her experience and knowledge, Esther would actually get nervous prior to presenting, despite her meticulous planning. Those fortunate enough to attend were aware of the quality of these lectures and of their privilege in taking notes from a living legend. After each of her lectures, Esther eagerly reviewed her course evaluations. In 1982, she wrote a letter to a friend, exclaiming

If I can't type even as well as usual, it is because my head is whirling (and a bit enlarged, I might add) after reading the evaluations!! You know how much I love that they say things like "changing my profession from cleaning woman to preventive therapist."

For those who knew Esther well, especially of her propensity for saving and documenting absolutely everything, it will come as no surprise that she guarded a sizeable folder containing some of her treasured continuing education evaluations. The word *excellent* appeared ubiquitously, and the written comments clearly demonstrate the level of self and personality that Esther's work exuded as well as the extent to which Esther's presentation impacted the lives of her students.

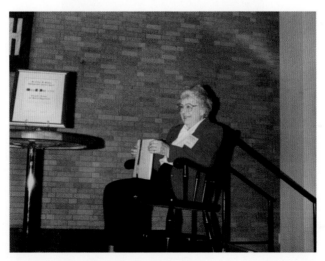

FIGURE 12.11: Esther on the stage, 1994.

❧ THE IMPACT SHE CREATED WITH ❧ CONTINUING EDUCATION COURSES

Although most attendees commented on her warmth and overall positivity, and others fixated on the humor and sense of fun and excitement she brought to her work, the unanimous reaction to her lectures was one of reverence.

❝ The keys of knowledge you opened to me led me to a new world," "It was an honor to be in the same room with Dr. Esther Wilkins," "I feel renewed," "I could have listened to her all day."

"It was an honor to hear her speak," wrote many students, all of whom experienced a renewed sense of devotion to the profession and a desire to achieve personal growth through the positivity with which she approached her work. Esther relished this feedback and treasured each index card, each carefully folded and catalogued piece of paper, stored in individual folders in a closet in her office. Esther commented in interviews conducted with her as well as in her own reflections that the best part of offering continuing education around the country and the world, making friends, especially with dental hygiene students, was her favorite part. In 1994, in a letter to a colleague, she reflected on the importance of her presentations to others and to herself.

It was an unparalleled feeling for her to receive a follow-up letter or an email from a student, expressing gratitude. After receiving one such email in 2009 from an attendee in California, Esther reflected,

this one brought cloudy damp eyes—it is so encouraging to know that sometimes we can plant a seed or two. Some people don't take the time and trouble to write, or they don't have anything to "take home" because they are just getting their credits for licensure or seeing their friends. But sometimes, such as this, I know I am not going nuts over this book for nothing!

Joyce Turcotte described making her initial invitation for Esther to speak in Connecticut:

❝ I called her on the telephone to introduce myself. Some were surprised that I would just pick up the phone to call, as if I had dialed a god. Little did I realize the impact of that phone call. I had called a queen, the queen of dental hygiene! She was very curious about whom I was, what I do, and so forth. Anyone who has ever chatted with Esther knows they are in for an education. She taught me more about continuing education from that conversation than I could have dreamed of. Joyce described the energy Esther puts into the experience. "Once we arrived at the meeting site, she kept me on my toes. It was never too late at night or too early in the morning to double-check the meeting room arrangements. Esther would have the hotel staff move tables, chairs, audio visual equipment, registration tables and so forth until she was pleased with the setting. She always offered her opinion, because she had more experience than anyone, so if you're smart, you'll listen to her and learn."

Joyce recalled her trepidation in driving Esther from the train station to present her course "for fear of being associated with the potential ill fate of Esther Wilkins."

A former student met Esther in Chicago in 2008 and reminded her of a story of when she attended a continuing education program in which Esther was presenting in 1996. "An attendee began leaving the room before the presentation was over, so Esther said, *Oh, don't leave now; there is a good part coming up*. No one remembers whether the person sat down again or not, but it did amuse the audience!"

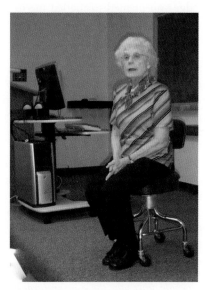

FIGURE 12.12: Esther in Chicago, 1996.

Although it takes a tremendous amount of time and effort to present a continuing education course, the rewards were beyond worth it for Esther. She stirred up energy in the profession as Beverly Whitford recalled after driving to Tufts with a colleague for one of Esther's 2-day periodontology courses in the 1960s. "One day was didactic and the other day clinical. I was in awe of this tiny blond lady who was a dynamo in the classroom. She opened my eyes to the use of curettes and inspired me to constantly research the most current dental hygiene standard of care." Beverly also noted that this renowned presenter of such valuable continuing education programs is also a down-to-earth person. While preparing a presentation with Esther for the Connecticut Dental Hygienists' Association, this dental hygiene icon said upon her arrival, *after the course, let's you and I go for a beer!*

This generosity of spirit and boundless energy are consistent themes in letters from colleagues and former students, many of whom had become close friends with Esther. Despite her fame and endlessly busy schedule, she set aside time for the people in her life, responded diligently to every colleague, and even provided one-on-one assistance to students completing their dissertation and master's theses. Over the years, many students sought, " . . . [Esther's] wise counsel on matters related to issues in [their] professional life," and thanked her for " . . . the clarity [she] brought to [their] writing" (Watterson, 2009, p. 1). As Lana Crawford expressed, "Esther always [had] room for one more . . . She [had] an open heart . . . and friends all around the world [and did] a remarkable job of keeping up with them!"

Lana, who remained one of Esther's close friends, painted her as a figure whose reputation made them seem almost unapproachable. Her first meeting with Esther was wrought with nerves, but Esther's ease and natural ability to socialize immediately put them at ease.

❝ The first time I worked up the courage and took a friend, Jan Schoen, to approach Esther was at the International Federation of Dental Hygiene 14th Symposium in Florence, Italy, in the Summer of 1998. We went to a beautiful villa on a hillside outside of Florence by bus. Esther and Wilma Motley were seated by each other during the banquet. Wilma was also a distinguished dental hygienist, loved and well respected in the dental community. I boldly introduced myself to both of them and they kindly posed for a picture. I remembered showing the picture later to friends who were amazed that I had been on such sacred ground between Esther and Wilma!"

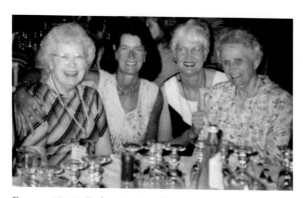

FIGURE 12.13: Esther, Janice Schoen, Lana Crawford, and Wilma Motley, Florence, 1998.

Esther often co-presented with other dental hygiene educators and professionals. One of the early continuing education programs in which Esther shared the stage was at her alma mater, Forsyth, in 1973, in a program entitled "Current Preventive Concepts in Dentistry." She frequently returned to Forsyth to present continuing education programs. In 1978, she and several other women dentists presented a program entitled "Women in Dentistry." The coordinator thanked her by letter for "giving the students, especially the male students, a firsthand view of some of the problems that women face in the dental professions."

One of her close collaborations was with colleague and lifelong friend, Anna Pattison, a friendship which lasted for many years. They presented together for many International Dental Seminars, including one notable 2009 seminar in Salt Lake City. For many dental hygienists practicing in the 1970s and 1980s, it is highly likely they took at least one of Esther and Anna's courses. For several years in the 1970s, they shared an office at Tufts

Dental School when Anna accepted an assistant professor position in the Periodontology Department. Together, Esther and Anna began their work for their preclinical course and the first incarnation of the handbook (*Clinical Periodontics Handbook*).

As editor of *Dimensions of Dental Hygiene*, Anna referred to Esther as "down to earth, funny, and full of useful information" in her "From the Editor" comments for the 2008 edition (p. 1). In reflecting on her presentation in San Francisco for the International Dental Seminars, she described Esther as "A Living Treasure." Anna said she learned something new from Esther after each program she presented.

There were occasional challenges to Esther's continuing education circuit, and some of these moments in which the program did not run smoothly are memorable. When she arrived to present at an event in Philadelphia, for instance, there were no rooms available, so she presented her course in a tent with students packed in to be able to see. Sometimes, there were technical problems or inclement weather, and the occasional miscommunication, getting to various cities which led to a myriad of other calamities. As Anne Guignon related in her 2001 *RDH Magazine* article,

> " somehow, [Esther's] accommodations for one program were some distance away from the place where the program was being presented. No one had made arrangements to get Esther there. While taking the conventional sidewalk route, she decided to save some time and go as the crow flies, proceeding to hike through a field of weeds. With dusty shoes and a few blades of grass and burrs in them, Wilkins presented one of her legendary programs" (p. 2).

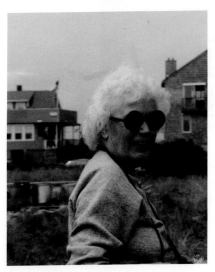

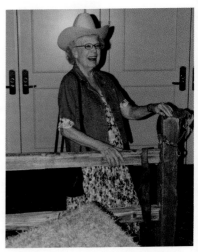

FIGURE 12.14: South Dakota, 1990.

FIGURE 12.15: Esther in the cowboy hat, 2001.

During an interview conducted by Ann-Marie DePalma in 2002, Esther shared that her most embarrassing continuing education moment was while taking a break from the podium. While she was in the restroom, it was discovered that her microphone was still on, but fortunately several people overheard her and came running to rescue her.

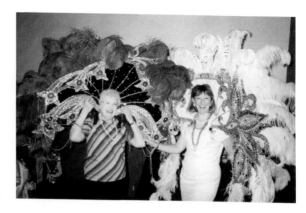

Figure 12.16: Esther and Tonya Ray in costume, New Orleans, 2010.

In 2008, Esther was en route to Dallas when her flight was canceled, but she was determined to make her destination and run her course. After some charming negotiation, she made it to Dallas via Puerto Rico. Without a bit of stress, she had a 4-hour layover in Puerto Rico and as she simply put it, *I arrived on time and my friends were waiting for me.* While an adjunct faculty member at Forsyth, Tina Daniels was preparing to travel to Quinsigamond Community College in Worcester for one of Esther's courses.

"On a cold winter day in Boston, Massachusetts, three Forsyth faculty and I loaded into my car (a red four-door Fiat) to travel to QCC. As we were almost ready to leave, someone said, 'can one more person ride in your car?' To my surprise, it was Dr. Esther Wilkins [who was] getting into the front seat with me! I could barely think, let alone drive. Somehow, we made it to Worcester safely; I survived the class. Thinking only about Dr. Wilkins riding back to Boston in MY car! We then heard a thump, thump, thump. I had a FLAT TIRE . . . with Dr. Esther Wilkins in my CAR! I pulled off the highway as far onto the curve as I could; we all piled out of the car to take a look. Esther took charge, and asked the big question, *do you have a Triple A card, dear?* I was so embarrassed to answer, no, I don't. In the era of NO cell phones, no Triple A card, what does one do or say? Esther said, *don't worry, dear . . . we will use mine.* Off she went up the hill to a house and knocked on the door; she asked to use the phone, Triple A came, the tire was fixed and we returned safely to Boston."

In 2002, Esther presented to dental hygienists in Italy. In her Christmas Letter of 2003, Esther expressed her excitement and what continuing education adventures she enjoyed:

One of my trips to give cont. ed. was to Albuquerque at the time of the big air balloon festival in October—what a special thing that was to see!! . . . They surely made a gorgeous sight. And then on a brief trip to San Francisco for a program. I walked over the Golden Gate Bridge!! I've been talking about that for years . . . Now I have the fever to do more bridges—so have on my list for the next trip to NYC to "do" the Brooklyn Bridge!!

Esther did indeed get to Niagara Falls the next year when she presented programs in both Niagara Falls and Ottawa, and she did indeed walk across the Brooklyn Bridge.

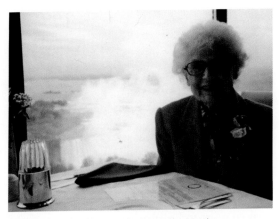

FIGURE 12.17: Esther, Niagara Falls, 1994.

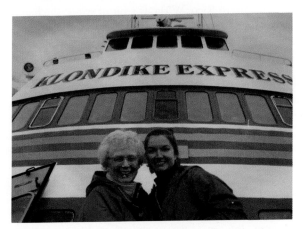

FIGURE 12.18: Esther and Pat Cohen on the Klondike Express, Alaska, 1995.

Esther also *was on an excursion boat on the Mississippi River . . . and I visited 2 miles high and learned to cast—but of course I never caught anything* (Christmas Letter, 2004). And in 2005, *our beautiful country gets bigger and bigger the more you see of it.* Another memorable trip involved travelling to Alaska with Pat Cohen, where after a seminar they borrowed a large van and took a little road trip looking for floating chunks of ice from the glaciers.

Esther learned through experience not to take on more courses than were manageable, although occasionally she was persuaded.

❝ During one week in May, [Esther] spoke at two events: the annual meeting of American Association of the History of Dentistry [AAHD] in Boston, where she discussed the history of Tufts University School of Dental Medicine, the Forsyth Institute, and Forsyth School of Dental Hygiene [now MCPHS]. The second engagement was the 40th anniversary and all-class reunion for the Quinsigamond Community College Dental Hygiene program in Worcester" (Massachusetts

College of Pharmacy and Health Sciences [MCPHS], 2008, p. 32). According to this interview, Esther said that managing a schedule of multiple bookings was *fun!*

In yet another busy week, Esther recalled,

Trudy Sinnett was in Birmingham, Alabama, at the University and I gave the course on one day. Then she and I drove North to Montgomery, and then I had to get up and give the course all over again the next day. I was bushed! By 1:30 to 2:00 I was saying to myself, "No, I already said that!" That could be the last time I ever consented to do two whole days one right after the other. I've done half days right after each other, such as one in New York City and the second day up the Hudson in June of 2009. In her Christmas Letter that year, she expressed, Gosh, I didn't realize there were so many until I went through the calendar!! I loved every one. Traveling is great. The people are great.

The courses were in later years spaced out more appropriately. Despite limiting her travel due to physical discomfort and needing to work on the 11th edition of CPDH, by the end of 2009, she had presented in Phoenix, Moline, Denver, New York City, Toronto, Anaheim, Baltimore, Springfield (Missouri), Hickory (North Carolina), and San Francisco.

The courses Esther offered varied according to the needs of the programs she visited, as well as her desire to inspire curiosity. Several focused continuing education courses in a row stood out for her as exemplary of the breadth she was trying to achieve: "Keys to Management of the Patient with Risk Factors for Periodontal Infections" (Utah Dental Hygienists' Association, October 26, 2001), "Instrumentation for Periodontal Assessment and Nonsurgical Therapy for Dentists and Dental Hygienists" (Massachusetts, Tufts University School of Dental Medicine, November 16, 2001), and "Perio Maintenance Isn't Just Recall" (Missouri, Greater St. Louis Dental Hygienists' Association, April 2, 2002).

Although she wasn't willing to name a favorite course, there was a particular story attached to three unconnected courses she taught in Memphis, which for her would always remain one of her most memorable experiences. The first time she visited Memphis was with her friend, Nancy Williams, who brought her to see Elvis's mansion on their way back to the airport. Esther reminisced with a wink, *I looked through the famous gate and took a picture.* Previously, Esther had described her fandom in a letter to friend, Connie Johnston: *Not to the point of going to Graceland every August to join the candlelight memorial, or anything silly like that!! But just a warm love for the danceable music he made.*

On their second trip to the city, Nancy arranged for a tour of Graceland, as she herself had lived in the city for many years and had never been, without realizing how eventful this would be for Esther. The climax came with Esther's third trip to Memphis for an entirely different continuing education course:

As I finished just before the attendees left for lunch, the Department Head got up and made a couple of announcements and then said, "We want to start right at 1:00 so be sure that you are back on time." I was back early to get my visual aids and slides in shape for the afternoon. Just about one minute of one, the lights seemed to dim when suddenly there was music in the background, the lights went off, and out came Elvis from between the curtain and the stage!!! He sang and talked—called me by name and thanked me for going to his house when I was in town before—and then he got me on stage, went down on a knee to sing to me. Everyone was howling and screaming; it was so exciting!! He stayed about 15 minutes and then left singing, "Love Me Tender, Love Me True—Never Let Me Go." It was just about the best course I ever gave. I thought we never would get settled down for the rest of the afternoon. Esther related the story as vividly as if it was yesterday; she did treasure her memorable moments, including *that whole wonderful day in my life.*

Just as CPDH was both an imperative source for students and labor of love for the author, her continuing education courses had a significant impact on the students and faculty who attended them; these in turn led to many solid personal and professional relationships for Esther.

❝ It was not until about 1976 that I actually met Esther," recalled Pat Ramsay. "I was the newly installed ADHA District I Trustee and had been asked to speak at the Student American Dental Hygienists' Association Northeast Regional Conference that was held at Forsyth. The keynote speaker was the renowned Dr. Esther M. Wilkins. This was my first opportunity to experience Esther's enthusiasm when addressing students. As I sat, I proceeded to worry about how I was ever going to follow the great Dr. Wilkins at the podium. Here she was, a legend sharing her wisdom and experience with all these students. Finally, it was my turn to speak. I approached the microphone and realized that the only way that I could manage this was to make light of the situation. I stood before the audience of several hundred dental hygiene students from throughout the Northeast and my words were: 'I feel like I have finally come of age now that Esther Wilkins is my opening act!'"

As a dental hygienist, Beverly Whitford attested that among the continuing education course she thought had the most impact was

❝ a periodontal course given by Dr. Esther Wilkins around 1970 at Tufts Dental School . . . I remember how impressed I was with Esther both as an educator and a wonderful human being. Her periodontal course was a turning point in my dental hygiene career, as it opened my eyes to contemporary dental hygiene practice of that time. As a 1959 graduate, we were taught to use scalers only. Working below the gingival margin was a 'No-No'! What we were 'trained' to do back in those days was really a 'Dental Manicure.' Being introduced to Gracey curettes and venturing into the sulcus widened my clinical world. This experience also made a statement to me about the need to constantly pursue continuing education to stay abreast of current advances in the profession."

Donna Homenko recalled the day when she finally shook the hand of her idol and had her book signed after one of Esther's continuing education courses in Toledo in 1981.

❝ True elation can only describe the experience—I had met the guru of Dental Hygiene—my chosen profession!" She invited Esther to present at Cuyahoga Community College. "When she arrived at the airport, we started the whirlwind trip, visiting the students at two of the community colleges, professional colleagues, dinner with the CDHA Board and then the course began next day, followed by dinner, visits to the health museum and a quick tour of Cleveland. Needless to say, we were exhausted as we waved goodbye to Dr. Wilkins at the airport; she was smiling and going strong!"

In the 1980s, Esther traveled to Columbia, SC, for the first of several courses hosted by Frannie Tompkins at Midlands Tech.

❝ When you had Esther presenting a CE at your college, two things happened: (a) You felt like you were putting together a mini-accreditation manual with Esther making changes weekly (in the days before computer), and (b) You could count on a packed house. Esther delivered on both counts." Frannie said, "that was when we really found out what a down-to-earth person Esther is. She, of course, insisted we call her 'Esther.' One of the things we were learning was the removal of perio packs, so Esther had us place two packs in each other's mouth. That happened to be the day we had planned to take Esther out to dinner for seafood. Have you eaten seafood with a eugenol period pack in your mouth? Esther enjoyed her food that night!"

Several years later, she returned to Midlands Tech to present another continuing education course, and according to Ms. Tompkins,

❝ being the drawing card that she is, the auditorium was once again packed! The president of the College was so impressed—I believe it was the largest CE attendance ever—that he came to meet Esther and afterwards wrote a letter about the great seminar." Esther left a lasting impression at Midlands Tech, as Wana Millan recalled in describing her first continuing education course with Esther as speaker. "We went into the room, and there she was, wearing a light green dress, and had a drawing board beside her, and she just sparkled. She had me captivated with her boundless energy, and I was swimming in the sulcus, along with all those bad bacteria and microorganisms that inhabit the world that I had chosen to live in for the rest of my life."

It is a recognized ritual that when Esther arrived at a city, someone had to take her to a grocery store so she could purchase her essentials, which included orange juice and whole milk (to go along with the package of oatmeal she brought with her). In addition, she usually flew home with tasty leftovers, usually in the form of a sandwich, from the weekend away.

Former student, Daughn Thomas, described a visit Esther made in 1996 to the Bronx, New York, to attend a luncheon in her honor. Esther was given a tour of Spanish Harlem, and then to Hostos Community College in South Bronx, where students and faculty greeted her with a beautiful bouquet of flowers, a big banner welcoming her, and "an arrangement of books representing each edition that created 'a kaleidoscope like-effect.'" Esther then had an opportunity to observe dental hygiene students with their patients, which she always enjoyed when visiting dental hygiene programs around the country. She signed autographs, exuded an energy that spoke to multiple generations, and reminded students of the contributions they would make in the future as dental hygienists. Daughn recalled how evident it was that Esther "inspire[d] students to elevate themselves to a higher level."

Esther's memorable speeches and the energy with which she delivered them have been recounted by friends and colleagues. At the Mount Wachusett Community College's pinning ceremony, Esther's remarks as keynote speaker included, *remember how your instruments looked? So shiny! So many! And the first examination of another person's mouth? So Dark! Don't be afraid to be a perfectionist. In a precise profession like ours, there is no room for mediocrity!*

The dental hygiene profession and all its institutions reciprocated Esther's warmth and enthusiasm.

❧ AN ACCIDENT IN SOUTH CAROLINA ❧

On October 26, 2006, directly following a presentation she made at the ADHA state association meeting in Charlotte, South Carolina, Esther had an accident. She had finished dinner with a group of friends, she was packed and ready to go home, and while leaving through a darkened restaurant instead of through the lobby, Esther lost her balance and fell on the right side of her body. She struck her head on the floor, and her hip was broken. Her arms were full, she lost her balance, she thought the floor was wet, and she caught herself on a chair leg. Up until this fall, at age 90 years old, Esther had not broken anything. She remembered asking *where are my glasses and where is my pocketbook?* Someone found both for her. She was in too much pain to move, but she was okay if she kept still. There were about a dozen people around her at that point, and someone called 911. She remembered the feeling of being taken out on a stretcher, and she never lost consciousness. In summation of this 2006 continuing education course, Esther declared,

I stayed longer than I had planned in South Carolina!

Her surgery took place the next evening, and Esther woke up with Frances Tompkins sleeping in the chair next to her bed; she slept there every night, after which Esther referred to her as *her angel*. She took Esther's laundry home every day and returned it the next day. Three of her "angels" (Fran Tompkins, Gloria Carbine, Tammy Byrd, Beverly Dunbar, and Brenda McCarson) spoke with personnel to inform them of exactly who they had as a patient and how to take care of her.

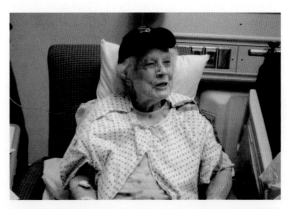

FIGURE 12.19: Esther in Red Sox hat, South Carolina, 2006.

Esther did not let this ordeal faze her, as Esther's niece, Betsy Tyrol, related,

❝ One Saturday in October of 2006, I got an early morning call from South Carolina. A woman from the Dental Hygiene School where Esther had just given a workshop was calling. She, along with a few others, came to be called by Esther as the South Carolina 'angels.' She informed me that Esther had broken her hip and was scheduled for surgery that day. Immediately, there was a faint voice in the background and the phone was handed over to the person in charge—Esther herself. She sounded weak from the medication and pain, but wanted to tell me she was okay."

❝ As the next few weeks unfolded, the fact that she was okay was obvious. By Monday she was on the phone again, telling me what she needed from her apartment and what I needed to do when I was there: who to call, what to cancel, what bills to pay and how to water her plants. By Wednesday I was checking and sending emails, packaging up chapters and mailing them to the rehab hospital, for of course, she was transferred earlier than usual to rehab. I was informed that she would have several weeks in rehab before being transferred to a rehab hospital in the Boston area; her stay was far shorter than the average stay. I continued to travel back and forth to the apartment to carry out instructions. There was always a long list of what needed to be done, for of course the book revision was in full swing and already behind schedule."

❝ All of a sudden, Esther said she was being discharged and wanted to know when I could pick her up at the airport. I told her any day but Tuesday and, of course, that was the day she came home. The Esther Network swung into action. A ride was available, food was purchased, and help was there to get her into the apartment and to bed was ready."

Esther owed a great deal for her recovery to her South Carolina "angels." They screened calls, took messages, cut her hair, brought flowers, arranged for transportation, and essentially provided 24/7 service to their celebrity visitor *so I could get better and stronger faster!!* Her angels created a scrapbook of pictures from her rehabilitation, which Esther considered one of her most prized possessions. *Fran was the most attentive angel of all, her and her dog.* Fran remembered she answered Esther's phone— "and the phone did ring quite often! She was even on two phones at one time!"

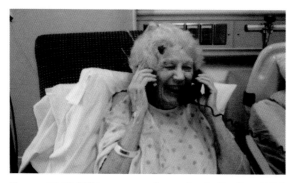

Figure 12.20: Talking on two phones, South Carolina, 2006.

227

Fran said Esther did not let a broken hip get her down for long.

❝ She was proofing the 10th edition chapters and even allowed me to read one chapter and critique it! It was a real WOW experience to be able to spend time with Esther. If Esther tells her side of this story, she will probably include the 'tough love' times that I 'encouraged' her to take care of herself when she got home.❞

Esther was extremely flattered that students came to visit her in the hospital and asked her to autograph their books.

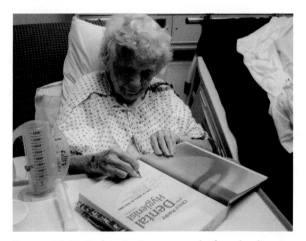

FIGURE 12.21: Esther signing autographs from her hospital bed, South Carolina, 2006.

ADHA had announced her fall on their Web site, as well as the American Academy of Dental Hygiene (AADH) Web site. The caption included a message from Margaret Lappan Green then ADHA president. "I know that dental hygienists across the country will join me in keeping her in our thoughts and prayers during her recovery" (ADHA, 2006, p. 1).

Esther was in the hospital 5 days before going to rehabilitation at HealthSouth Rehabilitation Facility in Columbia, South Carolina, on Wednesday, October 11. She was dedicated to her recovery and remembers being a particularly dutiful patient and *did everything they told me to do.* While recovering, she worked on three chapters of CPDH, which had been packed in her suitcase for her trip home from South Carolina. The Book traveled with her in various stages, regardless of the unexpected delay. Chapter contributor Karen Raposa remembered that to her amazement, 2 to 3 weeks after Esther's surgery, she received a handwritten letter from Dr. Esther Wilkins. According to Karen,

❝ this was no ordinary 'Handwritten Letter' . . . this was a 'Business Letter' to provide me with her thoughts and requests for additional revisions to the chapter I had sent her about a week prior to her injury. My jaw was on the floor! This lady never ceased to amaze me. She was sending me the revisions from her hospital bed! Once again, you just don't see that level of determination in many individuals in our society today." Karen says she will save that letter for her lifetime, as it is a "classic."

Esther travelled back to Boston, and when she arrived, Forsyth classmates Pat Ramsay, Jean Conner, and Marian Carone Clark picked her up at the airport. They brought a very exhausted but mending Esther home, and her niece, Betsy, arrived the following day. Betsy described Esther's recovery:

> I arrived on Wednesday morning to find her already up and around the apartment with her walker. Nothing was going to stop her from finishing the book. We had to cancel some of her speaking engagements, her course work, and other plans, such as the theater and lectures she wanted to go to, but she was on for The Book."

> She didn't want help, such as a cleaning lady or meals, other than those friends and I could provide. She didn't want someone overnight, except for those nights that I stayed. We adapted her apartment—switched the beds, installed grab bars in the bathroom, and picked up rugs and other things in the way of the walker. Food was on bottom shelves, along with the few dishes she needed. The pathway to the computer was cleared and she was in business. I did the grocery shopping and the laundry and ran errands. The Esther Network helped with all of that as well. New clothes, for various occasions, were purchased, tried on and returned. Outfits went to the tailor, since she had lost weight."

> After the initial visit with a new doctor, during which she took charge of most everything, she started physical therapy. She didn't have the therapist come to the apartment—she took a cab. After a short time, she would walk from the therapy over to Tufts and pick up a cab there. At least that can be done all inside—remember this is November now."

> As she progressed, and very quickly—the doctor was amazed at her determination and rapid recovery—she continued to be single minded in her efforts on the book. There was no nonsense in her approach. She was going to recover and as fully as possible. As with everyone, there were good days and bad days, but the bad days were not for complaining. They were for overcoming."

Betsy concluded,

> everyone who visited had to look at the x-rays to see the pins. They had to have a laugh or two. Plants, flowers, and gifts of food arrived regularly. The cards had to be put in a huge basket there were so many."

In November of that year, the plans for her 90th birthday were announced, which included a celebration at the Yankee Conference in Boston in January given by Hu-Friedy. A small celebration was planned for her actual birthday on December 9 at Anthony's Pier 4. By then she was walking with a cane, and Mary Dole commented that Esther was "queen for a day" and that there was an apparent "warmth and love that [everyone had] for Esther."

Betsy's story continued,

❝ after the Yankee conference, she was just about self-sufficient again. The doctor discharged her from physical therapy and saw her only once after the winter. She started up her workshop schedule and her course work at Tufts. The book revision was delayed, but not for long. A year and a half later, she is doing floor exercises, driving, and contemplating the next step in her career.❞

Esther was calm as a cucumber throughout the whole process.

Following her accident in South Carolina, many of Esther's friends grew concerned for her and the intense recuperation process ahead of her. Soon after, Pat Ramsay rejoiced,

❝ feisty lady that she is, she was up and about long before her friends or doctors thought she would be. Those of us who know her and love her are well aware of her stubbornness (of course, she would call it being determined). However, it was this characteristic that helped her get through that terrible period in her life.❞

Esther actually enjoyed the rehabilitation process and was slightly disappointed when her sessions were over; she liked being able to exercise and get stronger every day. As Esther wrote in her Christmas Letter of 2007, *into physical therapy, where as an A student, they told me to go home and do my exercises. Compliance? So-so.* Experiencing such intense recovery following her accident prompted her to make exercise an integral part of her life, and she eventually developed a twice-weekly regimen with a personal trainer, Karen.

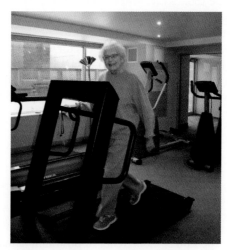

FIGURE 12.22: Esther on the treadmill, 151 Tremont Street, Boston.

Esther continued to receive cards, letters, emails, and packages for months after her accident. A particular mammoth card came from the Fones School of Dental Hygiene in

Bridgeport, Connecticut, signed by all of the students. On the second anniversary of her accident, Esther wrote a poem of thanks to her caretakers:

The Anniversary

On special anniversary two
I come with many thanks to you!!
We can recall that evening well,
That fateful Friday when I fell.
October 6, two oh oh six
The day put Esther in a fix.
Wondering how all this could happen to me
Next day I went down for surger-ee.
An Angel stayed each night on the cot,
To watch me, tend me and sooth me a lot.
Every day up to walk, a push by P. T.
Impossible progress?? Was it really me??
I moved to the rehab for OT and PT
My angels came daily to help referee!
My new home was Re-hab in South Carolina
Where tis said that nothing can be fine-ah!
How soon could I walk and how soon would I dance?
They pushed and they pulled—I had not a chance!
The mail began coming from far wide and near—
The grapevine of friendship to me is so dear.
In 2-3 weeks I was checked out to leave—
Took extra big suitcases: you wouldn't believe
The Carolina Angels to my plane they did go
They helped me so much—I do love them so!!

(WILKINS, 2008)

Due to the accident, Esther claimed The Book was *behind whatever schedule it was supposed to be on, and stayed behind all year. I finally sent the last of the proofreading 2 days before Thanksgiving.* It had been a most unusual year for Esther, *the first of its kind for me,* as until that day, at 90 years old, she had never even been hospitalized nor broken a bone. Ever the optimist, Esther always found something positive in any situation, *now that I walk with a cane, I generally got a seat on the subway, even in a full car!*

❧ ESTHER'S CONTINUING EDUCATION ❧ COURSES RESUME

Another entire book could be written on the 1,000 continuing education courses offered, the accolades Esther received, and her thousands of adoring fans. "Her depth of commitment to advancing the prevention of oral health and the optimal treatment of periodontal and dental diseases is unmatched. Her unique mastery of dental hygiene's body of knowledge has established Wilkins as the true leader of our profession" (Pattison, 2013, p. 13).

Esther's continuing education presentations reduced in number the last 6 years of her life; yet, she continued to advise, communicate, and share her knowledge through emails, telephone calls, and notes. She enjoyed the many requests for interviews, asking for reflections on her life and her professions, and she enjoyed attending the few events that were held locally in Boston, including reunions at Simmons, Forsyth, and Tufts. Retirement was not an option in her opinion.

I have never been in favor of complete retirement. When a friend said she could hardly wait to retire, move to Florida, and play golf every day, it sounded quite unappealing to me.

As one would expect, Esther continued to be passionate about her own continuing education, not limited to the dental profession. She read voraciously the newspaper and journals that came daily, clipping the articles she wanted to study later. She called herself *somewhat of an addict* by remaining on so many mailing lists. She was like a sponge for learning, and her energy level to keep active and involved remained high until the last few years of her life.

The author had the pleasure of accompanying Esther, Pat Cohen, and author's husband, Andy, to the 2009 Issam M. Fares Lecture, sponsored jointly by Tufts University Department of History and the Fletcher School, where the Right Honorable Tony Blair was speaking. Although the only available seats were in the back section, we were ushered to the eighth row of the VIP section. It seems there were many Tufts community members in the audience, and Esther was held in as much high regard by the dental community as she did with dental hygiene.

Esther believed in continuing to learn, not just to renew a license but to learn for the sake of learning. She sought for her students, her colleagues, and herself to expand understanding of multiple topics, from keeping up with new research, politics, the economy, to what is happening in the world and communities. She advocated strongly for being active.

Esther repeatedly insisted that there be a chapter in her biography devoted to continuing education. She considered her efforts in these programs one of her most valuable contributions, and it was essential that it be recorded with proper weight.

❝ I truly enjoy being part of an essential profession that focuses on oral disease prevention and health promotion. The continuing education programs I hold give me particular pleasure because they provide me opportunities to meet students and dental hygienists around the world" (Esther, as cited in Ray, 1996, p. 9).

CHAPTER 13

Memberships, Associations, Honors, Honor Societies, Awards, and Consulting and Review Boards

If you read about her accolades, you will find the list unending,
With just a glimpse you will know that more awards are pending.
Distinguished alumnus, excellence in hygiene, faculty awards,
Honorary memberships, degrees, and trophies she hoards.
Cynthia Biron (1997).

Throughout the years, Esther was active in numerous professional dental and dental hygiene organizations, including those in which she had been a member or fellow for over 70 years. She held office, served as editor, served on committees, initiated chapters, participated in presentations, and published in a variety of organizational publications dedicated to education, associations, scholarship, and advancing the professions in which she had been an active member: as a dental hygienist and as a dentist. As Esther related, *I never did win anything in elementary school or high school or college.* Being chosen to recite the Gettysburg Address at the Tyngsborough Memorial Day program at the town hall, when she was in the fifth or sixth grade was her first honor. *I didn't think of it as an honor at the time; I was terrified on the "big" stage.*

One could not quantify or list all of the honorary memberships Esther held in the various dental and dental hygiene societies and schools around the world. However, she treasured every one of them. But importantly, her most treasured awards were her students and their success as dental hygienists and dentists.

❧ MEMBERSHIPS AND ASSOCIATIONS ❧

An ardent proponent of memberships in professional organizations, Esther strongly encouraged colleagues and students to join as soon as they could and to remain active. Esther practiced what she preached.

American Academy of Dental Science

"If my estimate of woman's characteristics be correct, then there is much in dentistry which is not within the scope of the average woman. Woman is inexact. Like some other employments, there are things in dentistry to which a woman is manifestly not by nature adapted" (Kingsley, 1883, p. 15).

The Kingsley (1883) book was delivered before the *American Academy of Dental Science* (AADS). Of course, this content was dated before Esther Mae Wilkins, RDH, DMD, emerged on the dental scene and became a fellow of the AADS in 1979.

Esther was particularly proud of her membership in the AADS. Instituted in Boston, Massachusetts, on October 19, 1867, and incorporated on March 2, 1921, the AADS, the first honor society for dentists, aimed "to promote the cultivation of the science and art of Dentistry, sustain and elevate the professional character of dentists, and encourage mutual improvement, social intercourse, and good feeling" (AADS, 1884, *Preamble*, para. 1). A group of "highly respected, soundly educated, and ethically motivated practitioners, seeking to elevate dentistry to its highest potential, formed the American Academy of Dental Science" (Deranian, 2000, p. 1).

Noted fellows included Charles Eastman, Howard M. Marjerison (Tufts), Basil G. Bibby (Rochester), Dr. J. Murray Gavel, Dr. Henry Bigelow (surgeon at Massachusetts General Hospital who had introduced ether anesthesia to the world), James B. Gallagher (1968, Esther's husband), honorary fellows Thomas A. Forsyth (benefactor of Forsyth Institute) and Dr. Oliver Wendell Holmes ("poet, writer, teacher and physician who had an avid interest in dentistry," Deranian, 2000, p. 1). The primary aim of the academy was "the elevation of dentistry through education" (p. 1).

From the very beginning of the organization, members were named as "fellows," and stipulations were established that required that active fellows chosen for membership would reside in the New England states and have graduated from a college in good standing with a "recognized medical or dental degree" (AADS, 1884, *Constitution, Article III, Membership, Sect. 2*). Associate fellows do not reside in New England but qualify otherwise, and honorary fellows are distinguished in their professions. Admission of members was clearly outlined. Dues were required, *or you didn't get to hold office or vote!* All proceedings and business were conducted for the welfare of the academy. Rules of order were followed; a code of ethics was created, outlining the maintenance of professional character and the duties dentists had to their patients, the community, and the art of dentistry; and meetings were held monthly, with one yearly meeting.

The organization met 4 times a year, twice in the fall and twice in the spring, in addition to the March Business Dinner meeting at the Harvard Club. In order to be admitted, AADS members need to support an application, and a by-law requires a minimum of 5 years of practice and contribution to the field. There is no limit per year on how many new members are admitted. For instance, there were 17 members admitted in 1979, and in 2008, there were none.

James. B. Gallagher, Jr., of 7 Melrose Street in Boston, was admitted to the academy on November 4, 1968. The nomination for Esther M. Wilkins Gallagher was signed by her husband, James B. Gallagher, and Dr. Aligardas Albert Yurkstas. Esther was admitted as a fellow to the AADS on April 4, 1979, the first woman fellow to the academy. It continued to be one of her proudest accomplishments. Esther served as corresponding secretary since taking over the office in 1988 from her husband, Jim, when he passed away. The by-laws were revised in 2004 with regard to positions. Essentially, Esther's position was responsible for letters and other communications addressed to the academy. When the 2000 millennium edition of the constitution and by-laws were written, the copies were brought to the academy meeting. Esther, a member of the Constitution, By-laws, and Code of Ethics Committee, received the first copy because they said she did the most work! As thoroughly as Esther did everything else, it is not surprising that she fulfilled her role with dedication. Esther served as corresponding secretary, as well as a member of the Executive Committee from 2009 until 2016. Esther was actually quite a history buff. It thrilled her to go back and see what had been, how organizations came into being, and review the key individuals who made that history.

Records were kept with precision and diligence since the organization's founding. *The Book*, as Esther called it, the original 1867 constitution and by-laws, dates, and signatures, handwritten by each fellow who was admitted, is a large, leather-bound, gold-leafed volume, housed in the office at the Harvard Club. Esther brought the book home with her in April 2009, with the express purpose of professionally preserving it to prevent additional wear and tear that was evident through the years. As is Esther's style, she researched thoroughly the companies that could truly understand its value, treat it with respect, and assure *that it stayed around for many more years.* She decided upon G. V. Black, located in walking distance from her home in Boston. Esther let me hold the book, guarding me at all times, as I carefully turned the pages of the historic list of original, handwritten signatures of members of the academy for each new year. Grinning but still watching me like a hawk, she said, *there are some very famous dentists in that book! It's quite an honor to be in it!* It was quite a visit to history in reviewing each of the handwritten names of new members as they were admitted into the academy, as they have done since its inception in 1867, over 140 years ago.

Esther spoke fondly of the AADS and described the *old days* when there was a formal ceremony for new members. *Lately, it has become more informal and depended on who the chairman was at the time.* Rarely did Esther miss a meeting, even as it became more difficult for her to leave her home in her later years. Several academy members came to pick her up for meetings and bring her home, for which she was *very grateful.*

American Academy of Periodontology

Although busy with a new edition of her own textbook every 5 years, Esther still found time to edit nearly 200 abstracts for periodontal postdoctoral students at Tufts each year from 1968 through 1988, while Dr. Timothy Leary was editor. She also personally wrote 10 to 12 articles published in the *Journal of Periodontology* since joining the academy. Founded by two women in 1914 and expanded from 17 members in 1914 to approximately 8,000 in 2008, the American Academy of Periodontology's (AAP's) mission is to "advance the periodontal and general health of the public and promote excellence in the practice of periodontics" (AAP, 2018, p. 1).

Esther earned a certificate in periodontology from Tufts University School of Dental Medicine in 1966, and the specialty has been the topic of quite a few Continuing

Education lectures she presented around the world. In his 2006 nomination letter to the AAP in 2006, Dr. Robert J. Rudy (Tufts University School of Dental Medicine) said she "exemplified many of the characteristic most admired by the profession."

Esther was awarded a fellowship from the academy on September 16, 2006.

American Association of Women Dentists

One of the oldest organizations to which Esther belonged is the American Association of Women Dentists (AAWD), which was founded in 1892 in Philadelphia with only 12 members whose purpose was to form a society of female dentists who "could strengthen themselves by trying to help one another" (AAWD, n.d., p. 1). This original group was called the Women's Dental Association of the U.S. and was changed in name to the AAWD in 1921. Committed to dentistry, the organization continues to support women in the profession, provide mentoring opportunities, and serve as a "national network for employment opportunities and scientific exchange" (AAWD, n.d., p. 1).

Esther had been a member of the AAWD since 1952, over 64 years, and a member of the Massachusetts Society of Women Dentists since 1965, having served on many committees and as president from 1970 to 1972.

American Dental Association

Upon graduation from Tufts Dental College in 1949, Esther became a member of the American Dental Association (ADA) through its Massachusetts Dental Society, Metropolitan District. She served on the Local Arrangements Committee at the Annual Session when it was in Boston in 1990 and was a prevention program participant in 2005. The ADA, whose membership exceeds 150,000, turned 150 years old in 2009. It was founded in 1859 in Niagara Falls, New York, by 26 dentists who sought to establish a dental society and who represented the various dental societies operating in the United States at the time. Its membership represents more than 70% of the dentists in the United States, "making it the world's largest and oldest national dental association—America's leading advocate for oral health" (ADA, *150 Years*, 2009, p. 1). As a long-standing organization, it has amassed an extensive library of dental literature, and operates a charitable foundation that provides grants for scholarships, education, research, and assistance.

Esther was a strong proponent of membership in professional associations, and in 2000 wrote,

> *It's unfortunate that all dentists, dental hygienists, assistants, and technicians are not members of their individual professional organizations. Dentists must be the leaders and set the example for the entire team. I have never been able to understand dentists who do not recognize the significance of membership.*

Esther was a very strong advocate of water fluoridation, and she amassed in hard copy form what is essentially the complete history of the topic; the ADA is a major and vocal proponent of fluoridation.

American Dental Education Association

Esther had been a member of American Dental Education Association (ADEA) since 1951. *The American Dental Education Association has been a significant part of my life for many years.* During the first year Esther was teaching in Seattle, she and other faculty members attended the ADEA meeting in Colorado Spring, Colorado.

> *At that time there were less than 40 dental hygiene schools in the USA, only one of which that was not in a dental school. The group of dental hygiene educators that might attend was small. Few of the schools had a budget to support the dental educators, let alone including attendance for the dental hygiene faculty. During that period of time the program for accrediting schools, and the development of the national board for dental hygiene licensure were developing. Those of us that were able to attend over the years developed a close-knit group with long-lasting friendships . . . Perhaps my ramblings can illustrate my deep feelings about belonging to ADEA and its importance to me.*

This organization is "the voice of dental education" (ADEA, 2009) and states its mission as addressing contemporary issues "influencing education, research, and the delivery of oral health care for the health of the public" led by individuals and institutions, both in Canada and in the United States. Founded in 1923 in Nebraska with 47 member dental schools, currently every dental school in the United States is a member of ADEA, with 46,000 students and 12,000 faculty members. Active in the ADEA, Esther held offices in the section on periodontics from 1992 to 1995, including secretary, chairperson-elect, and chairperson.

Nominated by Mary Littleton of Hu-Friedy, on November 2011, ADEA announced that Dr. Esther M. Wilkins was the recipient of a Gies Award for vision, innovation, and achievement. "The William J. Gies Award is the ultimate recognition of exceptional contribution to and support for oral health and dental education. On behalf of the entire Hu-Friedy Family, I nominate Dr. Esther M. Wilkins for the Dental Educator Achievement Award." The award was conferred on Dr. Wilkins, the William G. Gies Award for Achievement—Dental Educator, at the ADEA Annual Session in Orlando, Florida on March 19, 2012.

The Gies Award began in 2008, named for dental education pioneer, scientist, and educator, William J. Gies, PhD, to honor both individuals and organizations exemplifying dedication to the highest standards of vision, innovation, and achievement in dental education, research, and leadership. The awards are presented by the ADEA Gies Foundation, the philanthropic arm of the ADEA. This award has "emerged as the preeminent recognition of exceptional contributions to and support of oral health and dental education" (Gies Award Brochure, 2016). Upon receiving the award, Dr. Wilkins said,

> *it is truly an honor which is very special, and I am humbled as I think of all the great educators in dentistry and dental hygiene who have received [this award] before me. Thank you for recognizing me. The Gies Awards are the highest awards given by this organization, so my feelings of having been selected for one of them are very humble.*

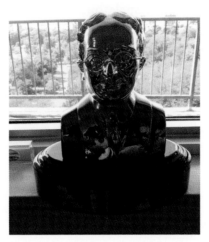

FIGURE 13.1: The Gies Award.

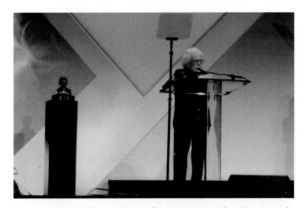

FIGURE 13.2: Esther at the podium receiving the Gies Award.

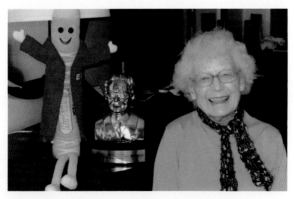

FIGURE 13.3: Esther and the Gies Award statue.

Pam Quinones, ADHA president in 2012, congratulated Dr. Wilkins:

❝ This recognition honors her continued efforts to highlight the importance of education in preventive health and in moving the dental hygiene profession forward. I can think of no one more deserving" (ADHA, 2012, p. 1).

Esther's Gies Statue is permanently displayed at Tufts University School of Dental Medicine.

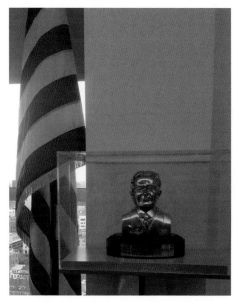

FIGURE 13.4: Esther's Gies Award statue, Tufts University School of Dental Medicine, 2017.

American Dental Hygienists' Association

Dear to Esther's heart was her long-standing association with the ADHA (see Chapter 8). An entire chapter is devoted to the organization in this biography. Founded in 1923, ADHA aims to improve the oral health and overall health of the public, increase awareness of and access to care, and serve as a means by which dental hygienists can communicate and work with each other. One of the major mechanisms for this information exchange is the *Journal of the Dental Hygiene,* to which Esther contributed over the years, as well as having served on the editorial board for 7 years. In addition, she was District I Trustee from 1945 to 1950 and served on numerous committees throughout the span of her career. The year Esther graduated from Forsyth School of Dental Hygienists in 1939, she became a member of ADHA.

Forsyth Dental Hygiene Alumnae Association

The first Forsyth (then Forsyth Training School for Dental Hygienists) Alumnae Association meeting was held in Boston, at Forsyth Dental Infirmary for Children on January 15, 1918, and recorded by Miss Keenan, Secretary from Foxboro (Forsyth, 1918, p. 285).

Esther graduated from Forsyth in 1939 and had been a member of the Alumnae Association ever since. Esther had commented that it is one of the few associations with regard to accurate recordkeeping on the graduates and the addresses and contact information for them. *They don't lose many alums.* Notably, Esther was very proud and pleased that a graduate of Forsyth in its earlier days is currently the president of the alumni association at the Forsyth School, now at Massachusetts College of Pharmacy and Health Sciences (MCPHS). Esther was also a strong supporter of the Forsyth School of Dental Hygienists as an active member of the alumni association (see Chapter 11).

International Federation of Dental Hygienists

Esther was a life member of International Federation of Dental Hygienists (IFDH), an organization formed in 1986 in Oslo, Norway. The IFDH is an international, nongovernmental, nonprofit organization without ties to any political, racial, or religious group, which aims to unite "dental hygiene associations from around the world in their common cause of promoting dental health" (IFDH, 2008, p. 1). Guided by a code of ethics and governed by a house of delegates that meets every 3 years, in conjunction with the International Symposium of Dental Hygiene, the IFDH aims to increase the professional profile and visibility of dental hygiene education, support the development of research and technology by dental hygienists, networking, and strengthen collaboration with other dental organizations around the world. IFDH currently has members in 28 countries. The MDHA aimed to "assist in promoting the art and science of dental hygiene, elevate and sustain the professional character and education of the dental hygienists, promote mutual improvement, social intercourse and good will; disseminate knowledge of oral hygiene, enlighten and direct public opinion in relation to oral hygiene and dental prophylaxis; to represent, to have cognizance of and to endeavor to safeguard the common interests of the dental professional" (Mass. Dental Hygiene Association, 2006, para. 1).

The Symposium is organized and hosted by a different country selected by the IFDH. Esther looked forward to attending these meetings for the educational sessions, paper presentations, poster presentations, exhibitors, and collaborative and networking sessions (see Chapter 8).

Massachusetts Dental Hygienists' Association

Although the Massachusetts Dental Hygienists' Association (MDHA) was founded earlier (Esther had been a member since 1939), it was officially incorporated on May 19, 1944, by 11 dental hygienists practicing in Massachusetts. The MDHA is part of the ADHA, representing District 1 on the board of trustees.

Esther was the chair of the MDHA convention held in May 1942 at the Hotel Statler in Boston. As long-time friend Mary Dole recalled,

❝❝ it was my first convention as a member of MDHA. I had the opportunity to meet Esther with whom I was so impressed by her efficiency and knowledge in organizing this convention."

As Esther had Wednesday afternoons *off* while working in Manchester-by-the-Sea, she often took the train up to Boston and *went to Dr. Gavel's office to meet Trudy about 5:00. With others, especially Edna Bradbury, we would plan big time activities for the MDHA* (Esther's acceptance speech, Gavel Award).

Esther Wilkins served as president of MDHA from 1944 to 1945 and was 1 of the 11 members who sought and received incorporation by the State. Esther was vice president when Edna Bradbury was the president of MDHA (and later ADHA). Esther remembered Edna fondly as a very charming woman, stately, who presented new ideas and, as Esther related, *was not afraid to open her mouth.* She added, *she was a beautiful woman.*

Mary Dole, also active in MDHA for many years, recalled this special group of dedicated dental hygienists: "Trudy Sinnett, a classmate of mine at Forsyth, was involved in the Association and who invited me to serve with her in various capacities in dental hygiene." Mary paid "special tribute to these dental hygienists who were really the foundation of what our association stands for today. They are: Charter Members Marion Coye MacCormack, Elta LeBlanc, Ann Wiltshire Buchanan, Gladys Flint, Isabel Kendrick, and Marion Kenney." Mary recalled that "these dedicated members gave of their time to the association strictly on a volunteer basis without any compensation."

About the time Esther was leaving her practice in Manchester to begin dental school in 1945, still very active in the MDHA, she completed *The 1945 Survey of Dental Hygienists in Massachusetts*, "the most complete survey in the history of the Association, and the findings were quite revealing" (Motley, 1986, p. 13). The survey "dealt with the annual work output, age groups and years of service, income and hours, and the education of dental hygienists in Massachusetts" (Motley, 1986, p. 143). Perhaps, in retrospect, this foreshadowed the impact Dr. Wilkins would have on the dental hygiene world through the "bible" that would be published 14 years later.

Esther served on various committees and held all state offices through the years with MDHA, which elevated her to the level of life member, awarded in 1964, "for long standing loyalty and interest" (MDHA, 1964, p. 7) in the MDHA.

When Esther graduated from Tufts Dental School, the MDHA held a reception for her, with Dr. J. Murray Gavel as a special guest (see Chapter 5).

Massachusetts Public Health Association

Working for a healthy Massachusetts, the Massachusetts Public Health Association (MPHA) was founded in 1879 and is the oldest public health organization in the United States. Its membership is dedicated to serving as a vehicle for timely communication and action on important health issues of statewide concern and for advocating for the rights of all to health care, especially individuals who are "vulnerable to disparities in health status because of race, ethnicity, class, gender or sexual orientation" (MPHA, 2018, para. 3). "The mission of MPHA is to prevent disease and injury by promoting laws, policies, and programs that protect the health of our families, communities, and workplaces" (MPHA, 2018, para. 2). Esther had been a member of MPHA since 1970. She was also a fellow of the American Public Health Association (APHA).

Omicron Kappa Upsilon

Esther was elected to Omicron Kappa Upsilon National Dental Honor Society and served as secretary in 1954. Founded in 1914 at Northwestern University Dental School with the intention of forming an honor society similar to other universities, devoted exclusively to dental students, Omicron Kappa Upsilon (which stands for conversation, teeth and health, and conservation) prides itself in the high ideals it set for its members, its position of leadership, innovation, research, and the art, science, and literature of dentistry. Membership is limited to those elected by the faculty and who meet established criteria for scholarship and character. These include charter, alumni, faculty, and honorary members.

The number of colleges has expanded through the years, now totaling 72 charters. Esther belonged to the University of Washington charter and was its secretary from 1955 to 1961 and later to the Xi Xi Chapter of Tufts University, where she served as vice president in 1975, president-elect in 1976, and president from 1977 to 1978. Never known for just attending meetings, her active membership in this honor society included roles as a board member and committee member, including constitution and by-laws revision in 1977 to 1979 and 2006 to 2007.

Organization for Safety and Asepsis Procedures

Esther was a member of Organization for Safety and Asepsis Procedures (OSAP) since its founding in 1985. It is a nonprofit organization made up of clinicians, educators, researchers, policymakers, and industry representatives who are dedicated to advancing and "promoting evidence-based infection control and safety policies and practices in dentistry" (OSAP, 2009, para. 2). Esther published in the organization's *RDH Special Supplement* in January of 2006.

Simmons College Alumnae Association

Esther became a Simmons alum when she graduated with a bachelor of science degree in general science in 1938, had been a very active member all her life, and served as class agent for the Class of 1938. Catherine McCarthy Murphy remembered, "before our 35th Simmons reunion another classmate, Mary Connolly Mastroianni and I became Co-Vice Presidents of our class. At the 40th reunion we moved up to President and Esther became Vice President for the 45th; she then became President for our 50th reunion in 1988."

For the 50th reunion, Simmons opened up the dorms for them (the 50th class) to stay. The rooms were barren, no curtains, but they gave them sheets. Lighting was poor, so Esther took a few lamps from another room; Esther recalled, *it was a very old dorm!* Esther spoke about the importance of her 50th, as she was in China the days before.

> *I didn't do the last section of the tour in a boat down the river, because my Simmons reunion was coming; so it was all planned in advance that I would go home from Shanghai. I had*

a little tour of the city and took the plane home alone. Though I was fairly bold most of the time, that airport and getting checked out was pretty scary!! But I got home that Friday before the reunion on Saturday.

Simmons's 70th reunion, Class of 1938, was celebrated in 2008 with *ladies* who worked together in the alumnae association: Ruth Nute (library), Catherine Murphy (general science), Esther (general science), and Mary Mountford (library science). *I'm one of only a few on two feet to speak at my class reunion [70th] in 2008.*
Catherine remembered one particular reunion meeting when Esther and her husband, Dr. James Gallagher,

❝ stopped by for a quick visit at our home in Medway. He was a happy and friendly man and was very interested in our reunion plans. In fact, he made a wonderful recording of songs that were popular during our college days. He brought the recording to our 45th reunion and played it for us to enjoy during our evening."

Tufts University School of Dental Medicine Alumni Association

Tufts University was founded in 1868. Tufts Dental Alumni Association, membership of which exceeds 7,000 alumni, states as its purpose to "maintain and promote good relations among its members, to promote good spirit towards the school, and to work in cooperation with the administration, faculty, and students for the welfare of the school and its betterment" (Tufts University School of Dental Medicine Alumni Association, 2018, para 1). As a graduate of Tufts Dental School, Esther became an alumnus and active member of the association since 1949, upon graduating from Tufts University School of Dental Medicine. Her alumni committee services included Instruments (1970 to 1975), Promotions (1972 to 1974), By-Laws (1976 to 1977), Clinics (1974 to 1987), and Infection Control (1987 to 2002). Esther also served as one of the four co-chairs for the Class of 1949, at their 60th reunion from Tufts in 2009 (see Chapter 5).

❧ Honors, Honor Societies, and Awards ❧ (in Chronological Order)

Theta Sigma Pi

Theta Sigma Pi is a women's national journalism society. Esther was chosen as one of eight women to receive the Matrix Table as a woman of achievement, awarded at the 21st annual banquet held in May of 1952 at the Olympic Hotel in Seattle, Washington. Esther was recognized as a pioneer in her work with the curriculum at the University of Washington. According to the newspaper reporter who covered the event, "her work has drawn national attention" (Brazier, 1952, p. 19). All eight of the recipients received "engraved silver bonbon dishes wrapped in circular plastic boxes to resemble wheels" (p. 19).

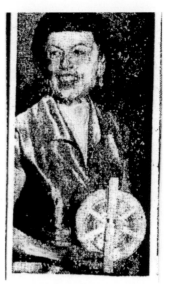

FIGURE 13.5: Esther with Matrix Award, 1952.

Omicron Kappa Upsilon

Founded in 1914 at Northwestern University Dental School, Omicron Kappa Upsilon is a national honorary fraternity of dental students. According to the organization's Web site, the name in Greek terms is "Soteria for conservation, Odous for teeth, and Hygeia for health" (Omicron Kappa Upsilon, 2009, p. 1). Omicron membership standards are "to encourage and develop a spirit of emulation among students in dentistry, and to recognize in an appropriate manner those who shall distinguish themselves by a high grade of scholarship" (p. 2). There are currently (2009) 70 chapters (58 active) of this honor society, a chapter in every dental school in the United States, 2 in Canada, and 1 in Puerto Rico. Membership is determined by a ballot system for those in the upper 20% of the graduating class who demonstrated high scholarship throughout their dental school training or as dental school faculty who have made an outstanding contribution to the "art, science, or literature of dentistry" (p. 2).

Nominated as a faculty electee at the University of Washington in 1954 into the Sigma Sigma Chapter, Esther was the first woman fellow and *was immediately elected Secretary*. When Esther moved back to Boston, she transferred her membership to the Xi Xi Chapter (Tufts University School of Dental Medicine) in 1967.

Northeastern University

In 1975, Esther was appointed as a senior lecturer, Health Sciences, at Northeastern University in Boston. In 1990, she received a recognition award for 15 years of Teaching at Northeastern.

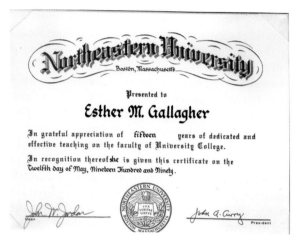

FIGURE 13.6: Northeastern University Award, 1990.

International College of Dentists

Officially begun on December 31, 1927, the International College of Dentists (ICD) was incorporated in the District of Columbia. Membership is based on a review of nominations "of the well qualified and capable." Both Esther and her husband, Jim Gallagher, became fellows in the ICD on the same day in 1972.

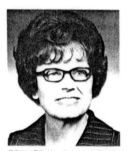 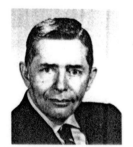

ESTHER W. GALLAGHER
Boston, Mass.

JAMES B. GALLAGHER, JR.
Boston, Mass.

FIGURE 13.7: Esther and Jim photographs, fellows, International College of Dentists, 1972.

The Convocation and Induction ceremony was held in San Francisco on Saturday, October 28 in the Imperial Ballroom of the Hilton Hotel. Dr. Wilkins *was asked to wear a dark dress and shoes and Jim dark hose and shoes, a dark suit, and a rather conservative tie.* Membership is by invitation only, and becoming a fellow is an honor bestowed on a dentist who has "made significant contributions to the profession, the community, and their families" (ICD, 2009, p. 2). There were 157 inducted in 1972, only 3 of whom were women. Jim said he thought it was the first husband–wife team to go in together, as far as anyone knew.

Esther was proud to be a member of this international organization whose objective is to advance the profession of dentistry around the world. Fellows wear a lapel pin (a small replica of the college key), a cap (collapsible style with gold bullion tassel), and a gown (gold and dark green) made of fine grade, mercerized poplin with lilac velveteen trim, with black velveteen bars on sleeves, and a 3-inch gold band below bars (ICD, 1973).

Esther was granted life membership in the ICD in 1989 and the ICD Distinguished Service Award in 2013 at the Yankee Dental Congress in Boston. The president of ICD that year, Joseph Kenneally, DMD, presented the award. "Nearly 150 national and regional leaders in the dental profession attended the ceremony, and when [Dr.] Kenneally asked who had either taught with Esther, been one of her students, or learned from her textbook, more than 90 percent of the hands in the room were raised" (Tufts University School of Dental Medicine, 2013, p. 3). "Dentists touch many lives, but teachers touch so many more," said Kenneally. "Esther Wilkins spent her life shaping the lives of those like us" (p. 3) (see Appendix J: Acceptance Speech, Receiving the ICD, Distinguished Service Award, 2013, accessed via the online e-book).

According to Demers (2013), 30 years earlier, Dr. Kenneally had been one of her students at Tufts.

❝ I spoke for a few minutes describing her career and why she was presented the award. She's 96 and hard of hearing, he explained. She looked at me and finally said, *are you done?* She then proceeded to deliver a 20 minute, off-the-cuff speech about herself and the changes she had seen in her some 60 years in dentistry. She was really

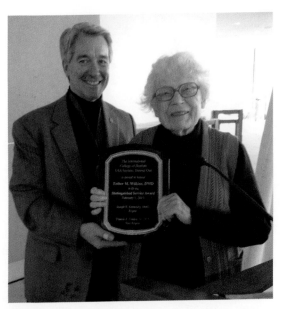

FIGURE 13.8: Dr. Wilkins and Dr. Kenneally, International College of Dentists, Yankee Dental Conference, 2013.

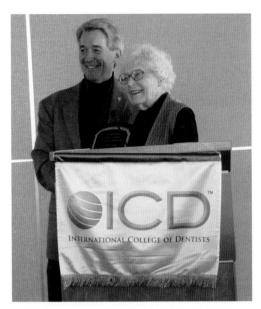

FIGURE 13.9: Esther receiving the International College of Dentists Award, 2013.

entertaining and funny, and the applause from the assembled guests was spontaneous and genuine. She thanked us, grabbed her walker, and went back to the table"(p. 6).

The American College of Dentists

Esther has been a fellow of American College of Dentists (ACD) since October 23, 1998. With the intention of addressing problems that faced the profession of dentistry and to "raise the standards of dentistry, to encourage graduate study, and to grant fellowships to those who have done meritorious work" (p. 1), the ACD was founded on August 20, 1920. It is the oldest national honorary organization for dentists and whose members exemplify "excellence through outstanding leadership and exceptional contributions to dentistry and society" (American College of Dentists, 2018, p. 1). The mission of the College emphasizes excellence, ethics, professionalism, and leadership in education. Fellowship in the college is awarded to those whose work has been meritorious. Fellowships are through nomination only and Esther was nominated by a former student from Tufts in the 1980s, Barbara Kay, who is a practicing dentist. The fellowship awarded to Esther M. Wilkins reads "this testimonial is given in recognition of services and devotion to the advancement of the science and art of dentistry."

Pierre Fauchard Academy

Pierre Fauchard Academy is an international dental honorary society with 10,000 fellows, serving "community, country, and profession" (Pierre Fauchard Academy, 2018) in many parts of the world, including the United States, South America, Europe, Asia, Canada, and Australia. Its administrative offices are located in Las Vegas, Nevada.

Founded in 1936 by Dr. Elmer S. Best, in memory of the father of modern dentistry, French dentist Pierre Fauchard, the academy fellows are distinguished in the profession of dentistry in their dedication to education and research, their noteworthy contributions that could serve as role models for others, and their upholding of the founder's objectives of integrity and ethics. Nominated by professional leaders, fellows must distinguish themselves through "contributions to dental literature, service to the profession of dentistry, and service to the general community, thereby bringing credit to dentistry" (Pierre Fauchard Academy 2018, p 1).

Esther was elected in 1974 as a fellow to the academy, which is an invitation-only honor for those whom others in the field have determined to be outstanding in dentistry.

Sigma Phi Alpha

Sigma Phi Alpha is the National Dental Hygiene Honor Society, which represents scholarship, leadership, and service in the field. It was founded in 1958 by members of the Section on Dental Hygiene Education of the American Dental Education Association, who through Sigma Phi Alpha sought to "enhance the dental hygiene profession's role and image in the delivery of quality healthcare to the public" (Sigma Phi Alpha, 2017, p. 1) and encourage members to advance the profession and image of dental hygiene through their achievements. According to Wilma Motley (1986), the group of dental hygienists, planned for a national dental hygiene honor society.

On March 24, 1958, their activities culminated in the establishment of Sigma Phi Alpha (Motley, 1986, p. 18). Founding members were Dr. Esther Wilkins (Sigma), Margaret Bailey (Kappa), Evelyn Maas (Alpha), and Janet Burnham. Margaret, Evelyn, and Esther were the first three presidents. Dr. Wilkins (third president) and Margaret Bailey (first president) drew up the by-laws, back in 1958. Esther had fun remembering the writing process. Margaret called Esther on the phone.

> *She was the Director of Dental Hygiene at Temple University and I was in Seattle: so when she called me, it was evening to her, but I was right in the middle of my afternoon clinic teaching!*

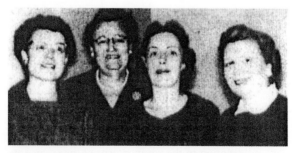

Figure 13.10: Founders of Sigma Phi Alpha: Wilkins, Bailey, Burnham, and Maas, 1958.

Membership in this honor society is composed of both educators in the field of dental hygiene, as well as students with high scholastic achievement who graduated from accredited dental hygiene programs. The organization provides scholarships and promotes educational programs at conferences.

The organization has developed several membership levels: (a) charter memberships; (b) faculty members who teach in accredited dental hygiene schools; (c) alumnae members of graduates of dental hygiene programs; (d) transfer members; and (e) nonvoting members, who are those recognized as having made an outstanding contribution to the profession of dental hygiene in the area of educational or community service.

Esther became a charter member of Sigma Chapter (University of Washington) in 1958, a charter member of Pi Chapter (Forsyth) in 1960, and was elected as the third supreme chapter president from 1960 to 1961. Patricia McCullough designed a key and seal for the society in 1958. Sigma Phi Alpha: Sigma (Sophia) meaning wisdom; Phi (Philanthropia) meaning human feeling and action, and Alpha (Arete) meaning valor and virtue, making up good character (Sigma Phi Alpha, 2017, p. 1).

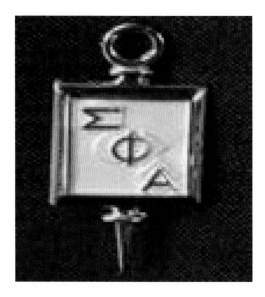

FIGURE 13.11: Sigma Phi Alpha pin.

Long-time friend, Barbara Schulze, commented that Esther

    was always at the helm providing educational programs for the advancement of dental hygiene. She was the 'energizing bunny,' initiating the development and organization of Sigma Phi Alpha. Several dental hygiene school directors shared with her the grassroots endeavors that made SPA a reality." Once established, the Society's annual meeting, which included a luncheon, was held in conjunction with the American Association of Dental School's meeting (now known as the American Dental Educator's Association). In 1961, the meeting was held for the first time in Boston at the Copley Plaza Hotel. Forsyth's Pi Chapter of SPA, then a year old, was selected to sponsor the luncheon. Once Esther reached Seattle, she and Barbara became weekly pen pals. "Multiple pages of instructions began to flood my mailbox. The closer the event, the more the mail! Computers and email were not yet on the work horizon! Somewhere along the line she forgot my name! Would you believe that the first letter salutation was 'Dear Ruth!' We joked about it to this day."

Mary Dole was also a proud member of Sigma Phi Alpha and attended the annual luncheon at the Statler Hotel in Boston on March 27, 1961, when Esther was president. Mary remembers that it was $5.00 per person to attend.

Distinguished Lecturer in Residence

Esther was honored as a visiting scholar at Texas Women's University in Denton, Texas, on June 24 to 25, 1983, where she was named as distinguished lecturer in residence.

Dental Products Report

In 2011, *Dental Products Report* awarded 25 women for their "clear contribution to the dental community and the diversity their story would bring" (Mannion, 2011, p. 40). Esther M. Wilkins, RDH, DMD, was honored with this distinguished group of women for her pioneering contributions and devotion to the field of dentistry. In the interview conducted for the publication of the *Top 25 Women in Dentistry*, and the discussion related to *Clinical Practice of the Dental Hygienist*, Esther said,

❝ That gives me a special outreach in the efforts that are being made to educate all people, especially children, that a healthy mouth is necessary for a generally healthy body" (Wilkins, as cited in Mannion, 2011).

Wear Visiting Professor

Wichita State University, in Wichita, Kansas, bestowed upon Dr. Wilkins the honor of the Wear Visiting Professor on March 30 to 31, 1983. This honor is bestowed on a distinguished group of individuals, nominated by their peers, whose contributions are truly noteworthy. In a letter to Dean Sidney Rodenberg on September 7, 1983, after being notified of her award, Esther said,

Thank you for the honor and privilege of being selected as one of this year's Wear Foundation award recipients. I accept with humble pride, and hope that I can meet the needs and expectations associated with the appointment.

Massachusetts College of Pharmacy and Health Sciences

Forsyth School for Dental Hygienists became part of MCPHS in 2002 (see Chapter 11). Esther M. Wilkins, RDH, DMD, received two prestigious honors from MCPHS: an honorary Doctor of Health Science in 2004 and the College Medal in 2012 (see Chapter 11).

Massachusetts College of Pharmacy and Health Sciences University, Honorary Doctoral Degree (Doctor of Health Science), 2004

For her outstanding contributions to the professions of dentistry and dental hygiene, Esther M. Wilkins was awarded an honorary Doctor of Health Science degree from

MCPHS at the commencement exercises at the Bayside Expo Center in Boston, Massachusetts in 2004.

In presenting her degree, President Charles F. Monahan "recognized Wilkins' ongoing efforts to advance the profession of dental hygiene through scholarly research and her groundbreaking work to expanding the dental curriculum to include an understanding of the disease process, the presentation of dental caries, and the treatment of periodontal disease" (DentistryIQ, 2004, p. 1). Esther's "unselfish mentorship of students and colleagues has made her one of the most beloved figures in the profession" (Monahan, as cited in DentistryIQ, 2004, p. 1).

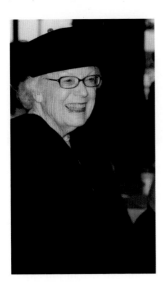

Figure 13.12: Awarding of honorary degree, Massachusetts College of Pharmacy and Health Sciences, 2004.

Esther was beaming as she received her degree, for which she was honored and quite proud:

> *It is an honor for me to accept this degree on behalf of all dental hygienists around the world. The impact of the meaning of such a beautiful honor reaches out to all.* She exclaimed, *we are proud that our Forsyth program has found a warm nest at MCPHS. I assure you . . . dental hygiene will play a significant role in the ongoing history of this College. We are all specialists in the great health sciences. We all have the same common goals related to the betterment and safeguarding of the health of all people.*

Massachusetts College of Pharmacy and Health Sciences College Medal, 2012

The MCPHS College Medal, the first of which was awarded in 2008, is "awarded in recognition of extraordinary service to the College in teaching, fund raising, administration, management, generosity and multiple labors within the College community and the health professions."

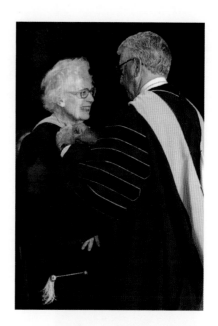

FIGURE 13.13: Receiving the College Medal, 2012.

Esther received this prestigious award at commencement on May 11, 2012:

"For her outstanding achievement in the practice and advancement of dental hygiene as a dental hygienist, dentist and educator for over seventy-four years; for her state and national leadership on behalf of the profession as President of Sigma Phi Alpha Dental Hygiene Honor Society, the Massachusetts Dental Hygienists' Association, and the Massachusetts Women's Dental Society, and as Trustee of the American Dental Hygienists' Association; for her authorship of two books, including the most widely used dental hygiene textbook in the world; for her ongoing efforts to advance the profession of dental hygiene through scholarly research and evidence-based practice; for her groundbreaking work in expanding the dental hygiene curriculum to include an understanding of the disease process, the prevention of dental caries, and the treatment of periodontal disease; for her unselfish mentorship of dental hygiene students and colleagues that has made her one of the most beloved figures in the history of the profession; for her generosity and dedication to the Forsyth School of Dental hygiene, her alma mater, as a Visiting Professor and as the primary benefactor of the Esther M. Wilkins Forsyth Dental Hygiene Clinic; and for her history role in helping to integrate Forsyth into the Massachusetts College of Pharmacy and Health Sciences; she merited the College Medal" (144th Commencement Program, MCPHS, 2012). (For Dr. Wilkins's College Medal acceptance speech, see Appendix I, accessed via the online e-book.)

Esther M. Wilkins Scholarship

MCPHS announced in 2011 the establishment of the Esther M. Wilkins Class of 1939 (Forsyth) scholarship, an endowed scholarship for dental hygiene students.

The Esther M. Wilkins—Restricted Scholarship Fund—Massachusetts College of Pharmacy and Health Sciences University

The Esther M. Wilkins Restricted Scholarship Fund is hereby established to provide financial assistance to students enrolled in the MCPHS Forsyth School of Dental Hygiene. The fund honors Forsyth's most distinguished graduate, Dr. Esther M. Wilkins, a world-renowned leader in dental hygiene and dental education, and author of the foundational textbook *Clinical Practice of the Dental Hygienist*, now in its 11th edition. The Esther M. Wilkins Restricted Scholarship Fund complements and extends the list of awards that reflect her extraordinary career, including the Esther M. Wilkins Lifetime Achievement Award, established in her name by the American Dental Hygienists' Association, and the Esther M. Wilkins Distinguished Alumni Award, which is presented annually to a Forsyth graduate who best reflects the leadership qualities that Dr. Wilkins has demonstrated throughout her professional life. Most especially, the fund represents the special bond between Dr. Wilkins and her Forsyth students, who continue to benefit from her example, mentorship, encouragement, and love.

Linda Boyd, Dean of the Forsyth School of Dental Hygiene at MCPHS, reflected on the importance of Esther Wilkins in this endowed scholarship: "Dr. Wilkins was a strong advocate for education through the many scholarship opportunities she created to support students. The fund she established supports dental hygiene students with generous awards, a legacy that speaks to her commitment to educating the next generation of dental hygiene students" (MCPHS, 2016c, p. 2).

Esther M. Wilkins Distinguished Alumni Award

The Esther M. Wilkins Distinguished Alumni Award was established in 1991 in honor of Dr. Esther M. Wilkins Class of 1939, the first recipient.

❝ Since 1992, the annual Dr. Esther M. Wilkins Distinguished Alumni Award has recognized and honored the achievements of Forsyth alumni across the profession of dental hygiene" (MCPHS, 2016a, p. 1). Criteria for the award include leadership, community service, personal education, professional contributions, impact on the profession of dental hygiene, participation in professional organizations, and dedication to the profession and to Forsyth.

❝ During the morning session of the Seventy-Fifth Anniversary Symposium, Dean Linda L. Hanlon presented an award to Forsyth alumna Dr. Esther M. Wilkins. "Dr. Wilkins is the recipient of the First Distinguished Alumni Award. This award was presented to Dr. Wilkins in recognition of her many contributions to the field of dental hygiene and specifically to the Forsyth School for Dental Hygienists. Dr. Wilkins is the first alumna so honored and all subsequent awards will be known as the 'the Esther M. Wilkins Distinguished Alumni Award'" (Forsyth Dental Center, 1992, p. 7). For subsequent awards, Esther served as chairperson and "outlined the format for all future recognitions" (p. 7).

Collectively, the awardees stand out as a "Who's Who" in the profession of dental hygiene. Beginning in 2012, the award was presented at the Wilkins Symposium, a continuing education program for dental hygienists.

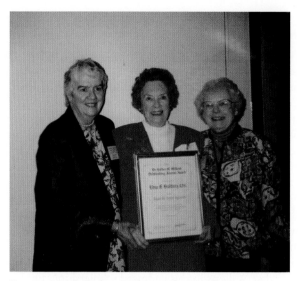

FIGURE 13.14: Barbara Wilson, Edna Bradbury, and Esther Wilkins.

American Dental Hygienists' Association

She was elected as life member in 1983. Additionally, Dr. Esther M. Wilkins received the Warner Lambert/ADHA Award (Educator) in 1988 for excellence in dental hygiene (American Dental Hygienists' Association, 1988). "She was in the first group of recipients—not a surprise to anyone," Helena Gallant Tripp stated, "it was a well-deserved award presented at the ADHA Annual Meeting and included a crystal obelisk and a check." The award was formerly named the Johnson and Johnson Award and was then named the Pfizer ADHA Award for Excellence in Dental Hygiene, awarded each year on the Sunday of the ADHA Annual Convention, designed to recognize dental hygiene practitioners who currently exhibit outstanding accomplishments in one of six practice areas (change agent, educator, administrator/manager, clinician, consumer advocate, and researcher). An award committee selects six distinguished dental hygienists per year, one from each category. Esther was the recipient of the educator category. Esther proudly displayed the Obelisk Award in her window overlooking Boston Common, capturing the morning light each new day.

When asked her most memorable dental hygiene experience, Esther answered, *receiving the ADHA award* (Hu-Friedy, 2009a, p. 1). When asked why she never served as president of ADHA, she responded that she became a practicing dentist and was no longer eligible to serve as president. It did not sway her dedication to the profession of dental hygiene or ADHA, and she truly enjoyed presenting the treasured award in person to each new recipient. Her generous contributions to fund this scholarship, Helena Tripp stated, "demonstrates her commitment to her students and to dental hygiene education." "Esther had sacrificed to put herself through school." Esther similarly wanted others to have that opportunity, also."

Esther was honored at the ADHA Annual Convention, held in Las Vegas, Nevada, on June 25, 2010, as the first recipient of the first Esther Wilkins Lifetime Achievement Award, "honoring the pioneering vision and enduring legacy of a distinguished career dedicated to the profession of dental hygiene." The award is sponsored by Colgate Professional Oral Care and hosted by *Dimensions of Dental Hygiene*. The award is "presented annually to recognize the distinguished career of a worthy individual who has consistently and effectively contributed to the enrichment of the dental hygiene profession" (Dimensions of Dental Hygiene, 2017). In her acceptance speech (see Appendix G, accessed via the online e-book), Esther said,

> *this is indeed a very great honor. In the future, some of you dental hygienists in this very audience will be standing here, as this award continues to be a special event at our ADHA Annual Meeting.*

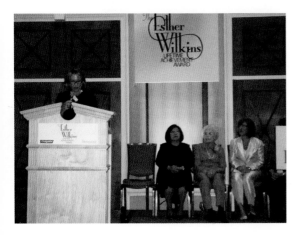

FIGURE 13.15: Lorene Kent, Dimensions, introducing Esther M. Wilkins Lifetime Achievement Award, 2010.

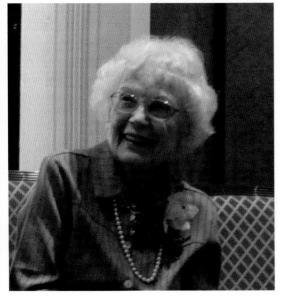

FIGURE 13.16: Esther Wilkins seated at Lifetime Achievement Award, 2010.

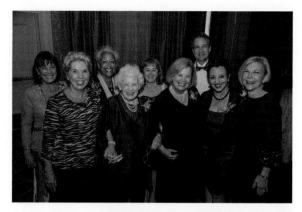

FIGURE 13.17: Esther, Denise Bowen, Phyllis Martina, Jill Rethman, Pam and Andy Bretschneider, Tina Daniels, and Mary Littleton, at the Lifetime Achievement Award, 2013.

The eighth annual Esther M. Wilkins Award was presented to Olga A. C. Ibsen at the ADHA convention held in Jacksonville in June 2017. Anna Pattison spoke about Esther's impact on the profession, as mentor and an inspiration to all dental hygienists, and Author presented a history of Esther Wilkins as trailblazer. A large poster located at the entrance of the reception depicted the 100 years of Esther's life encapsulating a century of relationships and an iconic personage.

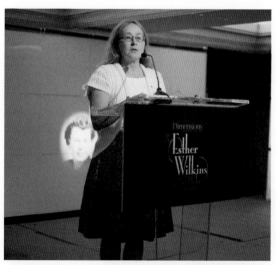

FIGURE 13.18: Esther Wilkins Lifetime Achievement Award Ceremony, Esther as trailblazer speech, Pam Bretschneider, Jacksonville Florida, 2017.

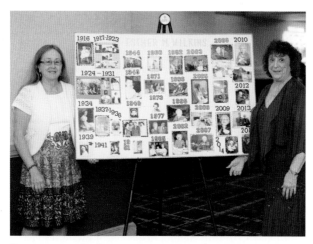

Figure 13.19: Esther 1 to 100 poster, Olga Ibsen and Pam Bretschneider, 2017.

Forsyth School for Dental Hygienists

In 1991, Esther was awarded the first Distinguished Alumni Award from Forsyth School for Dental Hygienists at MCPHS. The award was then named in her honor, the Dr. Esther M. Wilkins Distinguished Alumni Award, and it is awarded annually by the Forsyth School for Dental Hygienists at MCPHS. Each year, Dr. Wilkins proudly presented the award to subsequent recipients whenever possible.

International Federation of Dental Hygienists

Esther was presented an honorary life membership to the IFDH in July 1988 at their tri-annual meeting in Florence, Italy. "In Recognition of her dedication and contributions to dental hygiene throughout the world."

Tufts School of Dental Medicine Alumni Association

On April 30, 1994, the Tufts University Dental Alumni Association recognized Dr. Wilkins with the Faculty Award for teaching excellence. The award reads,

❝ Dr. Esther M. Wilkins, who has served as an inspiration to colleagues throughout her professional career. Throughout her teaching career, Dr. Wilkins has been known as a student advocate and a nurturing and caring instructor in the Department of Periodontology. In recognition of her service and teaching, she has been honored by numerous organizations and has brought distinction to herself and to her alma mater. Her compassion and dedication embody the professionalism that Tufts strives to instill in its dental students."

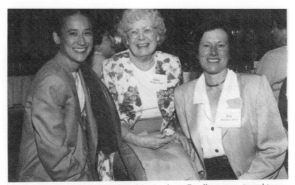

The Dental Alumni Association Award for Academic Excellence was given this year in honor of Dr. Esther Wilkins D49 at graduation. Former students from D79 Drs. Amerian Sones and Ann Sagalyn congratulate Dr. Wilkins (center) on her award.

FIGURE 13.20: Tufts Alumni Achievement Award, 1994.

Esther's husband, Dr. James Gallagher, also received this alumni recognition on April 12, 1986. The award is presented at Alumni Day at Tufts and is given to one faculty member and one staff member each year.

In June 2009, Dr. Esther M. Wilkins, DMD, was also awarded a special lifetime achievement recognition from the Tufts University School of Dental Medicine Alumni Association, six decades after her graduation from Tufts in 1949, for "groundbreaking strides" that she "made for women in the field of dentistry."

At alumni weekend at Tufts University School of Dental Medicine, September 8, 2009, Esther was again recognized for her contributions with a Certificate of Achievement, presented with sincere pleasure and pride, which included "in recognition for your many years of dedicated service to the teaching programs of the Department of Periodontology; enduring commitment to our students that enhanced their professional education and firmly established the national and international reputation at TUSDM as a center of excellence." The award was on behalf of "numerous students and a profoundly grateful dental school" (p. 2).

In 2011, Tufts University School of Dental Medicine honored Dr. Wilkins with the title of Clinical Professor Emeritus.

American Academy of Dental Hygiene

Esther became an honorary member of the American Academy of Dental Hygiene (AADH) in 2001, presented with a plaque by then President Barbara Murphy.

The AADH was founded in 1987 and has chapters in 12 states. Its goals are to foster continuing education in the profession, recognize excellence in the profession of dental hygiene, and recognize efforts to improve oral health. Essentially, as there is no national standard established for dental hygienists, the AADH accredits continuing education in dental hygiene, thus guiding a standard of excellence for the profession.

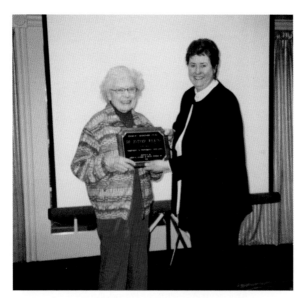

Figure 13.21: Barbara Murphy, American Academy of Dental Hygiene president, presenting Esther with membership plaque, 2001.

Dr. Wilkins described the importance of the academy:

❝ Being a part of the AADH gives me a great deal of pride. The Academy represents the highest in dental hygiene ethics and learning. After meeting rigid admissions requirements, each member is required to meet a standard of continuing education to maintain membership. The dental hygiene profession is a dynamic, growing health-care group, and high standards of self-motivation are needed to keep up with the new research, new inventions, and new methods. The members of the AADH are dedicated to this standard of learning and study. I admire, appreciate, and promote that in our profession" (Wilkins, as cited in Turcotte, 2004, p. 2).

American Academy of Periodontology

A fellowship was awarded to Esther M. Wilkins, BS, RDH, DMD, on September 16, 2006, from the American Academy of Periodontology (AAP). Fellows of the academy are chosen for distinguished service to the academy, and election is by the executive council.

Dr. Wilkins was one of six periodontists honored at the annual meeting of the AAP in San Diego that year with an AAP fellowship award, which is funded by Proctor & Gamble and recognizes distinguished service. Esther's award was presented by Kenneth A. Krebs, AAP president for 2005 to 2006 for her "devotion, time, and energy to the field of periodontology, including her service to AAP and dental and dental hygiene education"

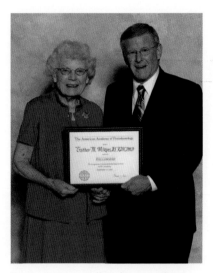

FIGURE 13.22: Fellowship award,
American Academy of Periodontology.

(Majeski, 2006, p. 55). Esther was particularly happy with the award and said: "I was especially pleased that Dr. Krebs mentioned my 45 years in dental and dental hygiene education" (Wilkins, as cited in Majeski, 2006, p. 55). Throughout her career, she acknowledged with pride at every opportunity her roots in the dental hygiene profession. As Barbara Schulze concluded her letter: "She never forgot her roots were in dental hygiene; she never lost her baby teeth!"

Dr. J. Murray Gavel Clinical Research Medal

Dr. J. Murray Gavel served as a trustee of the Forsyth Institute for 30 years and a long-time faculty member at Tufts University School of Dental Medicine. He passed away in 1999. Dr. Gavel had a group of students one day a week during Esther's school days at Forsyth; one day they were learning how to do laughing gas (nitrous oxide). He told Esther to be the patient, resulting in her being called "teacher's pet!" Esther described how Dr. Gavel was an active member of every organization to which he belonged and was president of many. Dr. Gavel was president of the Massachusetts Dental Society when Esther graduated from dental school. He and Esther had a contest of how many continuing education unit credits they could obtain; Dr. Gavel had over 100. She never did win the contest! Dr. Gavel was a very dear friend of Esther:

He devoted his whole life to his profession.

Esther M. Wilkins, RDH, DMD, ScD (hon.) received the coveted J. Murray Gavel Medal presented at the 15th annual Dr. J. Murray Gavel Clinical Research Lecture, at the Forsyth Institute, in Boston, Massachusetts, on November 3, 2008, surrounded by long-time friends, as well as colleagues, new friends, Forsyth Institute personnel, and members of the faculty and administration of Tufts University School of Dental Medicine and MCPHS

University. Greetings were sent from the Forsyth Institute by Philip Stashenko, DMD, PhD, and attendees were welcomed by J. Steven Tonelli, DMD, Chairman of the Dr. J. Murray Gavel Clinical Research Lectureship.

Once the Gavel Medal was awarded to Dr. Wilkins, Martin A. Taubman, DDS, PhD, senior member of the Staff Head, Department of Immunology, the Forsyth Institute, lectured on "Vaccine Therapies for Dental Caries Infection." According to the Forsyth Health Foundation, the Gavel Medal commemorates the achievements of a medical or dental researcher, educator, or practitioner who has contributed lasting and innovative benefits to mankind. The recipients also must represent the qualities on which Dr. Gavel stood.

Esther worked through numerous versions of her acceptance speech, making it clear what a great honor receiving the Gavel Medal is for a dental professional:

I am humbled, very honored, and indeed proud and appreciative to receive this beautiful medal in the name of my friend, Dr. J. Murray Gavel. Dr. Gavel was my friend, my teacher, and in many informal ways, a mentor.

Esther went on to talk about the long-time friendship she had with Dr. Gavel, beginning in her days as a dental hygienist in Manchester-by-the-Sea. Esther's friend Gertrude (Trudy) Sinnett was a dental hygienist in Dr. Gavel's dental practice at

the famous 198 Marlborough Street address. I had Wednesday afternoons off, and often took the train up to Boston, did my shopping, and went to Dr. Gavel's office to meet Trudy about 5:00 p.m. While at the office, we would have conversations with Dr. Gavel, who enjoyed teasing us and telling funny stories. Dr. Gavel was a one-day volunteer teacher at Tufts while I was a student there. Esther concluded her journey into the days of Dr. Gavel: *Thank you for this opportunity to talk with you for a few minutes to recall thoughts of my famous friend, Dr. J. Murray Gavel. I am very proud to receive this medal in his honor.*

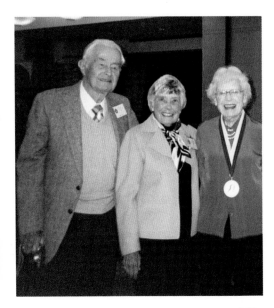

FIGURE 13.23: Esther receiving the Gavel Award, Warren and Mary Dole, Boston.

Dr. Wilkins continued to serve as an executive member on the Gavel Lectureship Committee at the Forsyth Institute, which offered clinical research lectures each year. In 2009, Esther wrote,

> *went to Forsyth last evening for the Gavel Committee. The next medal winner is a famous Harvard/Mass General Oral surgeon [Walter Guralnick] now 92. Good they are celebrating us old folks!!!* (email to the author, March 26, 2009).

City of Boston Resolution

Through the efforts of George Humphrey (then vice president for College Relations at MCPHS) in honor of Esther Wilkins's 90th birthday, December 9, 2006, this day became Esther M. Wilkins Day in the City of Boston, as issued by resolution by the Boston City Council, for Dr. Wilkins's contributions to the field of dental hygiene. Friends, colleagues, and students celebrated the occasion a day early on Friday, December 8 by officially presenting the proclamation to Dr. Wilkins in the Esther M. Wilkins Forsyth Dental Hygiene Clinic, at MCPHS. "Friends, colleagues and students celebrated the occasion a day early on Friday, December 8 by officially presenting the City Council's proclamation to Dr. Wilkins in the dental hygiene clinic that bears her name" (MCPHS, 2006, p. 1) (for photo, see Camire, 2006).

Simmons College

Esther became a member of Simmons College alumni upon her graduation in 1938 (see Chapter 2). She remained an active and generous alumnus for 78 years.

Nominated by Simmons Alumnus, Victoria Danberg, who said that "Esther has played a major role in changing the face of dental medicine, is a national and international icon in dental hygiene, is the most sought after speaker in dental hygiene in the world" and "has served as a role model and inspiration to generations of dentist, both male and especially female,"

Simmons College awarded Dr. Wilkins the Lifetime Professional Achievement Award in June 2011. In her acceptance speech (see Appendix H, accessed via the online e-book), Esther said *she was humbled to receive such a select award*. Once again thanking her hardworking mother who helped her and her sister *to learn responsibility*, she related the story of how she came to Simmons in 1934.

In an interview following the award, Esther said,

> *all things happened in my life because of my science background at Simmons College.*

In 2011, Dr. Wilkins created the Esther M. Wilkins Endowed Scholarship (Simmons College, 2017), which "is a two-part gift—Dr. Wilkins created a current use and an endowed option of the scholarship so students could benefit immediately." According to Esther,

> *There are plenty of students who could use some help; money counts.*

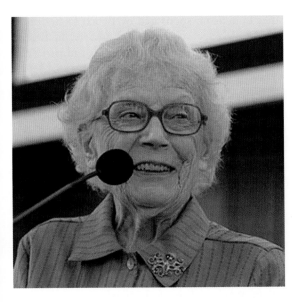

FIGURE 13.24: Esther receiving the Simmons Professional Lifetime Achievement Award, 2011.

Virginia Commonwealth University School of Dental Hygiene

Dr. Wilkins became an honorary alumna of Virginia Commonwealth University on September 19, 2008: *In grateful appreciation for 50 years of leadership, scholarship, and inspiration.*

The Lucy Hobbs Project

Nominated by Pat Cohen, Esther was selected in 2015 as a recipient of the Industry Icon Award, one of six categories, for the year's Lucy Hobbs Project Annual Celebration. She "showed the true qualities of what it means to be the Industry Icon within the dental industry by being a trailblazer who is consistently recognized and admired for your work."

The Lucy Hobbs Project is a national program that empowers women in dentistry to drive change and deliver success through networking, innovation, and giving back. The annual event celebrates professionals who embody the spirit of history's first female dentist, Lucy Hobbs. The eight recipients were chosen because they exemplified those characteristics and "whose unwavering professional dedication merits accolades" (Ceruti, 2015, p. 2). Lucy Hobbs "was denied access to education based on her gender, but persevered to learn dentistry through apprenticeship, and eventually graduated from the Ohio College of Dental Surgery" (p. 2).

Eight exemplary dental professionals received the award in 2015, which took place at the National Museum of Dentistry in Baltimore, those pioneers of change "who in some way have helped lead the change for women in dentistry and embody the project goals" (Aegis Dental Network, 2015, p. 1). Because travel proved challenging for Esther, representatives from Benco Dental traveled to Boston where Esther video-recorded her acceptance speech, which was shown on June 4 at the 2015 Celebration hosted by Benco Dental. At the Leading Ladies Luncheon, sponsored by Benco Dental, held as part of Women's Dental Summit 2015, Massachusetts Dental Society, in Boston in November 2015, Esther accepted in person the Lucy Hobbs Project Industry Icon Award.

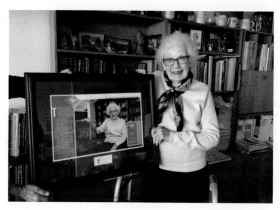

FIGURE 13.25: Esther with framed photo, Lucy Hobbs Award.

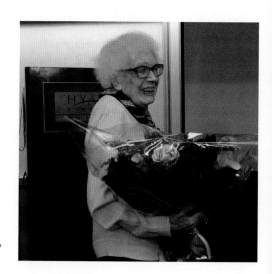

FIGURE 13.26: Lucy Hobbs Award
Women's Dental Summit luncheon, Boston,
presentation Benco, 2015.

The Dean's Medal, Tufts University School of Dental Medicine

Receiving the Dean's Medal at Tufts University School of Dental Medicine, established in 1996, is a prestigious honor, which recognizes "individuals who have demonstrated loyalty, service and generosity. Established in 1996, the Dean's Medal is the highest honor bestowed by the dean of a school at Tufts University and is reserved for those select individuals who had made significant contributions to their school and the greater community" (Tufts University School of Dental Medicine, 2016, p. 1). Dr. Esther M. Wilkins and Dr. Hilde Tillman both were honored with this award. Dean Huw F. Thomas, Tufts University School of Dental Medicine said,

“ Drs. Tillman and Wilkins enrolled in dental school when not even 2 percent of practicing dentists were women. Now, more than 50 percent of the dental students at Tufts are women. Drs. Tillman and Wilkins have been leaders in dental medicine, at Tufts, in their communities, nationally and internationally. They both exemplify the principles of leadership, humanitarianism and passion that we embody in our student” (Melanson, 2016, p. 1).

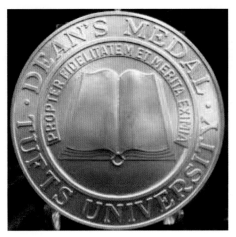

Figure 13.27: Tufts University School of Dental Medicine, Dean's Medal, 2016.

Esther's niece, Betsy Tyrol, accepted the award, which was presented posthumously on December 16, 2016, 1 week after Esther's 100th birthday.

❧ CONSULTING AND REVIEW BOARDS ❧

When you have had as much experience as Dr. Esther M. Wilkins, your expertise is tapped by a broad range of organizations and educational institutions. In addition to sharing her knowledge through continuing education offerings throughout the country, Dr. Wilkins served on review boards, editorial boards, advisory boards, and as a consultant.

She began as early as 1957, when Esther served the U.S. Public Health Service (USPHS) Dental Health, San Francisco Office, and as a consultant in School Health for USPHS Hawaii. In 1962, she served as a curriculum consultant in dental hygiene for the University of British Columbia and in 1964 at Diablo Valley College in Pleasant Hill, California.

In addition to curriculum advice, Dr. Wilkins provided expertise in the area of materials review, from 1969 to 1982, with the Bureau of Health Education, ADA, and as a member of the Exam Review Committee from 1970 to 1972 with the Northeast Regional Board of Dental Examiners.

Dr. Wilkins was particularly active as a member of various editorial review boards, which include *Journal of Periodontology*, *Journal of Dental Hygiene* (ADHA, 1976 to 1989), *Educational Directions* (ADHA, 1976 to 1982), *Dental Assistant Journal* (1991 to 1996), and *Dimensions of Dental Hygiene* (2002 to 2016).

Because both dental hygiene and dental professionals utilize a variety of instruments in their practice, companies that manufacture instruments and other products, as well as the government, sometimes ask practitioners to review products. Esther's opinions have been solicited by many companies and the U.S. Government, seeking her advice and occasionally endorsement (which she says she *did not do in fairness to everyone!*). She served in an advisory role for the U.S. Food and Drug Administration, for dental drug products, from 1973 to 1977; in product review, for Proctor & Gamble, Crest Committee, Cincinnati, from 1989 to 1992; and for Butler Brush Company, Chicago, product review, in 1992. In the 1970s, Esther collaborated with the Hu-Friedy Co., outlined specifications and requirements, which resulted in the TU-17 Explorer. She was awarded the Hu-Friedy TU-17 Explorer Innovation Award in May 2016. From 2003 to 2005, Esther served on the Oral-B Dental Hygiene Advisory Board.

Collectively, Esther Wilkins's contributions to the dental and dental hygiene professions certainly justified the accolades she received throughout her lifetime and beyond.

CHAPTER 14

Boston

Steady blue, clear view;
flashing blue, clouds are due;
steady red, rains ahead;
flashing red, snow instead
(or flashing red in summer, Red Sox game cancelled)
Flashing blue and red, when The Curse of the Bambino is Dead! (Desmarais, 2012)
(The Light on the Old John Hancock Tower,
as seen from Esther's Apartment)

❦ BOSTON, CAPITAL OF MASSACHUSETTS ❧

If you asked Esther what Boston was like, you would invariably receive first a smile, followed by an excited narrative of what the city offers and importantly what it meant to her, despite the Boston weather, which can change with the wind, and it often does. Esther compared Boston with her time in Seattle and said that *I lived in Seattle for 12 years and it rains more in Boston than it does in Seattle!* Boston was her hometown most of her adult life since she returned to Massachusetts from Seattle, Washington, to enroll in the postdoctoral program in periodontology at Tufts.

Boston, affectionately called "bean town," was founded by Puritan colonists on September 17, 1630, is about 90 square miles, and has a current population of 700,000.

Boston grew during this time, with roads (only 4 ft wide and unpaved), a cemetery, a marketplace, a "Frog Pond," taverns, churches, and a common area: Boston Common, the first public park in America, a green and flowering oasis, where the "militia drilled and the cattle grazed" (Ross, 1960, p. 36), and "a gathering place for expeditionary forces" (Friends of the Public Garden, 2005, p. 7). The Common, "the center stage of city life" (Friends of the Public Garden, 2005, p. 9), as well as the Frog Pond (which used to serve on occasion as an amphitheater in the 19th century), continued to serve as stops on Esther's personal tour for her visitors to the city, and she had a specific route to get there. She knew how to get around quite well in Boston and the shortest route to do so (to the chagrin of taxi drivers who were reprimanded for trying to take the long way around).

Friend, Kathy Bassett, related with laughter when, after a great evening visiting Esther and her City of Boston, they shared a cab back to her apartment and then to their hotel. "Esther kept right on the cab driver about the route he was taking and then demanded that he just *let us out here* if he was going to insist on taking us the long way, running up the fare, and not following her directions! Out we jumped and walked the remaining blocks and through the park back to her place. Esther really knows her city."

It is a captivating city, steeped in history, traditions, "firsts," and eminence: in dental science, medicine, literature, politics, the arts, and academic excellence. Tremont Street, a former cart path, seemed to be named after the mountain on Beacon Hill, "Trimount, Treamount, or Tremont" (Weston, 1957, p. 37). "The loftiest of its three peaks rising, a beautiful grassy cone, as high as the present gilded dome of the State House, topped by the beacon" (Bacon, 1916, p. 13).

Downtown Boston is not organized in any pattern at all; rather, it developed from roundabout and twisting paths that were walking ways or horse paths that seemed to be developed as needed around waterways or existing buildings or well-worn passageways, tunnels, courts, and small streets, a labyrinth, "interlaced in as meaningless a maze as one could hope to find" (Weston, 1957, p. 57). In fact, some of the streets, called "place" or "court" are little backstreets that go nowhere at all. Back Bay and South End are laid out in more of a pattern of triangles; the true Bostonian, however, "rejoices in the tangled sin-uosities" (Weston, 1957, p. 69), the "devious streets" (p. 93) or of the unorganized streets of other parts of Boston, the zigs and zags that is Boston.

Esther lived on Tremont Street, for almost 40 years, in a condominium with a distinctive burgundy awning, a revolving door, and a most pleasant front desk staff. Esther and Jim sought to rent a place with two bedrooms, a garage, and an elevator to accommodate Jim's disability. Built in 1968, the current building was a rented apartment building but was converted in 1984 to condominiums. Esther and Jim moved into 151 Tremont Street, Apartment 12N, Boston, Massachusetts, on July 10, 1978.

As reported in their 1978 Christmas Letter,

> *we've moved!! Now we are part of the Boston skyline, right in the heart of the historic down-town. Looking over the Boston Common, Public Garden, Back Bay, and the Charles River, we delight in the beautiful sunsets over suburban hills. We are just a few minutes' walk to school [Tufts] as well as everything else.*

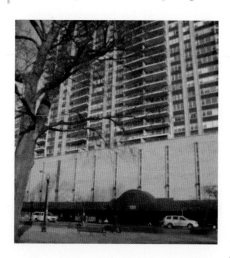

FIGURE 14.1: Gallagher residence, 151 Tremont Street, Boston, Massachusetts, 1978 to 2016.

Three of the four rooms overlooked Boston Common and provided a panoramic view of the city. One of the two bedrooms served as her office (for The Book) and one as a bedroom. There were two baths, one set aside for visitors and for hanging laundry, which Esther tended to do *Sunday mornings before others get up and use the machines* before her! It was spacious, 1,060 ft², but, as Esther was the first to agree, much of the extra space was taken up with book printouts, volumes of journals and books, and memorabilia from her many visits around the country and the world. If it had sentimental value, it was kept.

The views of the City of Boston from Esther's 12th floor condominium included breathtaking sunrises and sunsets, different during each season.

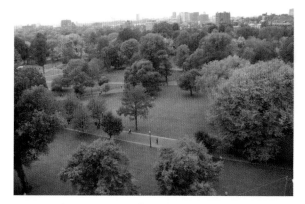

FIGURE 14.2: Boston view from the Gallagher condominium in autumn.

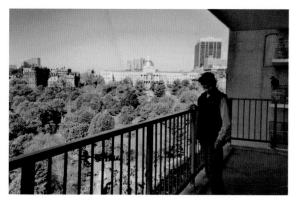

FIGURE 14.3: Esther on her balcony, Boston, 2012.

In view from their balcony were the skating pond on Boston Common (the center stage of city life), the State House on the right up the hill on Beacon Street (formerly called "Poor House Lane," Weston, 1957, p. 47), with former residents such as John

Hancock himself; Granary Burying Ground on Tremont Street which dates back to the 1660s (where the tombs and graves of Samuel Adams, John Hancock, and Paul Revere are located); the famous Brattle Bookstore on West Street (which at one time, according to Weston, 1957, housed 13 dressmakers, 4 lingerie shops, 8 fur stores, and 22 corset shops and which also included a foreign bookstore operated by Elizabeth Peabody and a meeting place of Margaret Fuller and her "conversations"); the Prudential Building is a short distance on the left; straight ahead in the distance is the Charles River (known as the People's River); and Boylston Street and Newbury Street just off to the left, the lights of which rarely subside in a city that consistently provides beauty and peace, in congruence with excitement and activity. Esther knew every street and every path to take to a specific destination, sometimes guiding you with her cane as you accompanied her.

Tremont Street, established in 1634, begins at Government Center and is in and of itself a historical Boston must-see on the hundreds of tours around the city. Esther often took visitors to the bronze ducks in Boston Garden, sculpted by Nancy Schon (Schon, 2009) and inspired by Robert McCloskey's now famous 1941 children's book. Esther delighted as she retold the story of a mother duck, Mrs. Mallard, and her children (Jack, Kack, Lack, Mack, Nack, Ouack, Pack, and Quack) on their trek from the Charles River.

Mary Dole related she was working as a dental hygienist at Charlesgate West in Boston the actual day in the 1940s that a mother duck, with little ducks lined up behind, crossed Beacon Street in Boston. One of the dentists returned to the office to inform the rest of the staff that the patients they were waiting for were late because Mrs. Mallard held up traffic as she made her infamous trek from the Charles River to Boston Garden. The newspapers covered the event for days! Esther bought endless copies of *Make Way for*

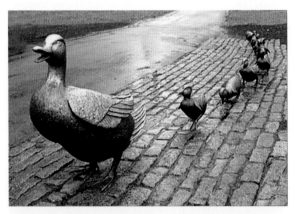

FIGURE 14.4: Sculpture of ducks on Boston Common.
(Used by permission of the sculptor, Nancy Schon.)

Ducklings, as she liked to keep it in the house to show guests, but she kept giving away her copy!

Tremont Street runs through the theater district of the city, crosses the Massachusetts Turnpike, through the South End, ending not far from the Esther M. Wilkins Forsyth

Dental Hygiene Clinic off Huntington Avenue. Tremont Street is bordered on the edge of Chinatown, where "colonial pastureland meets contemporary Asian culture" (Morgenroth, 2003, p. 3).

Chinatown didn't exist until the 1800s. Beach Street used to be on the ocean. The infamous "combat zone" was located not far around the corner on Washington Street (formerly called High Street) but is now part of the theater area due to rural cleanup. Up one street from the Park Street station, walking distance up the hill from Tremont Street where Esther lived is the State House, built in 1795 to 1797 by 24-year-old Charles Bulfinch, majestic with its golden dome and pine cone top. Inside the House of Representatives, high above the guest galleries is the famous Sacred Cod, a carved fish donated by Jonathan Rowe that signifies the importance of the codfish industry to the economy of the state. Esther gave tours of the Massachusetts State House as a guide in the early 2000s.

When Esther was walking in the area of the State House, she stopped people gazing at the famous dome and asked if they knew the significance of the gilded pine cone. At the slightest encouragement, they are told the story that it symbolized Boston's lumber industry and the State of Maine, which was a district of Massachusetts when the building was completed.

Located at 8 Park Street, the Union Club, built in 1905 has its own proud history, including the distinction of being the meeting place where the famed Saturday Club settled, its literary members including Hawthorne, Emerson, Lowell, Holmes, and Longfellow. Esther enjoyed dining at the Union Club, a membership-only, formerly men-only establishment two doors down from the State House. It has kept its old Boston charm, frequented by local dignitaries who hold meetings on the third floor or others conducting business on the "hill." Esther accepted any invitation for lunch from member Charles Monahan, president of Massachusetts College of Pharmacy and Health Sciences (MCPHS), although Esther commented, *they do not permit doggie bags!*

A short walk from Esther's home is the public garden, so picturesque in all of the four seasons. In its center, there is a suspension bridge which, according to Esther Forbes (1947), is a "microscopic copy of the Brooklyn Bridge" (p. 82) that goes over a small pond where all visitors to Boston should take a ride on the Swan Boats. Esther truly enjoyed the Swan Boats and often took her visiting friends to the boats. A bridge, measuring a few yards by about 100 ft in length, spans the water, from which one can

> " *Watch below a lazy pontooned vessel go with a stern like a swan and a man astride who peddles so passengers may ride as leisurely as potentates while it circumnavigates the tiny island and contoured pond back to childhood and dreams beyond. These are the swan boats and, if you please, Nothing is purer Bostonese"*
>
> (Westman & Kenny, 1974, p. 5)

One pleasant day, the author and her granddaughter, Sarah Anne, took a lovely short ride around the pond with Esther. The pond seems so much larger when one takes a first ride as a child. It is still a popular site in Boston, which Esther frequented with guests, and included the ducks, the Frog Pond (named, according to local lore because it was never known to harbor a frog), the skating pond in winter, and everything in between. Esther was quite fond of the cherry trees in bloom in spring in Boston Garden.

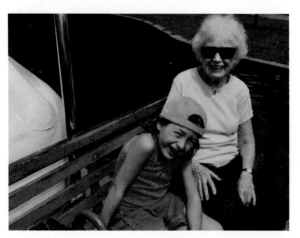

FIGURE 14.5: Sarah Anne Burns and Esther Wilkins, 2006.

You could see clearly the old John Hancock Tower from Esther's home and could tell the weather at any time from the flashing weather forecast beacon:

" Steady blue, clear view; flashing blue, clouds are due; steady red, rain ahead; flashing red, snow instead" (or the Red Sox game is cancelled). And in 2004, "the tower used flashing blue and red to commemorate the World Series win: *Flashing blue and red; the curse is dead!*" (Cornette, 2009, p. 1).

Esther loved Boston and she loved her home on Tremont Street, one she shared with husband, Jim, until he passed away in 1988. They both enjoyed so much of the city, despite the challenges. During the major blackout in the 1980s, Esther was flying in from a presentation in the Midwest, and she *had to walk up all 12 flights of stairs to her apartment.*

Much of the history provided about Tremont Street relates to the significance of the trolley that runs under it. The Tremont Street Subway was opened in 1897, the first subway (underground transit system) in North America and which now has 66 miles of track. It was at 124 Tremont, just a block or two down from Esther's home, that the bookstore of Ticknor and Fields once stood and where "William Dean Howells first met Mark Twain" (Harrell & Smith, 1975, p. 88). The Park Street Church is on the corner, with visitors such as Henry James and Henry Adams. Esther used the subway (the "T" for short) for transportation for many years, easily running up and down the stairs to the tracks. In later years, she took advantage of the elevators that had been installed in some of the stations. She delighted in telling stories of the people she met, especially those who did not give up a seat for her.

Boston is a walking city, and Esther took full advantage of her centrally located home to walk everywhere when she could.

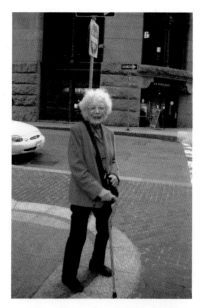

FIGURE 14.6: Esther in front of the Ritz Carlton, walking distance from Tremont Street, 2010.

❧ AMERICAN DENTAL EDUCATION ❧ ASSOCIATION ANNUAL MEETING, 1961, BOSTON

Boston served as a host city to the American Dental Education Association's Annual Meeting in 1961, which Barbara Schultz recalled as a perfect theme for the luncheon for which she was enlisted by Louise Hord. The luncheon was sponsored by Forsyth School for Dental Hygiene.

      ❝ Dr. Moody, a Boston University History Professor, was luncheon speaker, who highlighted historical events of the city. Freedom trail maps guided the visiting dental hygienists on a tour of the scenic and historical city route, but with no mention of the March winds! Heinz Company provided miniature bean pots!"

❧ FENWAY PARK ❧

Fenway Park, home of the Red Sox, was only a few trolley stops away from Esther's where in 2006, she attended a game with the author and her family. Beginning at Canestano's in Boston for a pizza and beer, several family members, who had never met Esther, were amazed that this tiny, famous, easy-going lady ordered a beer and drank directly from the bottle. They all then embarked on the walk to Boston's beloved Fenway!

273

Instead of the few cents she paid in the 1930s while attending Simmons, the box seats are now well over $100, and to make matters worse, it was raining and the Sox lost! Esther described how different it was yet the same from the last days she attended a game and commented in Esther style: *I think the 10 cent seats were closer!* She was a trooper, however, never complained, enjoyed the energy of the park, and had her picture taken with Wally.

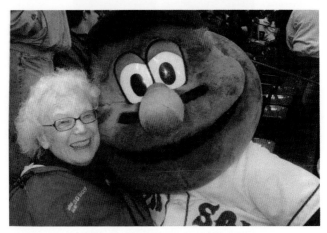

FIGURE 14.7: Esther with Wally, the Red Sox mascot, 2006.

❧ FIRST NIGHT AND OTHER ❧ BOSTON ACTIVITIES

The area of Park Street, Boylston Street, and Tremont Street is also often bustling. The very first "First Night" was in Boston, Massachusetts, in 1976, an event attended by 100,000 people, far more than the city had anticipated. The city had only seven police cars on duty that night. However, there were no arrests, no disturbances, and the example, perhaps, set the wheels in motion for other First Nights around the country.

The Parkman Bandstand, built in 1912 and renovated in 1996, in view of Esther's home, once included orations by Martin Luther King and James Michael Curley, and now serves as the venue for the summer Shakespeare and small-scale performances. Directly over the Bandstand, at 7:00 PM New Year's Eve, the children's fireworks are displayed. From Esther's balcony, a yearly tradition began for a small group of her friends. You could almost touch the sparks as they descended. It is truly magnificent, in the sky right over the Common.

In Jim and Esther's 1980 Christmas Letter,

the Christmas lights came on again . . . all over Boston Common, and signaled the official opening of the holiday season. It is nice of the City to decorate our front yard—some of you no doubt saw the picture of the lights last December—it was featured in TIME Magazine in a story of Christmas displays in various cities.

Esther was able to take advantage of other activities throughout Boston through the Alumni Associations of Simmons, Forsyth, and Tufts, such as museum tours, the Boston Symphony, Pops, and boat excursions.

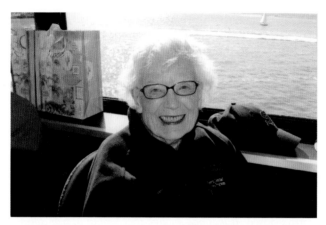

FIGURE 14.8: Esther on the Spirit of Boston, Boston Harbor, spring 2008.

❧ BOSTON TREE LIGHTING PARTY ❧

The official lighting of the Christmas tree, which took place in early December, ushered in the holiday season on the Common, a special event for both Esther and Jim, as it was located just below Esther's balcony looking toward the State House. About Christmastime during the 1970s and 1980s, Esther and Jim hosted an annual tree-lighting party *for the folks from Brant Rock*, Marshfield. Invitations went out, menus were planned, and the group (the Galligans, O'Neill's, Fords, Ames, Gallaghers, Stevensons, and Cohens) viewed the *big event* of Boston Common tree lighting from the Gallagher balcony. It used to be on a Sunday when the city would "turn on" the lights for the holidays (*until they changed it to Thursdays*). They would get together and just chat until the lights went on, and then everyone would leave. Esther continued the tradition for a few years after Jim died, but then the parties stopped, primarily due to the change of day, and it was too difficult for her friends to make it back to Marshfield later in the evening.

About 2000, the tradition changed to having a few friends and relatives over to view the tree lighting. During one of these yearly viewings, however, the call of nature and bad timing meant Esther missed the moment the tree was lit:

> *It was chilly but not bad, and we could hear pretty well. Suddenly, I decided I should go to the bathroom (or else) and was just about ready to get out there again when Pat Ramsay was hollering hurry up—so I hurried, but the lights were all on—and all I saw was the fireworks!!!*

❧ THE OAK BAR, ❧ FAIRMONT COPLEY PLAZA

One day, Esther called the author and asked whether she had read the *Boston Globe* article about the closing of the Oak Bar at the Copley Plaza Hotel, located not far from her home on Tremont Street. She explained that in the 1970s, she and Jimmy would go and listen to the piano player. Jimmy once wanted to ask for an autograph, but Esther said he was too shy. Esther wanted to go to listen just one more time. As one of her many skills is as a researcher, she sought out the name of one of the piano players (who taught music at Berklee College of Music), gave her a call, got the details, and reviewed the calendar for her open dates. On December 16, 2011, my husband and I took Esther to enjoy the music at Oak Piano Bar for one last time. I told Esther she could check one thing off of her "bucket list." She responded,

thank you, but I couldn't hear a thing!

She was not happy one of her beloved Boston landmarks was closing but even more upset when Woolworth's closed: *It was bad enough that Jordan Marsh closed, but Woolworth's?* The Oak bar closed in January 2012.

❧ BOSTON FRIENDS AND VISITORS ❧

Esther excitedly shared her beloved Boston with visitors from all over the world, going to restaurants, especially those close to her home, often taking home a boxed lunch that lasted the rest of the week, a few sugar packets, and an extra chowda! Many of Esther's long-time friends reconnected when they visited Boston. Lynda Sabat said that she got to Boston as often as she could, where she and Esther met "for dinner at Locke-Ober's to enjoy Savannah Lobsters and laugh about all the mischief we have been through."

Esther's Boston friends had the opportunity to see her quite often for small get-togethers, the symphony, parties, the theater, special occasions, or just for a visit. She delighted when friends who resided outside of the Boston area came to visit, so she could share her city with them.

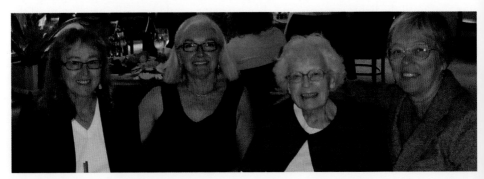

FIGURE 14.9: Pam, Pat, Charlotte, and Esther, Legal Seafood, Boston, 2012.

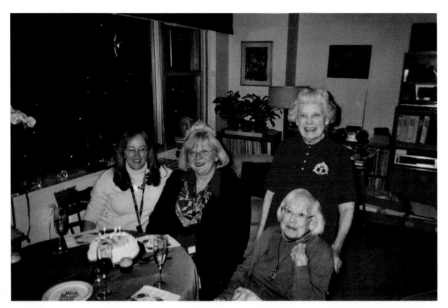

FIGURE 14.10: Laura Weinrebe birthday party at 151 Tremont, 2008: Pam Bretschneider, Pat Ramsay, Esther, and Laura Weinrebe.

✌ ESTHER'S CITY ✌

Having both the Park Street and Boylston Street Massachusetts Bay Transportation Authority (MBTA) stops within 50 ft of your front door proved quite convenient for Esther in getting around to meetings, the theater, the airport, the post office to mail off book chapters, her three colleges (MCPHS, Simmons College, and Tufts University), and everything in between. As she continued to teach at Tufts, the condo was convenient, as it is literally *just around the corner* on Kneeland Street.

Esther enjoyed the views of her city and the color changes of the seasons (vividly green in spring and summer, lined with tulips, and a white landscape in winter). She enjoyed pointing guests to the lights of Fenway Park a short distance away. The Citgo Sign that towers over Fenway Park and which can be seen from their Tremont Street condo was turned off during the energy crisis and was

turned back on in Kenmore Square. Jim fondly remembers watching it from one of his residences during dental school days (Christmas Letter, 1983).

As with most major cities, Boston offers innumerable choices for dining, from Italian food at the famous Boston North End to steaks at Locke-Ober's, to seafood on the pier, or one of Esther's favorites, Jacob Wirth's ("Jakes" to Esther). Although Esther would just as soon stay at home to eat, she did enjoy the fish (Jacob Wirth (2009), and of course, chowder ("chowda") from Legal Seafood. One of her favorite restaurants was Pier 4, located on the wharf in Boston. It was often Esther's first choice when visitors came to Boston and offered to take her out for dinner.

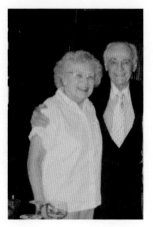

FIGURE 14.11: Esther with
Anthony Athanas, owner,
Pier 4.

It was also Esther's choice for a venue for her 90th birthday celebration.

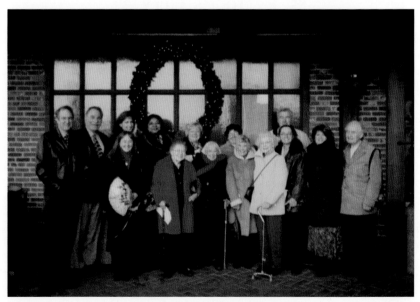

FIGURE 14.12: Esther's 90th birthday party, Pier 4, 2006.

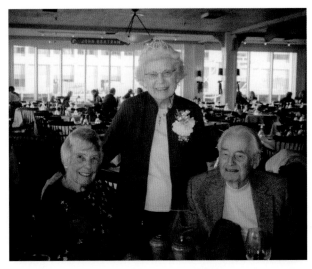

FIGURE 14.13: Esther's 90th, Mary and Warren Dole, Pier 4.

When Charlotte and Don Wyche came to Boston in 2013 for the ADHA convention, they joined Pat Ramsay and Bill, Pam and Andy Bretschneider, and Linda and Bob Boyd for dinner with Esther at Pier 4, because Esther heard the news that the restaurant was closing and she wanted to *say goodbye!*

Letting go of objects that represented memories for her were difficult. She rarely threw anything out. Years ago, Anna and Gordon Pattison were visiting from California and brought with them grapefruits. Jimmie later planted the seeds, and the grapefruit plant grew through the years, taller than Esther.

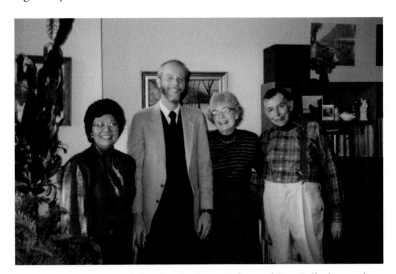

FIGURE 14.14: Anna and Gordon Pattison, Esther and Jim Gallagher, and the grapefruit tree.

After Jim died, the aging plant, now almost to the ceiling, began to brown and droop, despite her tending to it. During one of the author's weekly visit, Esther asked her to remove the grapefruit tree and discard it but to *do it quickly so she didn't see it go!* She insisted we never talk about it again.

❦ Clinical Practice of the ❦ Dental Hygienist and Esther's Tremont Street Home

The plan for one room for the book was modified, as it expanded through the years to the entire condominium. Catherine Murphy (Simmons Class of 1938) corresponded on a regular basis with Esther for over 70 years said that during one visit she made to Esther's apartment, "all the chairs were covered with an earlier revision of the book." A later holiday card from Esther noted that the chairs were now cleared for guests to use! This box and chair system was an effective process, a highly successful one through all 12 editions. There was definitely order, but most people just could not recognize what it was. She enjoyed saving the piles of years of journals, books with a story behind each one, letters and cards, plants, Jimmie's paintings, and the mementos from the places she's been and the people she has met. She surrounded herself with things she loved.

Esther's niece, Betsy, said that when her family was living in Brockton, Massachusetts, sometime in 1964, Esther stayed at their house while finding an apartment in Boston for September when Tufts classes began. Esther

> had the index to her book spread out all over the dining room—in alphabetic piles! My brother Rikk helped her with alphabetizing. I was not old enough apparently to be trusted with doing it accurately," she said in jest.

One might have thought that Esther's condo was cluttered, with piles and boxes and corners filled with journals, until week after week, when the years of her life are reconstructed and all those pieces were in those boxes, on those filled shelves, and tucked into little places, and she knew where every one of them was (sometimes after a little search and thinking about it), it became apparent that what was stored in those boxes were the essential pieces of her life: the memorabilia, the signed artifacts, photos, albums, and dusty awards. Despite the height of the piles, she knew where things were in those piles and boxes and could pull them out as needed.

❦ Esther's Passion for Boston ❦

When Esther was asked what it was about Boston she loved, she replied, *everything!* When you are from Boston, you feel it; it is part of your character, your existence. You cannot really put your finger on what it is, but it is part of you: it's deep-rooted and with a long history, its cultural traditions, its uniqueness, its activities, its exceptional loyalty to its sports teams, especially baseball, which Robert B. Parker (as cited in Howland, 1980) called "a religion for us" and "a sense of community and connection" (pp. 151), Boston's grace, its Yankee thrift, its special deference to the old and to the unique, its tucked away streets, its literary and academic excellence, its sunrises and sunsets, and what Ted Kennedy called "its irreverent charm." Bostonians, especially Esther, appreciated its marvel. She also represented the Yankee Bostonian women who "have always been noted for their independence, energy, public-spiritedness" (Sirkis, 1966, p. 21).

Esther's home, overlooking Boston's Garden, *went condo* in 1984, and Esther and Jim contemplated whether they could afford to buy it. Fortunately, they did (see Chapter 10). Not only did it prove to be an excellent investment in real estate, but it provided Esther and Jim a wonderful home over the years, accessible to public transportation, the colleges (Forsyth and MCPHS, Simmons, and Tufts), stores, restaurants, the airport, the subway, and breathtaking views of the Boston skyline. They even had an owl visit for a few days, hanging out on the balcony.

As the Gallagher condo window in the bedrooms and living room/kitchen faced Boston Garden, they were able to see the parades go by, including those by Boston's sports teams when they won the pennant, World Series, Super Bowl, Stanley Cup, or the basketball championship trophy. Wherever you stood in the condo, you would get to see a rainbow or a sunset, of which there are many, directly out her window, over the horizon, just over the Charles River. Esther enjoyed retelling the story of when Pope John Paul came to Boston in October of 1979 and spoke at the Gazebo, which can be seen directly from their balcony.

The highlight was the visit of Pope Paul October 1st, who passed right below our balcony on the way to say Mass on the Common (Christmas Letter, 1979).

In their Christmas Letter of 1980, Esther and Jim said,

" we had a box seat for Boston's 350th Birthday Parade, fireworks, and the huge cake on the Common. The Governor liked our location so much he set up his reviewing stand right across the street. Parades have been regular occurrences this year, including the 5 hour American Legion parade last summer."

Esther truly enjoyed living in Boston. The author had the good fortune to be invited by Esther to watch the Red Sox parades after their two World Series wins in 2004 and 2007 as they passed down Tremont Street in view from her balcony, the team finally winning the World Series after 86 years of no ultimate victory. Donned in our hats and tees and equipped with binoculars (I was reminded *not to change the settings!*), we could see more clearly Papelbon dancing the jig on the duck boats as they passed by. The trophy was held up high at the exact time they passed Esther's place; Ortiz seemed to look up and meet her blue eyes.

❧ DANCING, MUSIC, AND ART ❧

Although Jim and Esther had little leisure time, they spent it doing what they loved.

Dancing

Boston provided venues for the activities Esther and Jim shared, including dancing (especially ballroom), jazz, and art. As Esther related in their 1966 Christmas Letter, *here in Boston and Brant Rock we dance nearly every week and have been in a dance class (Jim is very proud of his Y.W.C.A. membership card).* The advantages and disadvantages of living in Boston: *A blizzard on blizzard turned Whittier's "Snowbound" into a commentary on current conditions. Although the snow cancelled out a couple of our Monday night dance classes at the "Y," our second love, the theater, flourished in the show-must-go-on tradition* (Christmas Letter, 1969).

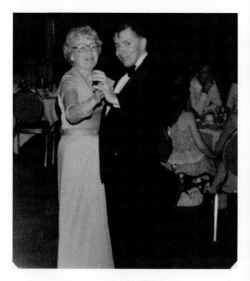

FIGURE 14.15: Esther and Jim dancing, senior class dinner at the Park Plaza, Boston, 1979.

After Jimmie passed away, Esther's passion for dancing continued.

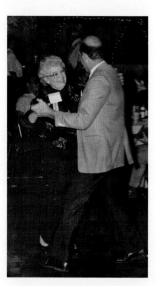

FIGURE 14.16: Esther dancing the polka, 1988.

If you ever attended an event in which Esther was present, you knew of her love for dancing and her frequent stepping out onto the dance floor.

❝ Esther was spotted in both Albuquerque (ADHA) and Chicago (UOR) this summer. Esther was treated like a rock star with hygienists waiting in line to have their photo taken with her. She was having fun on the dance floors at both events and seemed to have no trouble keeping up with the younger women" (Walters, 2008, p. 4).

As Carol Griffin reflected,

❝ the most fun of all is watching her 'outdance' everyone, watch other people marvel at her energy and tenacity to keep stepping out to the beat of the music." In concluding an *RDH Magazine* interview conducted with Esther in 2002, Ann-Marie DePalma advised, "if you don't already know this, she is great party lady! Get her on the dance floor and watch out" (p. 3).

Esther particularly enjoyed attending events where there was a dance floor, especially a formal gala at MCPHS each year. The gala gave Esther an opportunity to get on the dance floor, many taking turns as her partner.

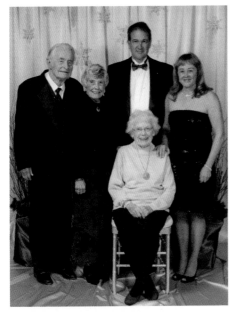

Figure 14.17: Mary and Warren Dole, Esther, and Pam and Andy Bretschneider, Massachusetts College of Pharmacy and Health Sciences Gala. (Used by Permission of Massachusetts College of Pharmacy and Health Sciences University.)

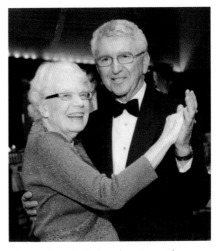

FIGURE 14.18: Esther dancing with President Monahan, Massachusetts College of Pharmacy and Health Sciences Gala. (Used with permission from Massachusetts College of Pharmacy and Health Sciences University.)

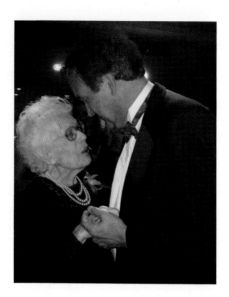

FIGURE 14.19: Esther dancing with
Andy Bretschneider, ADHA Annual
Session, Boston.

Music

Esther and Jim loved music. Together, they amassed a collection of jazz LPs of the *greats*, which were kept throughout their lives and left totally intact, like new, evidencing the care in which they were preserved.

> *The TOC offers a continuing source of entertainment. This summer the outdoor "Concerts on the Common" were in our front yard and could be heard if not seen (meaning that a tree blocked our view to the stage) and it was a pleasure to hear Ella Fitzgerald, James Taylor, Diana Ross, and other noted musicians* (Christmas Letter, 1981/1982).

Art

> *This fall, in addition to our most enjoyed extracurricular activities, the theater and ballroom dancing, we are enrolled in art classes at the Adult Education Center. Jim, who has been threatening to paint again after many years, is doing acrylics. And Esther—aggravated by the complications of getting satisfactory drawings done by the professional artists for the dental hygiene text revision, is in drawing class. Can't beat 'em—join 'em!* (Christmas Letter, 1970).

Continuing their tradition of involvement in the arts, the 1971 Christmas Letter brought news of Esther becoming

> " involved in needlepoint to the point of joining a class this fall. Up to then there was only one stitch (learned originally from Mrs. Baker in Manchester long ago), so it was a revelation to learn that there are some 150 stitches with their variations—of which 30 were included in the course. So as we go to press we find her working her Christmas sock, hopefully to be done in time to hang it up!"

As related in their 1972 Christmas Letter, hobbies and other activities, such as Theater Guild, continued.

During the summer Jim passed up picture painting for woodworking and made two handsome tall bookcases. The classic needlepoint chair seat cover started in January was almost finished in December.

It was announced in 1974 Esther had won a Blue Ribbon for her needlepoint pillow and Jim won first prize for his exhibited painting at the Marshfield Fair that year.

The 1977 Christmas Letter brought news of Jim's cabinet making,

a cabinet combination to house his records, record player, radio, tapes, records, old-time programs, recordings and big band recordings. In 1980, a particularly busy year for both Esther and Jim, they ended their Christmas Letter with *his every growing record collection of music of the 20s, 30s, and 50s, and a return to his artist's easel, provided some relaxation.*

Jim went to an outdoor painting class this summer and did a section of the historical Commonwealth Avenue Mall . . . that and several others were exhibited in October and someone wanted to by one (P.S. He wouldn't sell). In 1984, Jim attended a Wednesday morning class at the Brockton Art Museum and has made several great things—one especially to mention is a beautiful painting of Eagle Head and Singing Beach in Manchester by the Sea, that is in Manchester, Mass, where I worked as a dental hygienist with Dr. Willis, and "lived" on the beach every possible moment during those summers (Christmas Letter, 1984).

When Jim passed away, Esther continued her interest in the arts. As a theater buff with season tickets to the Huntington Theatre Company only a few trolley stops from her front door, Esther kept abreast not only of the shows in town but also the ones the *New Yorker* highlighted on Broadway and beyond. As her hearing was *slightly going* as time went by, she enjoyed reading the plays in advance of seeing them and often arrived at the theater early in order to take advantage of the *hearing devices* often offered by the theaters; she said she didn't like to miss a word. Esther and Pat Cohen shared third row mezzanine, aisle seats for many years.

❧ THE CHRISTMAS LETTER ❧

Jim and Esther began an annual coauthored Christmas Letter in 1966, the same year in which they married, while living at 27 Melrose Street in Boston. Each letter provided a detailed diary of the various trips, events, activities, publications, continuing education visits, conferences, and special events for the past year. Jim also utilized his artistry by adding appropriate hand drawings related to the year, including a Volkswagen drawing with a Just Married sign on the back. They both enjoyed sharing details of the year, from where they went, what they saw, what they did, the year's happenings, as well as the joys and challenges of life in Boston and Brant Rock, accompanied with Jim's drawings appropriate to the content.

Although the Christmas Letter continued after Jim's death, the letters became shorter, were often distributed late, and focused more on her adventures around the country with continuing education, white coat ceremonies, inductions, and later on, stories of technology, local events, and health challenges. The last official Christmas Letter was dated 2012, went out in 2013, and ended with the hope Esther would *graduate from the walker and ride the Boston MBTA using her cane!!!*

These valuable pieces of history captured the stories of Esther's life, carefully preserved and arranged chronologically in a manila folder tucked into the big brown desk in her office.

❧ BOSTON PUBLIC LIBRARY ❧

Never one to be idle, Esther began training as a tour guide at the Boston Public Library.

The "Beepul" as it was known years ago to college students, the Library building is nearly 100 years old and was the first truly public library in the USA. It has "Free for All" over the front entrance and is a National Historic Landmark. The beautiful murals and architecture are by many famous artists. Now under renovation—so when the front is open again with the lions on the grand stairway you will want to come and let me tour you through (Esther's Christmas Letter, 1993).

Grasping any opportunity to share information about oral health, Esther also volunteered at the Museum of Science in 1990.

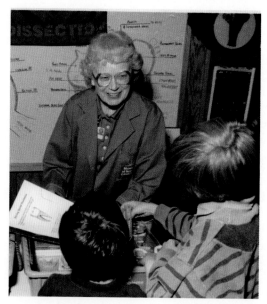

FIGURE 14.20: Esther volunteering at the Museum of Science, 1990.

Boston was Esther's city; she was passionate about it, dedicated to it, engulfed herself in its history, and shared her enthusiasm with anyone who would listen. She stayed in Boston as long as she physically was able. The condominium was sold in 2017.

CHAPTER 15

Brant Rock (Marshfield)

At my beach place, it was always fun,
even in deep fog when the place was quite enclosed.

Marshfield was a very special place for Esther, who recalled with fondness the many years she spent at their cottage. Jim and his first wife owned a home in the town and bought the cottage a short time before she became ill. She passed away about a year after they purchased the cottage; it was used very little at that time.

Before Jim and Esther were married in 1966, he brought Esther down to see his little cottage. At the time of Esther's introduction to the home, *the only furniture was two lawn chairs on the porch, and there was a single pot on the stove for making tea.* The one-level gable style cottage is located on Water Street in Marshfield, Massachusetts, in Bluefish Cove, Brant Rock, the fourth cottage up from the ocean, located directly on the river. Marshfield is about 30 miles south of Boston and has a population of about 22,000, and Esther was registered to vote in this beach town all her adult life. She kept the cottage primarily for the memories.

When Jim moved to Boston, he moved half the furniture from his downtown Marshfield house to the cottage and half to his apartment in Boston, giving life to the little cottage that Esther and Jim would soon enjoy together. As Jim described the cottage:

    "It is a delightful little home with the ocean [Massachusetts Bay] there a little left of the front; the beach grass and sand making a do-it-itself lawn; and the marsh with its ever-changing colors individualized for each season."

When not working or writing, Esther and Jim spent as much time as possible *down at the cottage* and beach. Esther said it was *just too hot to work on the book down there,* but they went down almost every weekend during the summers and *any time when Jim was off from Tufts.* She described how she enjoyed walking down to the beach and laying in the sun and how they went out dancing every Saturday night.

Occasionally, they would go to the cottage off season, as they did in 1969, as the cottage was winterized:

    "On a clear day from Bluefish Cove we can look across to Plymouth, and as we write this on Thanksgiving Day, we can't help but wonder why the Pilgrims went to all the trouble to go hunting in the deep woods for wild turkeys when right out in front was the big blue ocean teeming with lobsters. We wonder why didn't they have lobster—like we had this year! and what a giant beast it was—all 10 lbs. of him (or her as the case may be), enough for us and several starving Indians!!" (Christmas Letter, 1969).

As nothing is ever perfect, as reported in Jim and Esther's 1971 Christmas Letter:

" Our cottage and the delightful summer weather gave us a nice vacation. For a good part of four months many of our valuables (stereo, radio, etc.) were stored at the police station waiting for our housebreakers' cases (two—in May) to come up in court. As a result we had accessible windows chicken-wired, caged, etc. so now the front of the cottage looks like a pawn shop on Sunday!!"

They met and enjoyed the neighbors in the area, with whom Esther stayed in contact for many years, receiving neighborhood updates on the happenings of Marshfield. *The neighbors were nice*, Esther related. When they knew Esther and Jim were coming down, they prepared for their visit by opening up their windows of the cottage, as it *got pretty warm down there. They all looked out for each other.*

Paul and Pat lived next door. Pat was *quite an artist and displayed her work at the elderly center*, and Paul had a vegetable garden and shared his crops with Esther and Jim. The O'Neills lived four houses down, and Hank and his wife went dancing with Esther and Jim.

Esther joined the Friends of the Ventress Library in Marshfield, everyone attended the community meetings, and Esther was an officer quite often, 3 or 4 times as secretary for the Bluefish Cove Improvement Association. Jim and Esther's 1966 Christmas Letter proudly stated that they were

card-carrying members of the B.V.A. [Bay Village Association] and the B.C.A. [Bluefish Cove Association], important organizations which deal with such matters as rubbish collection, curbing of dogs, and neighborhood socials, and our red Volkswagen wears membership stickers for both. All of the Bluefish Cove Association tables, chairs, and a canopy tent were stored in Esther and Jim's garage, *as it was the only place dry and big enough.*

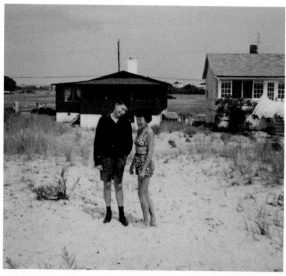

FIGURE 15.1: Jim and Esther, Brant Rock cottage, August 1967.

The last meeting of the 1991 season was held on the Gallagher porch. According to Esther, there were issues similar to those of the current day: the road, parking of visitors, and planning for the summer party held every year. Many a cookout, yard sale, Ladies Afternoons Out, and tent parties were held at Bluefish Cove during the summer months. For many years in December, Jim and Esther's Bluefish Cove friends joined them for the annual Tremont Street Tree Lighting Party (see Chapter 14).

❦ THE PINK PIANO (ESTHER'S STORY OF ❦ HER CHERISHED PIANO)

One Sunday at our cottage, the neighbors invited us over for a drink with her family. The family came out from all around and gathered about every Sunday and they had a lot of fun. So we went over and had a drink and everybody was busy talking and shouting and everything else and we were around on the porch. All of a sudden, Paul's older sister, there were 3 children in that family and he had a younger sister, too. The older sister who lived over in Marshfield Hills said out of the blue, "Anyone want a pink piano?" And I jumped up and I said "I do!" and she said "Fine, I'll give it to you for the price of the moving." And I said, Oh, that sounds wonderful, does it work? And we laughed and talked about it for a little while.

We arranged with the truck driver who would be moving it and they tried it and measured doors and so forth about getting it into my little cottage. The day came and over they came. They knew they couldn't get into the back door, so they went up through the sand to the front door near the front deck and they came in that way. They took the door off into the living room and just barely squeaked it through into the living room where they stood it up against the wall over the carpet, which means many years later the carpet had never been vacuumed underneath it. There it was; it was beautiful; it was about 100 years old and in pretty good shape, although it would need tuning, and I was delighted.

I still have the piano so my successors can offer it to someone for the moving after I'm gone. I won't part with it as long as I still have the cottage, but I won't want to take it out either. It's huge and it's beautiful and I had it tuned and it lasted a long time, in tune.

One summer day, while spending time in Brant Rock, Esther and Jim decided to have a breakfast party for about 10 to 15 people. As Esther had just procured the pink piano, she *used food coloring to make pink pancakes.*

The Annual Christmas Letter of 1967 provided more detail on the famous pink piano:

January brought the pink <u>piano</u>. Not just <u>any</u> piano, but a handsome pink one of ancient vintage (estimated by the tuner to be over 80 years). Jim started to learn to play and from "Let's go Fishing" in the Williams blue beginners book he has already advanced to a variety of nice-sounding pieces, including the Merry Widow Waltz, and Christmas Carols, especially Silent Night. We play four-hands, too, and have quite a repertoire. The piano didn't take up all our fun time—we continued our YWCA dance lessons (9 p.m. Mondays!) and have practiced on any moment's notice, especially Saturday Nights. As their 1968

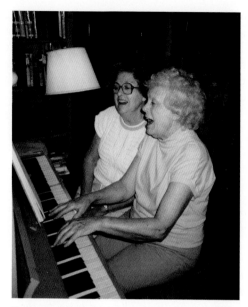

FIGURE 15.2: Esther and the pink piano, Brant Rock, 1991.

Christmas Letter reported, with Jim's ink drawing of the cottage on the top of the page: *Over all, the pink piano reigned supreme and Jim continues to practice—he is progressing to some sharps, flats, and more complicated cords now. And in 1969: Listen!! Hear the notes of "Silent Night" issuing from the pink piano (Jim says with him playing they're not issuing forth but being evicted). That's our mood music.*

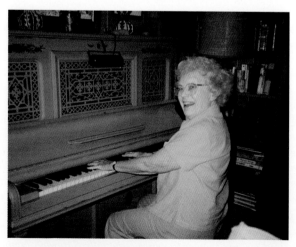

FIGURE 15.3: Esther playing the pink piano, 1968/1969.

Since Esther and Jim acquired the pink piano, it was used at the many parties held at the cottage through the years.

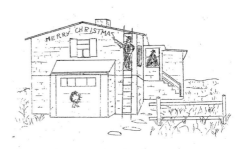

Figure 15.4: Jim's ink drawing, Bluefish Cove cottage, 1968.

❧ Gallagher Potluck Dinner ❧

Summer was a busy time at the cottage for the Gallaghers, as they held their annual picnic for their Tufts colleagues, cleverly named the Complete Denture Outing. Their colleagues all looked forward to the first Saturday in August when Jim and Esther Gallagher held their Annual Potluck Buffet Picnic, which began in 1974. Previous to this date, John Johansson, Tufts faculty, held an annual Plate-makers and Denturists Picnic at his home in Cohasset.

> *For the summers we have discovered the best way to get the cottage completely cleaned with all windows washed and the outside paint touched up in a hurry—have a party!!! So in 1973 we entertained the Lady Dentists' society and in 1974 some 60-plus assorted men, women, and children of the Department of Complete Dentures [Tufts] held their first annual picnic at our place. And what a day that was . . . weather just perfect and everything was heavenly. There is little doubt but that we have a second annual picnic in our future.*

RSVPs were required, and the festivities began in the early afternoon: *Come by 2-3 o'clock!* Cocktails began at about 5:00 PM, followed at 6:00 PM with the potluck buffet. Dress was very informal, as some of the activities involved swimming, sunning, and walking, and guests were asked *to bring your musical instrument to play for us or join while we sing.* The pink piano was inevitably used. Inclement weather did not matter, as Esther said, *we can all fit into the cottage.*

In the second annual picnic in 1975, the program included a Christmas in August:

> *Would you believe we haven't had a chance to take down the Christmas tree in Boston. Well, why not just dust the ornaments and have a Christmas in August party. Everybody bring a joke or white elephant, gift for the grab bag. Maybe Santa will show up to distribute them.*

The annual Complete Denture Department picnic continued for many years; only 1978 was missed due to Jim's accident in Ireland.

❧ NEIGHBORS AT BLUEFISH ❧ COVE, MARSHFIELD

Several of the neighbors looked out for the place when Esther and Jim were in Boston, working, teaching, or *Clinical Practice of the Dental Hygienist* (CPDH) writing. There was a Paul on either side of her.

> *Paul Alexander was the backbone of the group, a past president and a good friend to Jimmy. Paul and his wife were helpful to us, often gave us stuff to eat; Jim would enjoy anything she made. They looked out for us. Paul had lived the whole time since childhood in one of the cottages; the whole family boated, sailed, and fished. He passed away in his 90s, and Paul Galligan became my cottage watchdog.*

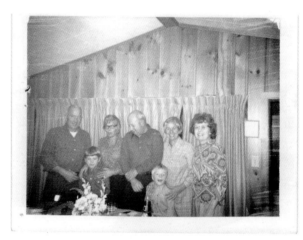

FIGURE 15.5: Brant Rock neighbors, 1969.

❧ BLUEFISH COVE LATER YEARS ❧

One day, Paul Galligan, who was retired then, called Esther after a storm and told her she had siding coming off the house and that she had bees. Esther insisted the story be included in the Brant Rock chapter:

> *At Bluefish Cove my neighbors on each side were named Paul. They were very kind gentlemen and always willing to help when I needed something done. Paul Galligan on the one side kept watch over the cottage and would call me if anything unusual happened. For example, in one of the big storms, he called to tell me that a section of the white siding had blown off, thus giving me a chance to call the company to plan the repair.*
>
> *One day he called and when I answered he said, "Esther, you've got bees."*
> *I said, I've got bees? He said, "yes, they come out from under the eave."*

I said, where? He said, "OK, stand in the street and look at the back of the garage. They go in and out right under that left upper corner."

I said, what do I do? He said "I've got someone for you. A couple of years ago, a friend over in the village had bees, so I called and asked her who it was. His name is John. Got a pencil? Here's the number."

So I called and made the appointment to meet me at the cottage. John came with his nephew and surveyed the situation. He studied the inside of the garage to see if he needed to open the wall lining. He decided they would go in through the hole the bees went in. He explained how they put a tube in and spray the channel with a chemical the bees would eat going in or out, which would poison them. His nephew dressed up in the protective cover-up headgear and proceeded. After a short time they were ready to leave, and I gave John the check.

He left saying, "you'll have no more trouble. You watch, and if any one bee goes in or out of that hole in three days, you call me and I'll come and do it over again for free." I thanked them and they left. Paul had been there and watched the whole process. He said, "I'll call you."

In a few days he called and said, "I watched. Two bees went in, but never did any come out" (The Bee Story, as told by Esther, January 18, 2009).

Many of the active neighborhood group members have since died, but Esther remembered them fondly and spoke highly of each of them. Esther and Jim very much enjoyed spending time with their Bluefish Cove neighbors. Some of the neighbors began to retire, and slowly, some of Esther's close friends and neighbors passed away. When her next-door neighbor Paul died, the sons didn't want to keep the house and they sold it, interestingly to another neighbor named Paul who became the official watcher of the cottage when Esther wasn't there. Many of the homes on the water have been rebuilt or floors added. Although the Gallaghers didn't "go up" to a second story, they did raise the foundation 2 ft in 1979, adding two rooms. As Jim said, "our little white princess now stands high above the water line." They also replaced the roof, built a deck, and got a new garage door *after the old one went kerplunk one summer day. Life at the seaside is tough on little houses.*

In 1986, they had an elevator lift installed, that Jim said "turned out to be a real fun thing." Instead of those 15 plus trips to tote things to and from the Voyager over the stairs, just load them on and ride up. (Of course, now Esther has to find another way to get her exercise!!)" In later years, Esther said the lift was essential to Jim's mobility into the cottage after his health began to decline, as well as she did in advanced age.

Esther exchanged Christmas cards with several of her Marshfield neighbors through the years. Friend Marie wrote in 2007

" every Christmas I remember the lovely tree lighting party you gave us. I thank you for that memory."

❧ MARSHFIELD, THE LATER YEARS ❧

Marshfield held many memories for Esther. She kept numerous artifacts at the cottage, such as the early print *Journals of Dental Hygiene*, along with many of Jim's paintings, and anything Esther *didn't want to throw out* that came from her Boston apartment.

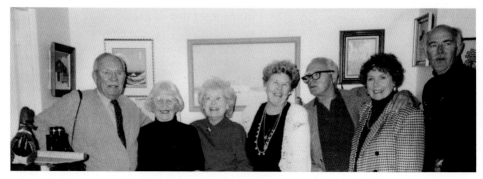

FIGURE 15.6: Brant Rock Christmas tree lighting, Boston, 1969.

Although Esther went to Marshfield much less often than the old days, primarily due to her writing, continuing education (CE) engagements, busy schedule, and the long drive, she enjoyed the peace and reflection. In her later years, Esther enjoyed going down to the cottage with her niece, Betsy. They brought lunch, often a cheese sandwich and bottle of milk, and sat out on the porch overlooking the dunes, occasionally sweeping the mice out, who decided to make their winter home in the basement garage.

During the last few years, when she no longer could drive, she asked to be brought to the cottage just to look around and maybe *clear out a few things*. On one such trip, the author and Esther stopped at the local grocery store (to be frugal) for a box lunch to each on the cottage porch, looking out across the beach grass towards the river.

Storytelling during the entire stay, from the elevator acquisition, to the pink piano, and the parties held on the beach, Esther showed a love for a place she enjoyed for so many years. The quest to clean out was short lived. As we sorted through the boxes on the shelves in the basement of the cottage, Esther gave detail on where each item came from: what was Jim's from his first marriage, which ones were wedding gifts, what could still be used, and what she kept for no apparent reason at all, carefully rewrapping them and putting them back on the shelf.

In retrospect and considering all that was left in her Boston apartment, untouched for years, it became evident that what was being kept were the memories. As with the scarves, autographed stuffed animals, theatre programs, long-playing records, and convention name badges kept in Boston, the silver-plated trays, Jim's paintings, lawn chairs long since unusable, and gifts still wrapped in tissue and in their original boxes in the basement of the cottage, Esther was unable to let anything go; she was holding on to the life she had lived, each item was cherished, holding its special place in her heart: *The ever-changing beauty of the marshes and the ocean, and that delicious sea air, are simply wonderful.*

The cottage was sold in 2016, after Esther moved to Laurel Place in New Hampshire.

CHAPTER 16

The Later Years and Reaching 100

When all is said and done,
Esther would like people to say:
She loved to dance!

D r. Wilkins continued to live up to her reputation as one of the most influential health educators of her time. The 12th edition of her text *Clinical Practice of the Dental Hygienist* was completed in September 2015, having celebrated its 58th year in publication.

For someone whose professional career had been so extensive, global, and multifaceted, Esther lived a very simple life. She commented that she never really took an official vacation except on her honeymoon in 1966. Travels in the United States and abroad were related to her book, associations such as American Dental Hygienists' Association (ADHA) and International Federation of Dental Hygienists (IFDH), or continuing education.

When asked why she kept so many items from her past, Esther responded,

I had many memories with each of those things and by giving them up, I would be giving away those memories. She began to move some of the items to her Marshfield cottage; little was ever discarded. On a trip to Marshfield, in our quest to clean out the basement, she set parameters: *When we go over the stuff in the basement, one thing there is my old ancient bicycle. It goes back to the 20s and 30s when I remember my father biking to work. There might be a way to fit the bike into my BIO—I'd like that! I can't imagine that my old treasure of an antique has to go to the dump!*

She was particularly fond of the Simmons songbook, which she kept since 1938. By keeping the things that she remembered, she could relive her life at any time.

Esther loved people and was a devoted friend, as evidenced by the many testimonials presented in this biography. As Beverly Whitford noted,

" she remembers names, she's humble, and doesn't flaunt her notoriety. She likes to be one of the crowd. Though her accomplishments through life were many, Esther remained quite modest. She was respected, admired, and adored by all who knew her and she had the utmost respect for the professions of dentistry and dental hygiene and those who chose to pursue them as careers. She had more friends than anyone I know."

One dear friend of many in the profession was Laura Peck Fitch (Forsyth Class of 1937), who was president of the Connecticut Dental Hygienists' Association at the same time that Esther served as president of the Massachusetts Dental Hygienists' Association. Beverly reminisced,

> ❝ I'm sure there are many interesting and amusing stories to tell regarding their working and traveling together during the early days of the American Dental Hygienists' Association. I bet they traveled wearing hats, gloves, and high heeled shoes. Esther and I shed tears together when I telephoned her in March 2008 to inform her of Laura's death."

Esther stood 5 ft, 2 in tall, was of small build, right handed, blue eyes, and she wore glasses since childhood and hearing aids later in life, *which sometimes were a minor inconvenience* (especially if she forgot to get fresh batteries). She had freckles on her arms that she attributed to the time she spent on the beach in Manchester, and she put on lipstick to talk on the phone. Esther never considered herself old, just aging, and she certainly met her 90s with a resume of endless accomplishments. Her life spanned 17 presidents of the United States.

Esther enjoyed a very healthy life. Other than the first broken bone she ever had with her fall in South Carolina, as well as a serious fall in her home town in 2012, she was hospitalized few times in her life: *tonsils (no overnight), vein-stripping in Seattle*, and cataract surgery in 2009. Lynda McKeown celebrated Dr. Wilkins's "boundless energy," and concluded, "what an amazing role model for healthy aging." Esther wrote about her long life in her 2010 article,

when pressed with the question of genetics, my personal pride led me to tell about my paternal grandmother who passed quietly away one month before her 100th birthday. She was a frail little old lady, but my memories are clear of her being busy sewing by hand and primarily, to help her many grandchildren get ready for back-to-school . . . My maternal grandfather lived into his late eighties, in spite of the daily evening pipe that filled the kitchen with smoke while he read the daily newspaper.

Anna Pattison described a typical Esther Wilkins day:

> ❝ I believe one of the secrets to her energy and longevity is her dedication to a healthy, daily routine. She starts with her morning exercises on a towel on the floor of her bedroom followed by breakfast. After working all morning on her book or teaching, she stops at 12 noon sharp to eat lunch. She continues to work on the book in the afternoon and might have an apple or orange for an afternoon snack. If she hasn't walked to the Tufts Dental School library to read reference articles for the book, she will go to the small exercise room in her building to walk on the treadmill. She is back in her condo for dinner. She rarely eats sweets. She is in bed by 9 PM and up at 5 AM to do her exercises. So, if you want to live to be 100 years old and stay fit, trim, and sharp as a tack, I am convinced that Dr. Wilkins lifestyle is the key" (Pattison, 2010, p. 8).

Esther's daily life was full. She was certainly not your average nonagenarian. It was filled with planning continuing education courses, managing her full calendar, doing her own laundry, cooking, cleaning, teaching, reading, and visiting. Until a few years ago, she had one-on-one, biweekly sessions with a personal trainer. She resolved to *get more exercise* and was conscientious not to miss a session with Karen in the exercise room in her building, unless she was out of the country or committed to a continuing education event.

On the way to 100, I am often asked how I have maintained my health into such an advanced age. The answer is to eat right, drink lots of milk, no smoking, top oral health with flossing and brushing at least two times daily, an apple a day, exercise as much as possible, drink fluoridated water, and the help of all my wonderful friends who contribute to my updating and attitude.

My morning starts with strengthening and stretching exercises, followed by a hot shower. Next is breakfast with orange juice, oatmeal, and coffee. Blueberries or strawberries are a rare treat on the oatmeal. Lunch is a sandwich, often cheese with lettuce, and milk. Dinner, accompanied by the evening news, varies between fish or chicken and includes vegetables, potatoes (especially baked because there are no dishes to wash), and salad. Saturdays, the traditional New England baked beans are on the menu. Sweets are always a no-no for obvious oral health reasons, as well as weight management.

Retirement is not on the list. The mind must keep busy and there is always more to be done in the promotion of oral health and prevention of oral diseases.

Esther's enthusiasm was noticed by everyone who met her.

“ It is her enthusiasm for her work and her drive to educate thoroughly as many people as she can about the power of prevention that has made her a celebrity, a 'shining star in dental and allied dental education' as Richard Valachovic, president of the American Dental Education Association's Gies Foundation, puts it” (Flaherty, 2012, p. 26).

Esther valued her friends quite considerably, some of whom received handwritten notes from her for 50 years. Once she mastered the typewriter (although with one finger at a time), she sent notes in typed form. Once the computer became an option and Esther grasped its many ways to reach out, she would write *lots and lots* of emails, sometimes beginning with *another little request, I need help, please,* or *just checking in.* As described by Pat Ramsay, “these emails always included several comments concerning ADHA, Forsyth/MCPHS, dental hygiene education in general, and friends whom we share. Esther's inquiring mind is always working.”

In her 90s and until 2011, Esther taught 1 day per week in the fall/winter at Tufts Dental School, walking the short distance from her home, as dedicated as she was when she began her career many years ago. She taught predoctoral students at Tufts periodontal instrumentation and instrument sharpening with Pat Cohen and Dr. Paul Levi. As Paul related,

“ when I called Esther to tell her that classes had been cancelled at Tufts one snowy day, she said she already had her boots on and was ready, despite the weather. It really took some convincing that it was Tufts Dental School, not Tufts University, so she decided it best not to go in after all. She figured she would never need the 'snow number,' so she *threw it away.*”

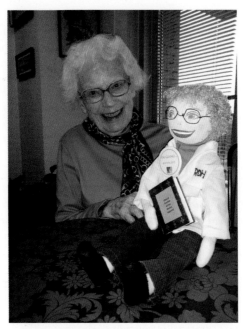

FIGURE 16.1: Esther and Esther doll, a gift from Charlotte Wyche.

Dr. Terrence J. Griffin, chairman of the Tufts Dental School Department of Periodontology at that time, said that "no matter where I travel, when people hear I am from Tufts, they ask about her. Even today, she has more energy in her little finger than you or I have together in our whole bodies" (Griffin, as cited in Camire, 2006, p. 2). As travel became more difficult for Esther, she gave up teaching at Tufts. Esther M. Wilkins, RDH, DMD, was awarded Clinical Professor of Periodontology Emeritus from Tufts University School of Dental Medicine in 2011.

❧ BIRTHDAYS ❧

Esther loved birthdays: hers and everyone she knew and called *dear*. A whole chapter could be written just on her 90th birthday, which lasted a whole year, to the point that Pat Ramsay commented, "enough! No more cake!" In addition to the lavish birthday held in Boston in conjunction with the Yankee Dental Conference in 2007, there were small celebrations with friends in various cities she visited in 2006, her 90th year, many cakes, balloons, and pictures with the woman of honor.

Well, my first fabulous birthday party was in the mountains of Colorado, where I participated in the annual meeting of CDHA, a couple of weeks before S.C. Of course, everybody makes me feel good when they say I don't LOOK 90 or on the phone I don't SOUND 90! (Christmas Letter, 2006)

An *RDH Magazine* article in 2007 described the wonderful party that Esther recalled as *a very special birthday*, sponsored by Hu-Friedy Mfg. Co., Inc., and Forsyth School for Dental Hygienists at Massachusetts College of Pharmacy and Health Sciences (MCPHS):

“ Hu-Friedy's special relationship with Dr. Wilkins has continued to grow over the years. Her guidance and support have enabled the company to achieve more. She helped direct Hu-Friedy toward better instrument design and stronger relationships with clinicians. In honor of her legacy with students, Hu-Friedy Manufacturing Company continues to endow five Dr. Wilkins Instrument Scholarships each year through the American Dental Hygienists' Association" (DentistryIQ, 2007, p. 1).

The party, which was held at Turner Fisheries in Boston, on January 23, 2007, was enjoyed by the many close friends of Dr. Wilkins, including Mary Dole (Forsyth Class of '41) and Bea Miller (Forsyth Class of 36). Speeches by representatives of Forsyth/MCPHS and Hu-Friedy told of the "shining accomplishments" of Dr. Wilkins in the field of dental hygiene and concluded with "goodie bags containing a Hu-Friedy commemorative Esther Wilkins Expro and a phone charm from Forsyth" (DentistryIQ, 2007, p. 1). Anna Pattison noted Esther was so busy enjoying her friends that she hardly had time to enjoy the food and birthday cake. Hu-Friedy continued to bestow upon Esther their thanks for her contributions to the dental field, including a lovely orchid plant sent to Esther each Christmas.

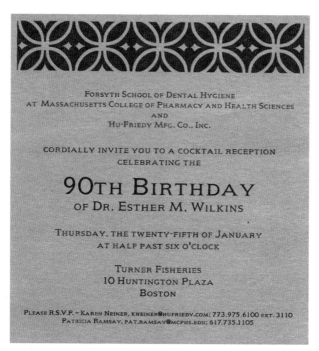

FIGURE 16.2: Hu-Friedy/Massachusetts College of Pharmacy and Health Sciences 90th birthday invitation, 2006.

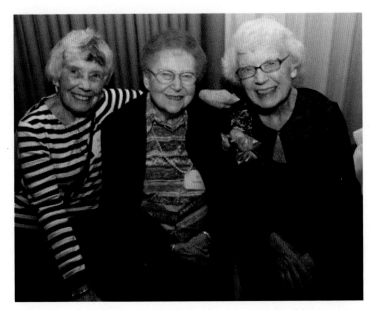

FIGURE 16.3: Mary Dole, Bea Miller and Esther, 90th birthday party, Boston.

Once all the parties seemed to subside, she continued to receive birthday cards every month for a whole year. Esther recalled that the very first birthday card was sent in June 2006 by Gail Cross Poline of Denver. Esther kept every card and occasionally pulled a few from the basket to read, smiling as she remembered the year of the 90th birthday. Esther remembers vividly that the first birthday cake *was at the Colorado State dental hygiene meeting high up in the Colorado mountains in late September 2006. It was a beautiful cake made by a dental hygienist.*

If Esther's birthday fell on a day she was presenting at a continuing education program, inevitably there would be a cake and celebration held. Esther's 93rd birthday in 2009 was spent in San Francisco. In early December, during her morning lecture break, a beautiful cake was brought into the hotel ballroom to celebrate Esther's 93rd birthday, accompanied by 400 serenading dental hygienists. Esther's 95th was a joint birthday party with long-time friend, Mary Dole, at the Wayside Inn, in Sudbury, Massachusetts.

A birthday venue Esther particularly enjoyed was Jacob Wirth's in Boston.

An additional 99th birthday was held at Forsyth, where the students and faculty presented her with a cake. According to Irina Smilyanski, Forsyth faculty member, "Esther pointed to the cake and said, *they put the candles upside down; it should be 66!*"

Esther remembered the birthdays of others, also keeping little 3 × 5 cards (that she maintained since the early 1950s) that reminded her of her friends' birthdays each month. She sent a handwritten card to everyone, delighting in their special day. As she began to age and her eyesight began to worsen, she communicated solely through email, and her contacts were limited to a few guests in her home.

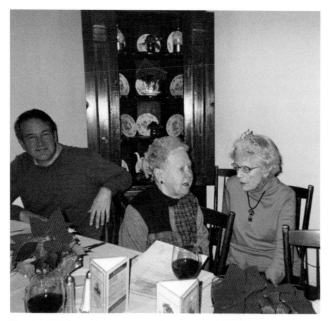

FIGURE 16.4: Andy Bretschneider, Pauline Redding, and Esther, Wayside Inn, 95th birthday, 2011.

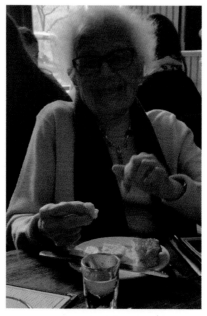

FIGURE 16.5: Esther blowing out candles, Jacob Wirth's, 99th birthday, December 2015.

❧ DISCIPLINE AND HARD WORK ❧

When I asked Esther in general how she gets everything done, she responded, *discipline!* Rarely, due to time, she would watch an old videocassette recorder (VCR) tape of *Jimmy Stewart or the other classics.* She would also occasionally listen to Elvis or Frank Sinatra on the CD player she received from friends on her 92nd birthday. Otherwise, she was reading, writing, teaching, and learning.

One discipline to which Esther was dedicated was exercise. Mary Kellerman, commented that if you wanted to find Esther at a dental hygiene convention, you had to get up early and go to the aerobic/yoga workouts: "She is always there in her jogging suit, to keep up her good shape." Esther believed that exercise, even for a few minutes, was necessary for good health and mobility through life.

❧ RESEARCH AND LEARNING ❧

Esther prided herself on keeping up to date with current events and new research, as she understood and recognized the talents of the people with whom she associated, and she tapped them on more than one occasion for information. Reading all the current literature cover to cover (preferring hard copy over electronic and disappointed many journals were *going digital!*), she placed her journals in binders and stacks and kept them for years and years, as

> *I might need an article in that pile.* She admitted, *it is something of an addiction that I remain on the mailing lists for journals and bulletins that allow continued learning. I have spent many years keeping in contact with the new research; changing viewpoints and terminology for patient instruction, and new products as new scientific information replaces the old. Perhaps my generation of biologic and other scientific terminology has long since been replaced with words and theories I may not recognize, but the challenge to learn what's new is still there.*

Lois Barber related,

> ❝when the American Heart Association had just introduced a new antibiotic protocol, I decided to introduce the specifics of the regimen as an educational message at the ADHA Product Presentation instead of the usual new product information. Esther came up to me afterwards, with a warm smile, saying *you beat me on that one.* Ever since, there has been an unwritten race for who can find out new gems of knowledge to share with colleagues first."

She just loved to be on top of knowledge in a variety of fields.

Through the years, Esther learned to get her email from a computer other than the one in her home (*amazing how much time letters and postage stamps and all that jazz used to take*), how to use PowerPoint, and use a flash drive instead of a CD. Lois Barber described that Esther's first PowerPoint lesson came in a hotel room in Orlando, Florida, after a continuing education course that Esther and Anna Pattison had presented.

❝ I was given the opportunity to start her transition from transparencies to PowerPoint slides. Although I had second thoughts about the impact of her losing her traditional wooden hand pointer, I knew she would embrace the technology. I felt very privileged to teach my mentor.❞

If Esther was busy or had a deadline or many plans for the day, she would be on the computer until 4 AM, if necessary. It is quite amazing that at her age, she was not only computer savvy but willing to learn new skills on the computer that could help facilitate projects. Most people her age don't even know how to turn it on. She even began using "tracking" for the 11th edition.

Esther had a thirst for learning and looking at topics with a different point of view. Daughn Thomas described Esther's visit to New York, when there was a Kwanzaa celebration taking place at the College:

❝ Dr. Wilkins had never heard or known anything about Kwanzaa. We explained to her what Kwanzaa meant to people of color and the 7 principles. Wilkins left there with a lot of knowledge about Kwanzaa and was very impressed.❞

Esther was very open to new information in any form. Her sharp mind continued to expand at every opportunity.

❧ A LEGACY FOR STUDENTS ❧

Perhaps the most significant influence Dr. Wilkins made in her lifetime was with students of all ages. She was convinced of the power of education and believed that all students deserved an opportunity to seek higher education. Discussions with current as well as former dental hygiene students and dental students (practicing dental hygienists and dentists) revealed a genuine appreciation for Dr. Wilkins's dedication to those entrusted in her professional care; she prided herself on their accomplishments, and they looked up to her as a mentor and major influence on their lives. Dental hygienists felt empowered by her to share what they know, to be heard, to what Kathy Bassett called "give back to dental hygiene." Esther once leaned over to her at a meeting with Dentsply executives, *you have important things to say, be sure they hear you.* Esther was passionate about dental hygiene, and she instilled that passion in others.

Esther was always thinking critically and asked the important questions. Laura Joseph said she would "constantly be the one to open up discussions and bring to light a different point of view." Jan Selwitz-Segal echoed others' comments about Esther's charisma as a mentor:

❝ Esther had a knack for bringing out the best in people. Her patience, confidence, and enthusiasm enabled others to accomplish truly challenging goals—a true master/mentor/guru!❞

Colleagues around the world reflected in their stories of the many incidences of care, concern, celebration, and support provided to them by Dr. Wilkins (although she insisted they call her "Esther"). When she attended any event (traveling to schools, colleges, alumni events, conventions, meetings, continuing education presentations, ceremonies, awards, pinnings, and dedications), sometimes to give a keynote address, sometimes invited every year (such as the 20 years to Bristol Community College in Massachusetts for her annual workshop with students), she became surrounded by admirers, seeking a discussion, consult, or photograph with her. It was quite a sight to witness.

She was not only recognized but also acknowledged as someone who has made a major difference in their lives and in the world of education, dental hygiene, dental science, and beyond. At Yankee Conference in Boston in 2008, Esther and the author came around the corner to get our coats at the convention center and were greeted by two faculty members who quickly arranged a photo shoot with adoring student fans. I took her cane and pocketbook and stood to the side, while Esther enjoyed the fun of her notoriety but more importantly, the students, who delighted in having their photo taken with their idol. One of the faculty members asked if I was Esther's personal assistant (seeing I was accompanying her and holding her belongings). I replied, "I am today!" Actually, I truly enjoyed being Esther's "date" at many meetings, reunions, and special events. She was great company, and the adoring fans always made it an exciting time.

Lois Barber recalled that dental hygienists flock around her "as her winning smile and warm welcome make you proud to be part of a profession of which she is both a foundation and a role model." She endeared herself to everyone she met because she had a genuine interest in learning about people.

Her continuous research in the health sciences advanced understanding for others. She certainly lived up to the expectations of John Simmons for women to make a difference in the world. She continued to acknowledge at every opportunity the significant contribution that her alma maters have made on her accomplishments, and she insisted on excellence and every student's potential to make a contribution to the world.

❧ Healthy Aging ❧

In response to the many requests for information on how Esther stayed so healthy, why her memory rarely failed her until her late 90s, and how she continued to live a long life, the following advice was offered by Esther herself: *Brush and floss thoroughly every single day; don't stress over anything which you have no control; eat oatmeal every morning and a glass of milk with every meal; eat few sweets; choose fish over beef; don't swear or smoke; exercise every day; be active and volunteer; laugh often; and dance!!*

In an article in *Dimensions of Dental Hygiene*, Esther described her perspective on the projected increased number of those who will reach 100 years old:

> *We all need to include daily physical exercise, a healthy diet without over-eating, restful sleep, and top grade oral hygiene as part of our lifestyle. Avoiding major risk factors is also important, such as traumatic accidents, tobacco use and exposure to second-hand smoke, alcohol abuse, lack of physical activity, risky sexual practices, and a diet that promotes over-weight or obesity* (Wilkins, 2010, p. 23).

Esther had no fear—of anything! Many years ago, she was on an airplane where they began taking names and addresses of passengers (before the days of manifest), as the plane was *severely bumpy*. Esther said that she really wasn't afraid; it isn't as if she had any control, so *why worry about it*. She rarely got upset or angry, although she did get irritated if something wasn't done quickly enough. However, she never had an unkind word for anyone; instead, she found something good to highlight, finding positive in even the most difficult situations, such as her accident. Students have asked for information about Esther's favorite things:

- *Color*: The color of the current edition of her book; and purple, the color of dental hygiene
- *Books*: *Make Way for Ducklings*; Robert Parker (Spencer) novels; classics such as *Moby Dick*; *The New Yorker* magazine
- *Foods and beverages*: oatmeal, Johnny Cakes, popovers, milk (powdered preferred), salmon and other fishes, hot dogs and beans (Saturday nights, of course), coffee ice cream, fresh fruits and vegetables, little baked potatoes, peanut butter (which her niece, Betsy, calls Esther's sixth food group because she loved it so much), fluoridated water, coffee (instant), leafy green lettuce, pizza, fresh vegetables, and anything anyone else made that she didn't have to cook
- *Entertainment*: Dancing above all else, the news, sunrises and sunsets, Elvis, old movies (classics, such as those with Cary Grant, Audrey Hepburn, Jimmy Stewart, John Wayne, Paul Newman, and Maureen O'Hara), music (Gilbert & Sullivan), theatre, entertaining her many friends!
- *People*: Her husband, Jim; her mother; her sister, Ruth; Dr. Frank Willis; Dr. Basil Bibby; Dr. Irving Glickman; Dr. J. Murray Gavel; early Lea & Febiger publishers; practicing dentists, dental hygienists, and dental hygiene educators; and students (she saved every little trinket they ever gave her)
- *Places*: Boston, Marshfield, Panama Canal, Beverly Hills, Florida Everglades, Ireland, New Zealand, Saudi Arabia, Japan, China, Israel, Mexico, La Scala (Milan, Italy), and Ayer's Rock (Australia)
- *Dental instrument*: The probe; Younger-Good 6/8

Although Esther edited much of this biography (of course), she did permit me to say that she maximized free opportunities and "waste not want not" was lived daily. She rarely threw anything away and preferred to either give it away or bring it down to the cottage. She was the queen of recycling, as evidenced by the extra meals enjoyed after taking home her leftovers. *After all, it can make several meals during the week and is easier than cooking.* She prepared most of her own meals each day, until her late 90s. Her trips to a wholesale club every few months allowed her at a bargain price to buy her bulk items: instant coffee, oatmeal, and powdered milk. She did not own a microwave in her Boston condo until she was in her late 90s; she preferred to warm things up in her oven. She did on occasion, use the toaster oven. The dishwasher, although it functioned, was used for storage of special dishes for company.

Esther recycled pretty much everything, long before it was fashionable to "go green." I received a thank you note once from her; it was actually a holiday card, with a *May all the magic of this special season be yours*. Esther thought it was a lovely card and didn't want to waste it, so she added "spring" in front of season; it was now a spring card (although it had a snowman on the front!). However, it was signed by Esther Wilkins, so the sentiment was valuable, regardless of the timing of the seasons. It also demonstrated, often quietly and without fanfare, her thoughtfulness. Rarely did she forget to send a birthday card to her special friends, and she saved every card and note she received.

Esther did not like to throw out clothes, because they had meaning to her. She said, *I had fun with it; so I don't want to part with it!* She also recycled plastic wrap, zip lock bags, tin foil, paper cups she picked up from various restaurants, napkins from everywhere she has ever gone, and stated that *slightly used paper towels are perfectly good to use again.* A mug was not discarded until it leaked, regardless of its color, chips, or cracks. Her niece cut her hair for her. Esther has been "going green" since she was *knee high to a paper hanger* (another Esther favorite saying!). Esther did her own nails and her own laundry. Her second bathroom (the one with the "floss" and "brush" embroidered pictures on the wall) served as a drying rack.

She walked to class at Tufts, to the post office, did errands, and the "T" (transit) was her companion quite often as it got her to where she needed to go. She would only use a vehicle when it was absolutely necessary, such as when the sidewalks were icy, or someone was picking her up. Esther epitomized Yankee Thrift and Boston's nickname of *The Walking* City, as the ultimate pedestrian commuter, still making the daily walk to Tufts or to get to South Station or other "T" stops until her late 90s when her balance became an issue, and she did not take naps (except for an occasional one *after a big trip when the plane got in late*) until her 90s.

Despite her busy schedule, Esther somehow found time to spend with friends, one of the most important facets of her life. Laura Weinrebe, a retired hygienist (Forsyth) who lived in Esther's building until moving to a nursing home in 2008 after a fall, was not in good health. She fell in her apartment in the same building as Esther lived and was hospitalized. After Esther investigated the name of the hospital and the room and exact address with zip, sent cards, and notified other friends in the building, she went to visit her. Later, she received a note from Laura's daughter-in-law, Agneta, who wrote

> " Dear Esther: Thank you for being such a good friend to Laura; you really cheered her up at the hospital" (May 6, 2008).

Esther said that Laura had a way to charm you, as once she wrote to Esther on the back of a left-over holiday card and said, "my short-term memory causes me more interesting things to do like write to you." There were many stories of Esther's compassion for others and, importantly, an effort and commitment of time to care for others. Barbara Posner Sommer remembered that on more than one occasion, Esther visited Barbara's mother who was ill and hospitalized: "It meant a great deal to me then; I have never forgotten it and it means every bit as much to me now when I think about it. Esther has a caring spirit."

❧ REVISITING TYNGSBOROUGH, 1972 ❧

Esther never forgot her roots and held her childhood in Tyngsborough in the palm of her hand, ready and eager to relate stories of her mother, sister, and cousins. In 1972, she and her sister, Ruth, and husbands took a trip back in time: As related in their 1972 Christmas Letter,

" the Wilkins Girls, Esther and Ruth, took their husbands on a nostalgic tour of Tyngsboro. The visit to the Winslow Grammar School was well documented by a photo of the girls playing hopscotch in that same old back play yard—a picture no doubt is sure to become a family conversation piece."

In 2012, during a visit to Tyngsborough during Memorial Day Weekend, Esther had a second fall (after her first fall in South Carolina in 2006). She was visiting her cousins when she stumbled on the outside stairs, suffering a fractured skull which resulted in a benign paroxysmal positional vertigo, which plagued her for the rest of her life. She suffered complete loss of hearing on the right side and increasing loss of vision on the right side.

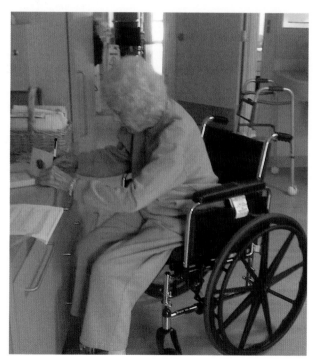

FIGURE 16.6: Esther in her wheelchair, rehab, 2012.

After spending several days in the hospital, she was moved to New England Rehabilitation Hospital in Lowell, Massachusetts, where according to Esther, *I became quite well known at the Rehab because I was the lady over in Room 250A who gets a big stack of mail every day. Those wonderful cards and letters were from many of you and I thank you over and over again* (Christmas Letter, 2012). Esther kept in good spirits, but due to vertigo, she transitioned from the cane to a walker to help keep her balance. She began relying on others and learning to accept the changes she was experiencing.

According to Anna Pattison,

❝ Esther expressed regret that she had to miss the American Dental Hygienists' Association Annual Session in Phoenix in June. She was also disappointed to miss *personally presenting the Esther Wilkins Lifetime Achievement Award to her longtime friend and colleague, Gail N. Cross-Poline, at the elegant ceremony presented by Dimensions of Dental Hygiene and sponsored by Colgate.* A video greeting from Esther in the hospital was shown at the ADHA Plenary Session on Saturday morning."

She was recorded for this video in her hospital room, as she sat on a wheelchair. She wrote the greeting out on a scrap paper, editing it, and practicing it, and she insisted she be helped with putting on her make-up, *so people won't see I'm weak.*

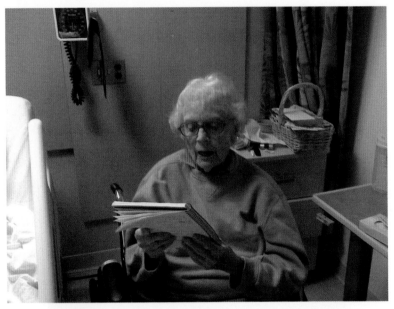

FIGURE 16.7: Esther reading for the video for American Dental Hygienists' Association, 2012.

Anna continued,

❝ it was most reassuring for everyone to see that our 'Matriarch of Dental Hygiene' was well on her way to recovery. As always, Esther continued to inspire everyone with her indomitable strength and ability to persevere in the most dire circumstances."

She was perturbed one Sunday that the therapists were *off*. She said,

this is terrible. If I don't get my exercise and walk every day, I will get behind. I just convinced one of the nurses to take me for a walk this morning.

After both accidents, there was an influx of well wishes, concern, and requests for updates on her progress. The whole dental community reached out. Caren Barnes wrote

> ❝ one thing I learned from her fall in SC, people overwhelmed her with visits and that might not be appropriate for a while. I know you and Betsy will be there to guard her privacy and visiting time. God bless you and our beloved Miss Esther."

Daily updates were sent to the dental hygiene and dental communities, and Web sites provided information on her status.

Esther was working on the 11th edition of her book when she was injured by this fall, although she could hardly wait to get back to work.

> ❝ Her single-mindedness, attention to detail, and enduring dedication to the profession was truly remarkable." Anna Pattison remembered, "similar to her first accident in South Carolina in 2006, she took great pleasure in reading the scores of cards and letters she received from dental hygienists and dentists all over the country."

She never threw any of them away, keeping them in a basket on the table in her sitting area, sometimes opening up a few years later, which brought smiles at all the well-wishes she had enjoyed.

Esther continued to dedicate herself to her own recovery through regular exercise and adherence to her physical therapy schedule.

> *Had a great class this morning doing my PT for my problems with that steady walking. I must do all my exercises very regularly so I can hope to get off the walker* (personal communication to the author, September 25, 2012).

❧ ON THE WAY TO 100 ❧

Those who spent time with Esther during her last decade noted a slowdown, and Esther herself was concerned she took a while to remember things sometimes. It was a bit disheartening, but in Esther style, she persevered, often with humor. She once wrote to me that *I'm not being very smart these days, if I ever am!*

Travel outside of her apartment became difficult, although she did manage to go down to the lobby to pick up her mail, speaking with the friendly front desk staff who were helpful and extremely accommodating to Esther, especially during those last few years of residency.

Although in her youth Esther loved to cook, she relied on Meals on Wheels for her lunches and dinners during the last 3 or 4 years of her stay in Boston. Although she offered them to visitors, they respectfully declined. Friends who visited from out of town brought a special treat to Esther in the form of Legal Seafood Chowder, Chinese food, McDonalds, or a home-cooked breakfast. Invariably, the friends received a thank you email, all caps and exclamation points for giving her a break from her delivery food. Her favorites were fresh produce during the summer, reminding her of when she and Jim grew tomatoes out on the condo balcony.

❧ LAUREL PLACE ❧

Esther moved to Laurel Place, an assisted living facility located on Lowell Road in Hudson, New Hampshire, in April 2016, located near her niece's residence. The facility has operated since 1951, with the principle to "provide innovative programs that assist in keeping our residents connected to their community" (Fairview Healthcare, 2017, p. 1). Her living quarters was a private suite, steps away from the dining hall, complete with flowers, white tablecloths, a remarkably supportive staff, and three meals a day. Esther chose to have breakfast in her room each morning and didn't seem to miss the "Meals on Wheels" meals she had been depending on for a few years.

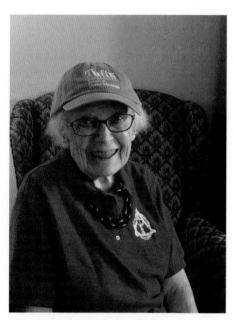
FIGURE 16.8: Esther with Tufts hat.

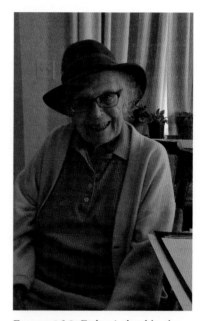
FIGURE 16.9: Esther in her blue hat.

Laurel Place suited Esther, as she could spend her time answering emails, catching up on journal reading, and taking a nap, without having to worry about cleaning, laundry, meals, and medical care. She enjoyed walking to the dining hall, with white tablecloths and centerpieces that aligned with the season. She often had breakfast in her room, but she primarily joined her tablemates for lunch and dinner, which included hot meals and coffee ice cream for dessert. Her suite included a small kitchen area, a foyer, and a large room for sleeping and sitting at her window in her favorite table and chairs brought from her

Tremont Street home. Outside her back door was an open-air, private patio. All editions of her book were placed on her bookshelf, along with other personal items.

Carolyn S. Beaulieu, activities coordinator at Laurel Place, reflected on Esther's residency:

❝ We welcomed Esther Wilkins Gallagher to Laurel Place Assisted Living. Though at first she was not particularly happy about her new circumstances she quickly became a very active member of our close-knit community."

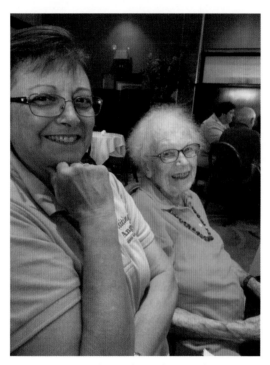

FIGURE 16.10: Esther and Carolyn Beaulieu.

❝ Esther was quite spry for her years. Even though she used a walker she would take part in weekly exercise programs, yoga and would do our hall station exercises with her assistants. When our new bus arrived we all wanted to get onboard for a trial run. Esther was one of the first to LEAP up the stairs to check it out. Everyone was amazed at her agility. Esther did not let her age stop her . . . it may have slowed her down but she kept busy both physically and mentally."

❝ Esther looked forward to playing Boggle each week with the group. She enjoyed games that kept her mind sharp but she also enjoyed games like Bingo where she could have her coffee, maybe win some change and socialize. Esther loved talking with the other residents as well as the staff. I looked forward to her wry humor on some topics and the twinkle in her eye when she was being 'politically incorrect.' She was outgoing and outspoken."

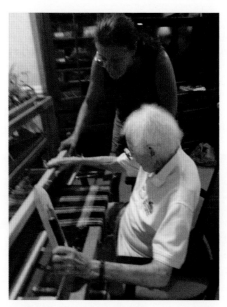

FIGURE 16.11: Esther weaving, Laurel Place.

❝Esther loved the idea of learning new things. She had enjoyed it when I performed a private 'concert' of the Appalachian Mountain Dulcimer for her. When I told her she could learn to play one along with other residents, she jumped at the opportunity. She quickly got the strum patterns of the songs and played along using a traditional turkey feather for her pick. She took great pleasure playing with our group for the memory care unit . . . taking the responsibility of being available for their listening enjoyment very seriously. When we had a weaver bring a loom to demonstrate, Esther was one of the first to get up and try it out. She had many thorough questions for the weaver."

❝Seeing the elderly with computers is still a relatively new concept for Assisted Livings but it is becoming more and more common. It was wonderful seeing Esther at hers. She was able to maintain her vital communications with people she knew professionally and personally. She never lost touch with her previous community when she joined ours. She had many friends who visited and many who dined with her. She made even more friends here." Carolyn concluded, "though we did not know her at the height of her successes we knew her and for that we are most are fortunate."

As her assisted living apartment was located on the first floor near the front door of the building, the visitors who came during Esther's stay at Laurel Place found her close by, often at her computer or small table she brought with her from Boston in front of a lovely window with bright sunshine streaming in. Her niece, Betsy, was a regular visitor, attentive and accommodating to Esther's needs and requests, helping her in her new environment.

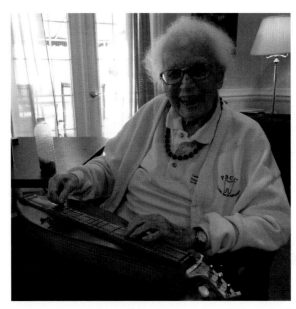

Figure 16.12: Esther and the dulcimer, Laurel Place, 2016.

Close friend Tina Daniels called Esther quite regularly, on a prescribed schedule that was convenient for Esther, which Esther looked forward to each day. Other visitors were also welcomed with open arms and a big kiss.

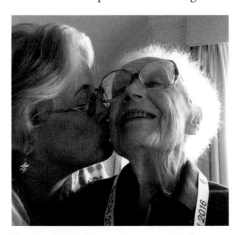

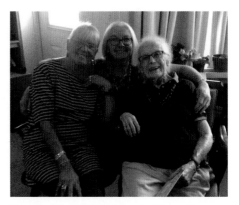

Figure 16.13: Nancy Barnes and Esther, Laurel Place, 2016.

Figure 16.14: Mary Rose Boglione, Pat Cohen, and Esther, 2016, Laurel Place.

Esther was well attended to at Laurel Place and the *caring angels* who tended to her needs, helping her with daily routines. She enjoyed telling them about dental hygiene and her career. They were respectful and very attentive and sometimes asked her dental health

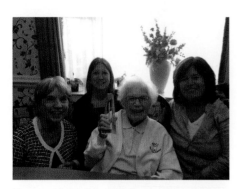

FIGURE 16.15: Mary Littleton, Karen Neiner, Esther, and Patti Parker with the TU-17 Explorer, Innovation Award.

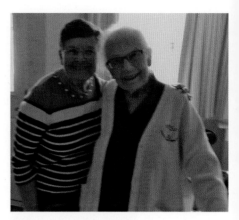

FIGURE 16.16: Beverly Whitford visiting Esther, Laurel Place.

questions for themselves and their families, in addition to asking for autographs. Esther suffered a bout of arthritis in her back, but she recovered and continued to engage in life at Laurel Place. Esther's first cousin, Weezie, was a resident of Laurel Place at the same time as Esther, to spend 2 weeks as a respite for her daughter.

During our semiweekly bio session at Laurel Place, Esther reflected on the various photos I brought to her, stimulating, and soothing at the same time, as she touched the photos and related stories about them. The Dove tree was one such memory, in which

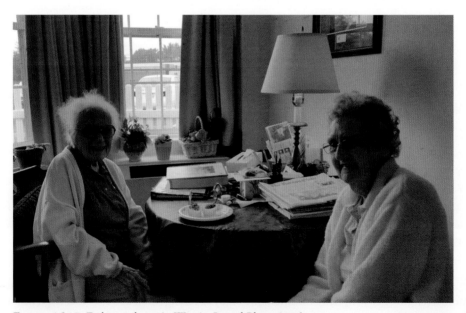

FIGURE 16.17: Esther and cousin Weezie, Laurel Place, 2016.

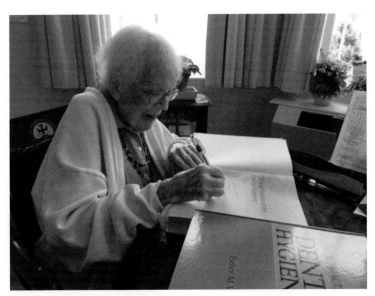

FIGURE 16.18: Esther signing *Clinical Practice of the Dental Hygienist*, Laurel Place, 2016.

Esther was introduced by Pat Cohen to this very special tree at the Arnold Arboretum. She had difficulty remembering, but gave me instructions to ask Pat to write about it; I was expected to report to her our conversation at my next visit. According to Pat Cohen,

> we made our annual visits there to catch the tree in bloom. It is quite amazing. The green petals are often palm size and they turn white at peak season. When gentle breezes kiss the tree, it seems that doves are flapping their wings. It is also called the handkerchief tree, because the leaves appear as white handkerchiefs waving."

Pat referred me to a Web site where I located photos to share with Esther, who perked right up when she saw them, memories started coming back to her.

Although becoming increasingly frail, Esther still took the pages of the biography and painstakingly made corrections and added missing commas. She looked forward to our meetings, not only to review the biography but also to share her day at Laurel Place. She enjoyed giving tours of her new home, at which time we were required to do the exercises along the way with her.

❧ 100TH BIRTHDAY CELEBRATIONS ❧

Esther was excited but a bit nervous about reaching 100 years old. She commented that her mind was sharp, but the rest of her was aging (she never used the word *old*). She depended on the walker for all travel and preferred to stay close to Laurel Place, rather than venture out and struggle with mobility. Several celebrations of her 100th were planned.

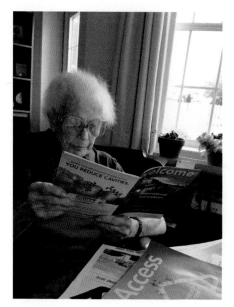

FIGURE 16.19: Esther reading a journal, Laurel Place, 2016.

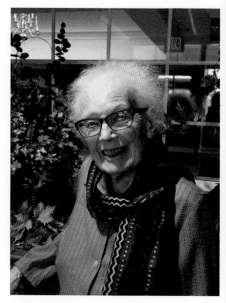

FIGURE 16.20: Esther fall photograph, Laurel Place, 2016.

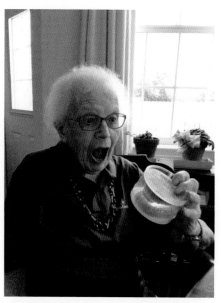

FIGURE 16.21: Esther, Laurel Place, Fall 2016.

Her last public appearance was at the 100th anniversary/Esther 100th birthday party held by MCPHS at the Marriott Hotel in Newton, Massachusetts. Her niece, Betsy, helped her plan her travel to the event.

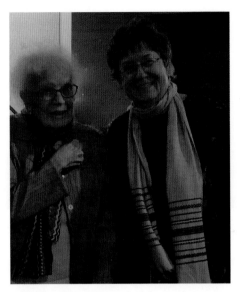

FIGURE 16.22: Betsy and Esther at the 100th Forsyth and 100th birthday reception, October 2016.

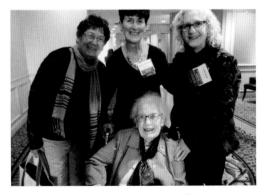

FIGURE 16.23: Betsy Tyrol, Mary Kellerman, Esther, and Linda Boyd, 100th birthday reception, October 2016.

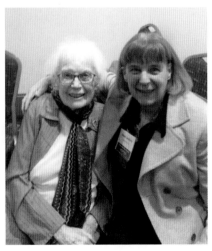

FIGURE 16.24: Esther and Susan Jenkins, 100th birthday, October 2016.

Esther's friends at Hu-Friedy planned a hundredth celebration on Esther's actual birthday, December 9, 2016, when she would turn 100 years old. A special group of friends were invited.

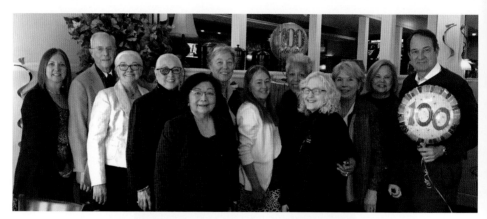

Figure 16.25: 100th Hu-Friedy party, Hudson, New Hampshire, December 9, 2016.

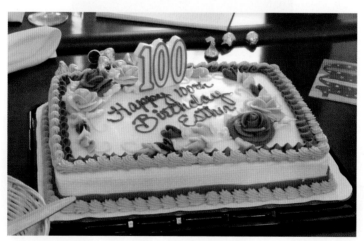

Figure 16.26: The 100th cake, December 9, 2016.

Esther's niece shared her reflections:

❝ Despite Esther's initial unhappiness with leaving her beloved apartment and her independence behind, it didn't take long for her to adjust to her new apartment and a new routine in assisted living. The one thing she looked forward to most was her upcoming 100th birthday."

❝ Lots of plans were underway to make it a really special time. Two parties were planned, one by Mary Littleton of Hu-Friedy. Her idea was to have a luncheon at a local restaurant on the day of Esther's birthday with only a very few of Esther's closest friends. As it had become more difficult to get out and travel any distance, this made a great deal of sense. Many of those invited had to travel a long way, some across the country. But all were eager to share in this special event."

❝ The second party was to be at the assisted living facility a week after the big day. This was for family and staff and residents of Laurel Place."

❝ Additional arrangements were made for those traveling a long way or those not included in the two parties to have a visit with Esther. Schedules were set up so that she would not have too many visitors on any given day."

❝ A third big event was planned by Tufts Dental School. Esther was chosen to receive the Dean's Medal in Boston, with a reception to follow. When she received word in November, she was thrilled."

❝ One more event should be noted. At the Esther Wilkins Symposium, held every year in October at MCPHS, a reception was planned to celebrate Forsyth's 100th anniversary. Esther was the guest of honor, with a tribute to her 100th birthday as well." With all the planning and excitement, Esther jumped right in with her opinions, wanting to know all the details and making sure that certain people were included. She also made sure that her wardrobe was set, favoring purple of course.

❝ Tina Daniels came first from Florida on the Wednesday before the Friday birthday. She spent the afternoon with her friend and mentor. On Thursday Charlotte Wyche came in from Michigan. She had time with Esther before dinner. That evening Tina, Charlotte, Pam, and I had dinner with Esther in the private dining room at Laurel Place. The whole facility was festive with holiday decorations. There were many smiles and much laughter with this small reunion, lots of reminiscing."

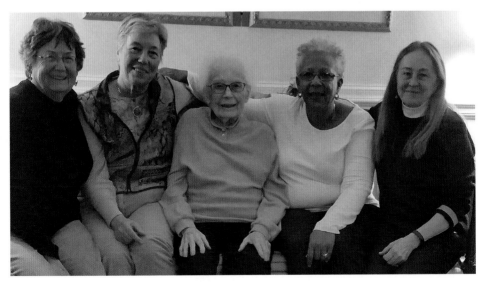

Figure 16.27: The last summer, Laurel Place, December 8, 2016: Betsy Tyrol, Charlotte Wyche, Esther, Tina Daniels, and Pam Bretschneider.

❝ Cards, flowers and gifts started coming early and seemingly never stopped."

❝ Sad to say, early in the morning of her birthday, Esther had a stroke. After an emergency room visit, she returned to Laurel Place and hospice was called. She lived for three more days and died Monday, December 12, 2016."

❝ She had spoken often of living to be 100. With all her determination, despite her increasing frailty, she succeeded in meeting that one last goal."

Esther enjoyed a poem by Johnny Ray Ryder, which was read at her interment:

But I have roots stretched in the earth,
growing stronger since my birth.
they are the deepest part of me.
I'm stronger than I ever knew.

✤ IN LOVING MEMORY ✤

The loss of Dr. Wilkins was profoundly felt in the dental communities. The grief was felt by many, and condolences came in from all over the world (see Appendix K, accessed through online e-book). (see MCPHS, 2016c).

❝ Esther Wilkins' spirit is with us and she is voice in our head pushing us to be the best dental hygienist we can be and continue to advance our profession," said Linda Boyd.

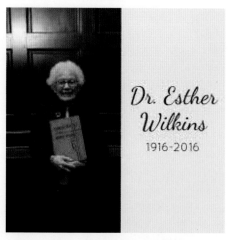

Dr. Esther
Wilkins
1916-2016

FIGURE 16.28: Esther and first edition,
Clinical Practice of the Dental Hygienist.

During her incredible career, which spanned 77 years, trailblazer in two professions, she met the challenges she faced and left the world a legacy, which will continue to inspire future generations throughout the world who will follow in her footsteps. The grand matriarch, a pioneer who loved her profession with untiring energy, who wrote the road map for practice, who insisted on excellence, will dance with us forever. She once said her words to live by were

life isn't about waiting for the storm to pass. It's about learning to dance in the rain.

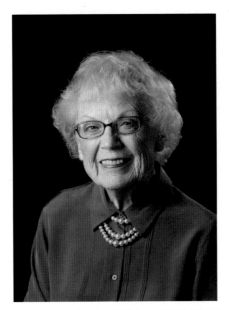

FIGURE 16.29: Esther Wilkins, RDH, DMD.

CHAPTER 17

Legacy of Her Friends and Their Stories

"She has more friends than anyone I know"
(Beverly Whitford, RDH, BS).

Friends were high on the important list for Esther. She held onto the close relationships she had with colleagues, friends, relatives, and students right up until her passing.

ℒ ORIGINS OF THE BIOGRAPHY ℒ

The author's friendship with Esther began in 2002. Charles Monahan, President of Massachusetts College of Pharmacy and Health Sciences (MCPHS), asked me to assist Dr. Wilkins in researching a few articles early in her revision of the ninth edition of *Clinical Practice of the Dental Hygienist* (CPDH). I was the director of Institutional Research at the College at the time. With the help of an incredibly talented library and learning staff at MCPHS, I learned to tap the resources of the medical databases available to assist Esther in her quest for new literature.

Through her guidance, I learned to understand the quality of the peer-reviewed articles Esther was seeking, began to review the articles for content for Esther, and sent her via hard copy the most current research on the particular chapters on which she was working. Esther smiled when I informed her I was learning through this process about a myriad of topics from patients with special needs, to the impact of cigarettes on the mouth and body, and how much a dental hygienist must know in order to educate his or her patients and practice his or her profession.

I am grateful for this experience and enjoyed the process once again for the 10th and 11th editions. For the 12th edition, she learned to access the articles herself and, of course, print them out for highlighting. Our close friendship and work on the biography continued until her passing.

The title for this biography was proposed and accepted on the first try! Usually, Esther went through a thorough investigation before making a decision or formulating a response to something important. But when I suggested to her that we seek input and present her biography from the perspective of her friends, Esther responded with a wide grin and said, *yes, I like that.*

Esther's friends were an important part of her life, keeping communication lines open (email, telephone calls, letters, and meetings), reconnecting if some time has passed, and looking forward to reunions at conventions or continuing education events. She would much rather talk to a friend at a reception than eat. When Esther suggested to Mary Dole that she wasn't sure anyone would want to read about her life in a biography, Mary told her,

> you just put your name on it, and that is all you have to do." She added, "I had no idea that I would be contributing to it, but I am very honored and trust that my comments will inform the dental hygiene profession as to what a good friend and mentor Esther has been to me throughout my career as a dental hygienist."

The letters that were sent for this biography thrilled Esther, who said in an email midway through the writing:

> *I don't believe I ever thanked you for undertaking this bio. When I see the interesting letters with their fabulous memory-inducing thoughts, I am so appreciative of what you are doing. Of course, no wonder my eyes get a little damp occasionally, especially when readings things like Ted [Hawaii] wrote. It's that big head swelling up and squeezing the juice out!*

What has amazed me through the process of writing her biography is the consistency in the immediate smiles and enthusiasm in respondents' willingness and eagerness to talk about Esther. It is almost like a reward, a special gift to get to talk about her and to be included in her biography. According to many of her friends, she always considered life half-full, was such a positive person, one who always lit up a room and a conversation. It has been an honor meeting many of these special people in Esther's life, several of whom have become close friends.

For her biography, Esther enlisted friends who are content experts, whom she recruited as contributors for her book, as she has developed a trusting relationship with them and tapped some of their strengths in specialty areas. Dr. Laura Mueller-Joseph worked with Esther on the last three editions of CPDH as a contributor for Chapter 1: "The Professional Dental Hygienist" and the treatment planning section. She related,

> at the time I could not believe that she was asking me to contribute something to her book and that she thought I had something relevant to add. I was simply honored and immediately said yes."

Dr. Mueller-Joseph also commented about her experiences working with Dr. Wilkins on CPDH:

> She was very attentive to detail. My colleagues and I often laughed when we would get an email from her, as it was usually too long and detailed, listing out all of the changes she would like incorporated into the chapter and questions regarding the layout and sending a snail mail to make sure they got them."

Laura did, however, say that she and her colleagues were "in awe of her talent to keep everything straight. She is a true icon representing the profession of dental hygiene."

There is often a story within a story, and the request for memorable Esther moments submissions began on a used piece of paper that happened to be in the front seat of her car when we were driving back from Marshfield. As the passenger, Esther began brainstorming (after she told me she could drive better than I was) about what would be *fun* and came up with the idea of funny stories. In 2008, a letter was sent to about 150 *close friends* who were asked to submit their stories for this biography:

> *This letter is a request for your insight into the impact of Esther's life on you. Can you remember a particularly enjoyable anecdote of a time you would like to tell us about? Did you attend any of Esther's classes or continuing education courses? Can you remember anything she said that was helpful, that made you laugh, that was significant to you in any way?*

It became apparent from the responses we received that Esther's energy amazed many: the planning, the travel, the presentations, the questions, and the autographs. As Gail Barnes recalled,

❝ her energy and stamina are astounding. One morning we met in the hotel hallway as we were both going to breakfast. Esther said that she was feeling a *little stiff and needed to jog*. Off she went, sprinting down the hall." In the preface to *Esther's Essentials: A Guide for Good Practice* (Wilkins, 2012), Tessie Lamadrid Black, Colgate's oral health advisor, called this little booklet a "testament to her legacy as one of the greatest dental hygiene advocates in history" (p. 3).

It has been a challenge incorporating all the accolades, and Esther never got tired of hearing them.

Mary Dole recalled that when she was hospitalized at New England Baptist Hospital,

❝ Esther made a great effort to visit me there and had that long walk up Parker Hill Avenue that is truly a hill to climb. I really appreciated that visit and, of course, our conversation evolved around dental hygiene, which made me more determined to recover fast to return to dental hygiene." Esther and Mary Dole had been friends since 1942. The sentiment of all the letters sent on Dr. Wilkins behalf is aptly presented by Wana Milam: "May God Bless her in life, as I know she has been a Blessing to others."

Tina Daniels, one of Esther's most revered friends, reflected on over 43 years of friendship with Esther, which she entitled *Talk Louder and Speak Up!*

❝ Reflecting on 43 years of friendship, I shared countless memories with my 'Esta,' as so fondly let very few of us call her. She once told me, *look at all we have in common, dear*. For example, both our father's names were Ernest. In 1966, the year I graduated high school, Esther married Dr. James Gallagher.

While we didn't meet until my senior year at Meharry Medical College School of Dental Hygiene in 1971, Dr. Esther Wilkins and I were predetermined to become friends."

❝I can still hear Esther's voice, a voice I heard almost every Friday and Sunday on the phone for the last 4 years of her life, telling me to *talk louder* and *speak-up*. Knowing her, she would say, *Tina, write about all the great discussions we've had about the dental hygiene profession.* We discussed my career as an educator, a career that she helped shape; she took pride in my experiences as well as her own, and I was more proud than any of my experiences that Esther had become an integral part of my life. In addition to her career oriented and driven self, Esther had a warm side that she rarely let anyone see."

❝I had the distinct privilege of hearing her speak about her early childhood— her teenage years, her mother and father, her sister and niece, Betsy Tyrol, to whom she introduced me to in 2004. We invested in one another's families; she shared her experiences with teaching Sunday school and with going off to college. I recognized her inclination for music, her determination in following through on everything she did in life. Esta and I talked for hours, whether at her little round table overlooking the Boston Common on the subject of Dr. Gallagher and her first love or sitting on my patio in Florida with the phone up to my ear, listening to her say *talk louder, speak up.*"

❝We compared memories of our many international trips together: Madrid, Spain, and Durban, South Africa. During the last five years of her life, our friendship deepened; we emailed frequently, sometimes more than once a day, and we laughed together on the phone as only old friends do."

❝When one had been asked to become a contributor to her textbook, it was critical to save Esther's emails. It wasn't a personal pastime, it was a must, to refer to her emails many times, reviewing her comments, as well as the edits, which were all a vital part of success in completing the challenging task of reviewing a chapter in The Book."

❝Being asked to write for her biography, I began looking back over my electronic files of Esta's emails. Over 10 years of being involved with editions 11 and 12, I have been through three PC's and two laptops, constantly saving messages from Esta. But nothing could prepare my surprise when I discovered that I had saved 398 emails in the last four years of her life."

❝In early 2016 emailing became more difficult for Esther, but she didn't quit, she didn't give up on sitting down at the computer, sometimes at 3:00 AM, to type what she was thinking. Daily routines began to change for her, but she refused to miss our weekly scheduled phone calls, which became vital to her last days, and she never got tired of asking me to *talk louder and speak up.*"

❝Most 98-year-old people would be in bed and asleep by 8:22 PM, but not our Esta. Let me share an example of her determination. Here is my favorite email of all time from my friend, Esta. She was up using the 'machine,' computer of course. Not only was she emailing, she had just finished reading chapters of the text to send back to Linda Boyd."

—Original Message—
From: Esther Wilkins <estherwilkins@comcast.net>
To: 'Tina R Daniels' <ernestinedaniels1.daniels@aol.com>
Sent: Wed, Dec 17, 2014 8:22 pm
Subject: RE: Today is Wednesday - From Tina_Dec 17, 2014
Hi Tina,
So cheered by your letter today—and here I am back at the machine.
Enjoyed your tree pictures. Very pretty on the email . . .
Yes, Pam was a real big help yesterday. She is used to helping her mother
So runs in and starts doing things.
It was good to see Betsy and I'm glad you called to say hello to her—
We drove to BJ's and CVS so caught up on errands.
I finished the third big reading and sent the package back to Linda today.
I am so sleepy that I can hardly keep my eyes open to write on the keyboard
so goodnight dear Tina with a big hug. esta

❝ At 99 years of age, she fussed at her inability to ride the stationary bike downstairs in her condo. And, of course, the biggest disappointment of all, her inability to walk wherever she wanted to walk in the City of Boston or take the train or even drive."

❝ Our weekly conversations were a vital part of her last days. We had serious discussions, we laughed at situations she would get herself into. I heard all about the PT guy, when he was coming or didn't come. The housekeepers, of course, as Esta always felt she could do without anyone around. One most surprising occurrence was when my Esta had me start sharing what the minister talked about each Sunday. I took the time to send an email on the central message and the corresponding scriptures. I learned it was best to email her a mini manuscript of the sermon. Before I started doing this, I realized trying to explain the sermon on the phone wasn't working. When she read the email first, I would listen and she would talk . . . most of the time, she would not have to say *talk louder and speak up!*"

❝ Even today, Esta's spirit is still very much present in my life's journey, just as it was right up to the few days before she ended her life's journey."

Ernestine [Tina] R. Daniels, RDH, BS

❧ Contributors ❧

Throughout this biography, you have been reading these stories from a remarkable set of family, friends, and colleagues who took not only the time to reflect on the impact of Esther on their lives but who also submitted many of the photographs included in her biography. I am sincerely grateful to Esther's army who responded to her request for stories. I wish she was here to see the final copy.

It seems appropriate to help you meet these men and women who played such an important role in Esther's life and who were kind enough to submit their recollections of life with Esther (my sincere apologies if I missed anyone who should have been included on this list):

Biography Content and Photo Contributors

Barber, Lois	Dominick, Christine	Lorman, Louise (Weezie)	Rudy, Dr. Robert J.
Barnes, Caren	Duchin, Dr. Sheldon	Machado, Kristen	Ryan, Peg
Barnes, Gail	Duncan, Teresa	Magoon, Barbara Connell	Sabat, Lynda
Barnes, Nancy	Faiella, Dr. Robert A.	McCleary, Emily Jean	Saito, Fumi
Bassett, Kathy	Fitch, Laura Peck	McKeown, Lynda	Schon, Nancy
Beaulieu, Carolyn S.	Furnari, Winnie	Milam, Wana	Schulze, Barbara
Bell, Christina Clarke	Gladstone, Rhoda	Miller, Beatrice	Selwitz-Segal, Jan
Biron, Cynthia	Griffin, Carol	Monahan, Charles	Silk, Claire
Boglione, Mary Rose Pincelli	Guignon, Anne	Mueller-Joseph, Laura	Smilyanski, Irina
Box, Suzanne	Hasegawa, Kumiko	Murphy, Catherine	Sommer, Barbara Posner
Boyd, Dr. Linda	Hatley, Gail	Neiner, Karen	Sones, Amerian
Bretschneider, Andy	Hempton, Dr. Timothy	Niemyski, Ann Marie	Spiegel, Doris C.
Bretschneider, Matthew	Homenko, Donna	Norris, Dr. Lonnie	Steffenson, Dr. Bjorn
Burnham, Janet	Hoviliaras-Delozier, Christine	Nunn, Lynn Hunt	Stenberg, Shirley
Burns, Sarah Anne	Ibsen, Olga A.C.	O'Loughlin, Dr. Kathleen	Strong, Roberta R.
Cataldo, Dr. Ed	Jasper, Barbara	Odegard, Astrid	Thomas, Daughn
Christiansen, Cassandra	Jenkins, Susan	Parker, Patti	Tillman, Dr. Hilde
Cohen, Pat	Joyce, Jonathan	Pattison, Anna	Tompkins, Fran
Cole, Marie	Kalis, Dr. Michelle	Pickett, Frieda	Tringale, Maria
Conner, Jean	Kellerman, Mary	Poline, Gail Cross	Tripp, Helena Gallant
Cortell, Marilyn	Kenneally, Dr. Joseph	Polydoroff, Susan	Tronquet, Alice
Crawford, Lana	Kenney, Marion	Quong, Dr. Ted L.	Turcotte, Joyce

(continued)

Croffoot, Connie	*Kent, Lorene*	*Rainchuso, Lori*	*Tyrol, Betsy*
Crow, Joanne	*Keylor, Rita Snow*	*Ramsay, Pat*	*Weiner, Jane*
Daniels, Tina	*Lampi, Janet*	*Raposa, Karen*	*Weinrebe, Laura*
Dawidjan, Barbara	*LePeau, Nancy*	*Ray, Tonya Smith*	*Whitford, Beverly*
DePalma, Ann Marie	*Levi, Dr. Paul*	*Reid, Sheila*	*Wilkinson, Linda*
Dinius, Ann	*Littleton, Mary*	*Rhodes, Marilyn*	*Wilson, Barbara L.*
Dolan, Alberta Beat	*Lorman, Janet Clark*	*Richman, Dr. Andrea*	*Wyche, Charlotte*
Dole, Mary			

To each and every contributor, I give heartfelt thanks.

❧ CONCLUSION ❧

One could sit down to reflect on one's life and ask what impact one made on the world; not so for Esther M. Wilkins, RDH, DMD, who wrote the definitive text on dental hygiene, trail-blazed through the professions of dental hygiene and dentistry, and made her mark when single-handedly in 1959 she became the Matriarch of Dental Hygiene, coined in 2009 by Mary Dole. "Who else fits this category?" She will be remembered fondly forever.

References

Aegis Dental Network. (2015). *National Museum of Dentistry hosts Lucy Hobbs Project opening reception.* Retrieved from https://www.dentalaegis.com/news/2015/06/4/National-Museum-Dentistry-hosts-Lucy-Hobbs-Project

American Academy of Dental Science. (1884). *Constitution, by-laws, and code of ethics of the American Academy of Dental Science.* Boston, MA: American Academy of Dental Science.

American Academy of Periodontology. (2018). *About the American Academy of Periodontology.* Retrieved from https://www.perio.org/about-us

American Academy of the History of Dentistry. (1970). Tufts centennial issue. *Bull Hist Dentistry, 18*(1), 14–26.

American Association of Women Dentists. (n.d.). *History of AAWD.* Retrieved from http://www.aawd.org/aboutus/history/

American College of Dentists. (2018). *American College of Dentists.* Retrieved from http://www.acd.org

American Dental Education Association. (2009). *ADEA dental education at a glance.* Retrieved from http://www.adea.org/publications/adedentaledataglance/Pages/default.aspx

American Dental Hygienists' Association. (1959). Clinical Pratcice [sic] of the dental hygienist. *Journal of Dental Hygiene, 33*, 47.

American Dental Hygienists' Association. (1988). *The Warner-Lambert/ADHA Awards Program for professional excellence in dental hygiene.* Chicago, IL: American Dental Hygienists' Association.

American Dental Hygienists' Association. (2006). *Esther Wilkins hurt in fall.* Retrieved from http://www.adha.org/enews/10252006.htm

American Dental Hygienists' Association. (2016). *About ADHA.* Retrieved from http://www.adha.org/aboutadha/profile.htm

Anderson, A. (2002). *New York World's Fair 1939–1940.* Retrieved from http://websyte.com/alan/nywf.htm

Bacon, E. W. (1916). *The Book of Boston: Fifty years' recollections of the New England Metropolis.* Boston, MA: Pilgrim Press.

Bailey, K. (1999). Pioneers and activists. *Dental Alumni Record, 3*(2), 16.

Bennett, B. (2005). Book reviews: Clinical practice of the dental hygienist. *Journal of Dental Education, 69*(12), 1393. Retrieved from http://www.jdentaled.org/cgi/content/full/69/12/1393

Biron, C. (1997). *A tribute to Esther Wilkins, RDH, DMD.* Retrieved from http://www.proofs.com/display_article/117955/56/none/none/Dept/A-Tribute-to-Esther-Wilkins,-RDH,-DMD

Brazier, D. B. (1952, May 7). Eight Seattle women honored at Matrix Table. *The Seattle Times,* p. 19.

Brown, R. W. (1952). *Dr. Howe and the Forsyth Infirmary.* Cambridge, MA: Harvard University Press.

Bussy, R. K. (1985). *Two hundred years of publishing: A history of the oldest publishing company in the United States. Lea & Febiger, 1785–1985.* Philadelphia, PA: Lea & Febiger.

Camire, C. (2006). *Grandmother of dental hygiene receives honor from Boston Council.* Retrieved from http://www.lowellsun.com/local/ci_4825569

Ceruti, K. (2015, April 17). Award winners walk in the footsteps of Lucy Hobbs. *The Daily Floss.* Retrieved from https://thedailyfloss.com/2015/04/17/courage-defines-eight-award-winners-who-walk-in-the-footsteps-of-dental-pioneer-lucy-hobbs/

Collins, J. (2009, May 24). Joseph "Bill" Landry helped put Tyngsboro kids on the diamond. *Lowell Sun*. Retrieved from http://www.lowellsun.com/ci_12441620?IADID=Search-www.lowellsun.com-www.lowellsun.com

Cornette, K. D. (2009). *Fenway facts*. Retrieved from http://www.redsoxdiehard.com/fenway/facts.html

DeAngelis, S. (2002). *Upcoming author's talks, Esther M. Wilkins, BS RDH, DMD*. Retrieved from http://www.library.tufts.edu/Friends/nl_Spring2002.html

Demers, D. (2013). *Dr. Esther Wilkins: The rock star of dental hygiene*. Retrieved from http://www.drbicuspid.com/index.aspx?sec=ser&sub=def&pag=dis&ItemID=314519

DentistryIQ. (2004). *Dr. Esther Wilkins receives honorary degree from Massachusetts College of Pharmacy and Health Sciences*. Retrieved from http://www.dentistryiq.com/articles/de/2004/07/dr-esther-wilkins-receives-honorary-degree-from-massachusetts-college-of-pharmacy-and-health-sciences.html

DentistryIQ. (2007). *Hu-Friedy and Forsyth honor Dr. Wilkins' birthday*. Retrieved from http://www.dentistryiq.com/articles/rdh/2007/03/hu-friedy-and-forsyth-honor-dr-wilkins-birthday.html

DePalma, A. (2002, August). Dr. Esther Wilkins. *RDH Magazine, 23*(8). Retrieved from http://www.rdhmag.com/display_article/152357/56/none/none/Colum/Dr.-Esther-Wilkins

Deranian, H. M. (2000). *American Academy of Dental Science*. Boston, MA: American Academy of Dental Science.

Desmarais, K. (2012, October 8). What is the rhyme for deciphering the weather lights on the old Hancock building in Boston. *Americaninno*. Retrieved from https://www.americaninno.com/boston/what-is-the-rhyme-for-deciphering-the-weather-lights-on-the-old-hancock-building-in-boston/

Dilts, E. (2015). The Lucy Hobbs Project 2015 winners. *Incisal Edge*, 41–57.

Dimensions of Dental Hygiene. (2010a). News. *Dimensions of Dental Hygiene, 8*(7), 18.

Dimensions of Dental Hygiene. (2010b). *The Esther M. Wilkins Lifetime Achievement Award lauds the mother of dental hygiene*. Retrieved from http://www.dimensionsofdentalhygiene.com/ddhright.aspx?id=8690

Dimensions of Dental Hygiene. (2017). *Dimensions* announces Lifetime Achievement Award recipient. *Dimensions of Dental Hygiene, 15*(6), 10.

Dimensions of Dental Hygiene. (n.d.). *News: Just off the press*. Retrieved from http://www.dimensionsofdentalhygiene.com/ddhright.asp?id=1310

Editors. (2001, June 13). It was 20 years ago that RDH came out to play. *RDH Magazine*. Retrieved from http://www.rdhmag.com/articles/print/volume-21/issue-1/feature/it-was-20-years-ago-today-rdh-came-out-to-play.html

Editors. (2008). 75 Years of commitment to care. *Journal of Dental Hygiene*.

Fairview Healthcare. (2017). *Mission statement*. Retrieved from http://www.fairviewhealthcare.com/index.php

Flaherty, J. (2012). *By the book*. Retrieved from http://now.tufts.edu/articles/book

Forbes, E. (1947). *The Boston book*. Boston, MA: Houghton Mifflin.

Forsyth, J. C. (1918). Forsyth Training School for Dental Hygienists: Alumnae Association. *New Jersey Board of Registration, 60*(3), 285–286. Retrieved from http://quod.lib.umich.edu/cgi/t/text/pageviewer-idx?c=dencos&cc=dencos&idno=0527912.0060.001&node=0527912.0060.001%3A2&frm=frameset&view=image&seq=323

Forsyth Dental Center. (1992, Spring). Esther Wilkins honored as outstanding alumna. *Forsyth Dental Center News*, 10.

Forsyth Dental Center. (n.d.). *Forsyth Dental Center booklet*. Forsyth, GA: Forsyth Dental Center.

Forsyth Institute. (2007). *Museum of Fine Arts, Boston and The Forsyth Institute agree to purchase of Forsyth Institute Building*.

Forsyth Institute. (2011). *Forsyth kids*. Retrieved from https://forsyth.org/forsythkids

Forsyth Institute. (2014a). *About Forsyth*. Retrieved from https://forsyth.org/about-forsyth

Forsyth Institute. (2014b). *Our history*. Retrieved from https://forsyth.org/our-history

Forsyth Institute. (2014c). *Research*. Retrieved from https://forsyth.org/research

Forsyth, J. (1918, March). Forsyth Training School for Dental Hygienists. *The Dental Cosmos: A Monthly Record of Dental Science, 60*(3), 285.

Forsyth Training School for Dental Hygienists. (1939). *Forsythian.* Andover, MA: Andover Press.

Friends of Hu-Friedy. (2017). *Student ADHA members from across the nation compete in board review challenge. 200 students participated in the Are You Smarter than Esther Wilkins? competition at ADHA CLL 2017.* Retrieved from https://friendsofhu-friedy.force.com/FOHF/s/news /a2H36000001xtGuEAI/dental-hygiene-students-from-across-nation-compete-in-board-review -challenge

Friends of the Public Garden. (2005). *Images of America: Boston common.* Chicago, IL: Arcadia.

Furnari, W. (2012, July). No matter how you say it, swear each year: The dental hygiene oath or the dental hygiene pledge. *Access Magazine.* American Dental Hygienists' Association.

Gladstone, R., & Garcia, W. M. (2007). Dental hygiene: Reflecting on our past, preparing for our future. *Access, 21*(9), 12–20.

Goodwin, C. G., & Wood, J. (2008). *A brief history of Simmons College.* Retrieved from http://my.simmons.edu/library/collections/college_archives/briefhistory.shtml

Gowan, S. T. (1977, June 23). Dental hygienists get latest information. *Caledonian Record*, p. 1.

Guignon, A. N. (2001, October). A funny thing happened on the way to the podium. *RDH Magazine, 22*(10). Retrieved from http://www.rdhmag.com/display_article/123997/56/none/none/Feat /-A-funny-thing-happened

Guignon, A. N. (2007). A letter to Dr. Fones. *Dental Office.* Retrieved from http://www.dentalofficemag .com/display_article/246287/56/ARCHI/none/Colum/A-letter-to-Dr.-Fones

Gwozdek, A. (2006). *The dental hygiene textbook.* University of Michigan.

Handelman, S., & Zero, D. T. (1997). Dr. Basil Bibby: Early fluoride investigator and intellectual provocateur. *Journal of Dental Research, 76*, 1621–1624. Retrieved from http://jdr.sagepub.com /content/76/10/1621.full.pdf+html

Harrell, P. C., & Smith, M. S. (1975). *Victorian Boston today: Ten walking tours.* Boston, MA: The Victorian Society in America/New England Chapter, the Victorian Society.

Hartley, M. (2006, July). Who are our da Vincis? *RDH Magazine, 27*(7). Retrieved from http://www.rdhmag.com/display_article/260176/56/none/none/Dept/Who-are-our-da-Vincis

Helm, M. R. (1993). Survival of the fittest: Dental hygiene's future evolves from its past. *Access, 8*(9), 25–32. Retrieved from http://www.adha.org/downloads/history/survival.pdf

Hine, M. K. (1989). *History of the American Academy of Periodontology, 1945–1989.* Chicago, IL: American Academy of Periodontology.

Horowitz, S. L. (1996). An interview with Coenrad F. A. Moorrees. *Journal of Dental Research, 75*(6), 1342–1345.

Hovliaras-Delozier, C. (2008). Esther M. Wilkins, BS, RDH, DMD: A mentor and icon in dental hygiene. *Access, 22*(4), 34–37.

Howland, L., Ed. (1980). *A book for Boston.* Boston, MA: David R. Godine Publishers.

Hu-Friedy. (2009a). *Esther Wilkins, RDH, DMD, personal questions.* Retrieved from http://www.hufriedy .com/opinionLeaders/opinionLeader.aspx??alias=wilkins

International College of Dentists. (1973, March). New Fellows, U.S.A. section: Inducted in 1972. *Newsletter*, 12.

International College of Dentists. (2009). *International College of Dentists: Worldwide Dental Association.* Retrieved from http://www.icd.org/home.htm

International Federation of Dental Hygienists. (2008). *About the IFDH.* Retrieved from http://www.ifdh .org/about.shtml

Jacob Wirth. (2009). *Jake's history.* Retrieved from http://www.jacobwirth.com/pages/history.html

Kingsley, N. W. (1883). *Woman: An oration delivered before the Academy of Dental Science.* Boston, MA: Thomas Todd Company.

Knothe, A. (2013, September 17). MCPHS University honors oral health pioneer. *Telegram and Gazette.* Retrieved from http://www.telegram.com/article/20130917/NEWS/309179655.

Lamson, D. F. (1895). *History of the Town of Manchester, Essex County, Massachusetts, 1645–1895.* Retrieved from https://books.google.com/books?id=WgIXAAAAYAAJ&pg=PA382&dq= But+the+same+tides+flow;+And+the+same+stars+glow;+And+the+waves+sing&hl=en&sa= X&ved=0ahUKEwi4tN-hqNrZAhXIdN8KHa1BDm4Q6AEILTAB#v=onepage&q=But%20 the%20same%20tides%20flow%3B%20And%20the%20same%20stars%20glow%3B%20 And%20the%20waves%20sing&f=false.

Learning dental hygiene. (1950, August 6). *Seattle Times,* p. 19.

Majeski, J. (2006). American Academy of Periodontology honors Esther Wilkins, BS RDH, DMD. *Access, 20*(12), 55.

Mannion, A. (2011, September). Top 25 women in dentistry. *Dental Products Report, 45*(9).

Mark, K. L. (1945). *Delayed by fire: Being the early history of Simmons College.* Concord, NH: Rumford Press.

Massachusetts College of Pharmacy and Health Sciences. (2002). A beautiful fit: Forsyth School for Dental Hygienists joins MCPHS. *The Bulletin,* 14–17.

Massachusetts College of Pharmacy and Health Sciences. (2005). Up and running: Esther M. Wilkins Forsyth Dental Hygiene Clinic dedicated at MCPHS–Boston. *The Bulletin, 30,* 20–22.

Massachusetts College of Pharmacy and Health Sciences. (2006). *Boston City Council honors Esther Wilkins.* Boston, MA: Massachusetts College of Pharmacy and Health Sciences.

Massachusetts College of Pharmacy and Health Sciences. (2007). Delta Dental makes $3 million gift. *The Bulletin, 32*(2), 27.

Massachusetts College of Pharmacy and Health Sciences. (2008). A special look at our distinguished Forsyth graduates. *The Bulletin, 97*(2), 30–32.

Massachusetts College of Pharmacy and Health Sciences. (2014). *Dental hygiene professionals gather at Esther Wilkins Symposium.* Retrieved from http://www.alumni.mcphs.edu/s/1022/index.aspx?sid= 1022&gid=1&calcid=3720&calpgid=1547&pgid=252&ecid=3941&crid=0

Massachusetts College of Pharmacy and Health Sciences. (2016a). *Alumni and friends.* Retrieved from http://www.alumni.mcphs.edu/s/1022/index.aspx?sid=1022&gid=1&pgid=2001

Massachusetts College of Pharmacy and Health Sciences. (2016b). *An evening with the stars.* Retrieved from https://issuu.com/mcphspublications/docs/ua_160314_springbulletin_vf3_issuu

Massachusetts College of Pharmacy and Health Sciences. (2016c). *Esther M. Wilkins DH '39, DMD, dental hygiene pioneer, passes at 100.* Retrieved from https://www.mcphs.edu/about-mcphs/news/ esther-m-wilkins-dh-39-dmd-dental-hygiene-pioneer-passes-at-100

Massachusetts College of Pharmacy and Health Sciences. (2016d). *MCPHS celebrates centennial anniversary of Forsyth School of Dental Hygiene.* Retrieved from https://www.mcphs.edu/about-mcphs/news/mcphs-celebrates-centennial-anniversary-of-forsyth-school-of-dental-hygiene

Massachusetts College of Pharmacy and Health Sciences. (2017). *The Esther M. Wilkins 11th Symposium.* Retrieved from http://www.alumni.mcphs.edu/s/1022/index.aspx?sid=1022&gid=1&pgid=1937& crid=0&calpgid=1186&calcid=2847

Massachusetts Dental Hygienists' Association. (1949). From D.H. to D.M.D. *The Bulletin, 14*(3), 2.

Massachusetts Dental Hygienists' Association. (1964). Life membership awarded. *The Bulletin, 30*(3), 7.

Massachusetts Dental Hygienists' Association. (2006). *Massachusetts Dental Hygienists' Association, overview.* Retrieved from http://www.massdha.org/about-mdha/overview.asp

Massachusetts Dental Hygienists' Association. (2018). *Massachusetts Dental Hygienists' Association, about us.* Retrieved from http://massdha.org/about-us/

Massachusetts Public Health Association. (2018). *What is MPHA?* Retrieved from https://mapublichealth .org/about/what-is-mpha/

McCloskey, R. (1941). *Make way for ducklings.* New York, NY: Viking Press.

References

Melanson, A. (2016, December 17). Late dentist from Chelmsford wrote the book on dental hygiene. *The Lowell Sun*. Retrieved from http://www.lowellsun.com/local/ci_30668063/late-dentist-from-chelmsford-wrote-book-dental-hygiene

Merrimack Valley Economic Development Council. (2009). *Tyngsboro*. Retrieved from http://www.merrimackvalley.info/facts_communities_tyngsborough.htm

Millstein, C. B. (1999). One Kneeland Street: Fulcrum in a century of definition. *Journal of the Massachusetts Dental Society, 49*(3), 27–30, 50–51.

Millstein, C. B. (2002). Inventing the Forsyth Infirmary. *Journal of the Massachusetts Dental Society, 51*(2), 8–13.

Millstein, C. B. (2008). *A thirty-year history of Tufts University School of Dental Medicine—1960–1990*. Tufts University School of Dental Medicine.

Morgenroth, L. (2003). *Boston neighborhoods: A food lover's walking, eating, and shopping guide to ethnic enclaves in and around Boston* (2nd ed.). Guilford, CT: Globe Pequot Press.

Motley, W. E. (1986). *History of the American Dental Hygienists' Association, 1923–1982*. Chicago, IL: American Dental Hygienists' Association.

Motley, W. E. (1988). *American Dental Hygienists' Association 75th Anniversary Scrapbook. Part 5: 1953–1962*. Chicago, IL: American Dental Hygienists' Association.

National Children's Oral Health Foundation. (2016). *America's ToothFairy*. Retrieved from http://www.ncohf.org/our-programs/esther-wilkins-education-program/

National Grange. (2011). *National Grange: American values, hometown roots*. Retrieved from http://www.nationalgrange.org/

For a complete history of the National Grange, see *People, Pride and Progress: 125 Years of the Grange in America* by David H. Howard (Washington, DC: National Grange, 1992; 336 pages, hardcover, bibliography and index, foreword by former U.S. Rep. Thomas Foley, former speaker of the house of representatives). Copies are available from the National Grange, 1616 H. St. NW, Washington, DC 2006.

National Weather Service. (n.d.). *NWS Boston—The Great Hurricane of 1938*. Retrieved from http://www.weather.gov/box/1938hurricane

Northeastern University Libraries, Archives and Special Collections. (2004). *Forsyth School for Dental Hygienists records*. Retrieved from http://www.lib.neu.edu/archives/collect/findaids/a79findprint.htm

Omicron Kappa Upsilon. (2009). *Historical review*. Retrieved from http://www.oku.org/oku/HistoricalReview.htm

Organization for Safety and Asepsis Procedures. (2009). *About OSAP*. Retrieved from http://www.osap.org/page/AboutOSAP

Pattison, A. M. (2007). Editor's note. *Dimensions of Dental Hygiene, 5*(3), 10.

Pattison, A. M. (2010). Editor's note: Happy birthday Dr. Wilkins. *Dimensions of Dental Hygiene, 8*(1), 8.

Pattison, A. (2013). Legends of the profession. Centennial celebration of dental hygiene, 1913–2013. *Dimensions of Dental Hygiene*, 12–13. Retrieved from http://www.dimensionsofdentalhygiene.com/print.aspx?id=16321

Pierre Fauchard Academy. (2018). *Dental profession news and information*. Retrieved from http://www.fauchard.org

Quinsigamond Community College. (2008). All smiles at dental program reunion. *QCC Connection, 6*, 4.

Ray, T. S. (1996). In the spotlight. *Practical Hygiene*.

Rice, L. (2016, December 28). Debbie Reynolds in 2015 interview: My life is golden. *Entertainment Weekly*. Retrieved from http://ew.com/movies/2016/12/28/debbie-reynolds-in-2015-interview-my-life-is-golden/

Ross, M. D. (1960). *The book of Boston: The colonial period*. New York, NY: Hastings House.

Schon, N. (2009). *Public art: Make way for ducklings*. Retrieved from http://www.schon.com/public/ducklings-boston.php

Sigma Phi Alpha. (2017). *History*. Retrieved from http://www.sigmaphialpha.org/about/history.htm

Simmons College. (1935). *Simmons College Bulletin, 28*(3–5).

Simmons College. (1938). *Yearbook of Simmons College, Microcosm, Class of 1938*. Retrieved from https://archive.org/details/microcosm1938simm

Simmons College. (2017). *Esther Wilkins '38, author of definitive dental hygiene text, creates $100,000 scholarship*. Retrieved from http://www.simmons.edu/alumni-and-friends/give/donor-profiles /esther-wilkins

Simmons College Library Archives. (2008b). *The presidents of Simmons College*. Retrieved from http://my.simmons.edu/library/collections/college_archives/president/index.shtml

Sirkis, N. (1966). *Boston*. New York, NY: Viking Press.

Stooksberry, D. (2004, July/August). *'Dental hygiene bible' author addressed BCD students*. Retrieved from http://webservices.bcd.tamhsc.edu/bdro/archives/2004/bdro_julaug2004/

Taylor, J. A. (1922). *History of dentistry: A practical treatise for the use of dental students and practitioners*. Washington, DC: Georgetown University.

Telegram. (2013). *Dental arrival*. Retrieved from http://www.telegram.com/article/20130921/ NEWS/309219984

Town of Manchester-by-the-Sea. (2017). *Singing Beach*. Retrieved from http://www.manchester.ma.us/ Facilities/Facility/Details/Singing-Beach-11

Travel Information Exchange. (2009). *History of Boston, Massachusetts*. Retrieved from http://www.newenglandtravelplanner.com/go/ma/boston/history.html

Tufts Dental College. (1949). *Explorer, 1949*. Boston, MA: Tufts Dental College.

Tufts-New England Medical Center. (1967). Dentistry-full-fledged member of community health team. *News, 4*(4), 3–7.

Tufts University. (2011). *Tufts man of the century, Dr. J. Murray Gavel*. Retrieved from http://dental.tufts .edu/1176818445905/TUSDM-Page-dental2w_1185977827512.html

Tufts University School of Dental Medicine. (1974). Alumni corner. *Alumni Notes, 4*(2), 7.

Tufts University School of Dental Medicine. (1990). *Universal procedures for infection control at Tufts University School of Dental Medicine*. Boston, MA: Tufts University School of Dental Medicine.

Tufts University School of Dental Medicine. (2013). Esther Wilkins. *News@TuftsDental*.

Tufts University School of Dental Medicine. (2016, December 16). Tufts University School of Dental Medicine honors trailblazers in their fields: Dean's Medals recognize two professor emeritae for decades of contributions to the school, accomplishments in oral health. *Newswire*. Retrieved from http://www.newswise.com/articles/tufts-university-school-of-dental-medicine-honors-trailblazers -in-their-fields

Tufts University School of Dental Medicine Alumni Association. (2018). *Alumni association*. Retrieved from https://dental.tufts.edu/alumni/alumni-association

Turcotte, J. (2004, August). The Academy. *RDH Magazine, 25*(8). Retrieved from http://www.rdhmag .com/display_article/209519/56/none/none/Feat/The-Academy

University of Washington, School of Dentistry. (2011). *News & events*. Retrieved from http://www.dental.washington.edu/about/news-amp-events.html

University of Washington, School of Dentistry. (2016). *Dr. Esther Wilkins, founder of UW dental hygiene program, dies at 100*. Retrieved from https://dental.washington.edu/dr-esther-wilkins-founder-uw -dental-hygiene-program-dies-100

Walters, P. (2008). Esther Wilkins spotted dancing the summer away. *Probe*, 4.

Watterson, D. G. (2009, December). Tribute to Dr. Wilkins: The grand matriarch is a treasure! *RDH Magazine, 29*(12). Retrieved from http://www.rdhmag.com/articles/print/volume-29/issue-12 /feature/tribute-to-dr-wilkins.html

Weston, G. F. (1957). *Boston ways: High, by, and folk*. Boston, MA: Beacon Press.

Westman, B., & Kenny, H. A. (1974). *A Boston picture book*. Boston, MA: Houghton Mifflin.

Wheeler, M., & Wheeler, W. C. (1914). *Dotty Dolly's tea party.* Chicago, IL: Rand McNally. Retrieved from http://users.clas.ufl.edu/jshoaf/jdolls/jdollwestern/dottydolly/index.html

Wilkins, E. (1946). Early Tufts Dental School women graduates. *Tufts Dental Outlook, 20*(3), 2–3.

Wilkins, E. M. (1948, June). A study of oral calculus. *Tufts Dental Outlook,* 21(4), 9–12. (Reprinted) *Journal of the American Dental Hygiene Association,* 22, 88, October 1948.

Wilkins, E. M. (1960). Are dental hygienists over-trained and/or under-utilized? *Public Health Dentistry,* 20, 78.

Wilkins, E. M. (1971–2016). *Clinical practice of the dental hygienist* (3rd–12th eds.). Philadelphia, PA: Wolters Kluwer Health/Lippincott Williams & Wilkins.

Wilkins, E. M. (2008, December). The evolution of dental hygiene. *Dimensions of Dental Hygiene,* 6(12), 12–14. Retrieved from http://www.dimensionsofdentalhygiene.com/2008/12_December /Departments/Guest_Editorial.aspx

Wilkins, E. M. (2009). *Clinical practice of the dental hygienist* (10th ed.). Philadelphia, PA: Wolters Kluwer Health/Lippincott Williams & Wilkins.

Wilkins, E. M. (2009, January). Guest Editorial: New face at the door. Access, *23*(2), 2–4.

Wilkins, E. M. (2010). On the way to 100: Maintaining health in mind and body. *Dimensions of Dental Hygiene,* 8(1), 20–23.

Wilkins, E. M. (2012). *Esther's essentials: A guide to good practice* (An educational Supplement to *Dimensions of Dental Hygiene*). Santa Ana, CA: Belmont Publications, Inc.

Wilkins, E. M., & McCullough, P. A. (1962). *Clinical practice of the dental hygienist.* Philadelphia, PA: Lea & Febiger.

Wilkins, E. M., & McCullough, P. A. (1964). *Clinical Practice of the Dental Hygienist* (2nd ed.). Philadelphia, PA: Lea & Febiger.

Wilkins, E. M., McCullough, P. A., & Stickels, C. (1958). *Clinical practice of the dental hygienist* (1st ed.). Philadelphia, PA: Lea & Febiger.

Wolff, C. W. (1999). Trail-blazer: At a time when women didn't have careers, Esther Wilkins wanted more—and got it. *Dental Alumni Record,* 3(2), 17–18.

Appendix A

Estherisms

❧ The Profession of Dental Hygiene ❧

Our American Dental Hygienists' Association is OUR professional organization; you will need it as much as it needs you. Hold hands and stick together, and say this often: I am a dental hygienist and I am proud of it! That's what ADHA is all about.

Each dental hygienist represents the profession as a whole to every patient he or she treats throughout the day.

I believe that dental hygienists not only need to wash their windows to see clearly their patient needs, but they must open the windows wide to affect the needed correlation.

Referring to patient care as tooth cleaning is very degrading. When you think of the scientific, biologic, process of treatment and care involved—and the high degree of skills needed to assess, plan, perform, and evaluate—and the time we spend learning how to use our fine delicate instruments—it is pretty sad to say it is just cleaning.

You must believe in what you are doing.

We can use our humor to learn and to teach, and to understand a patient's problem—our work is very serious, but we need to laugh, especially at ourselves.

We are fortunate as members of a health care profession to know the significance of oral health in lifelong health for ourselves, for our patients, and all people we can influence.

The window of opportunity for dental hygienists is wide open. Never before have so many different practice settings awaited those with a dental hygiene degree. Clinical practice in a private dental office is just one of so many options. From public health to alternative practice, it is possible to create the career you desire.

All dental hygiene career paths have one goal: to improve oral health. This is the basis of the dental hygiene profession, regardless of how individual professional destiny is fulfilled.

Dental hygienists are the *key* players in disease prevention.

As health care professionals, we are different. We must realize that people look to us for a particular kind of guidance and leadership.

In a precise profession such as ours, there is no room for mediocrity.

Our big challenge today is to accept the responsibilities that go with the opportunities that accompany our new equipment, facility, high-tech study and diagnostic methods, and applied scientific knowledge.

Access to care is a critical issue facing the profession and the nation.

The ultimate responsibility to our patients is the integrity we manifest.

The center of concern is your patients.

We are scientifically educated women in a scientific profession in a scientific age.

A dental practice isn't complete without a dental hygienist.

Being professional can be thought of in terms of actions and attitudes. We want you to like being professional. We don't want you thinking of it as "stuffy" or something that you have to put on a lot of fancy talk.

The dental hygienist's obligation is to see that no patient needs special rehabilitative dental or periodontal services because of any condition which could have been prevented by dental hygiene care.

Personal integrity, continuing competence, and a devoted belief in the worth of what we are doing—those are the keys in our professional quality control and professional growth.

Dental hygienists get farther and accomplish the most when they do it together!

Dental hygiene has jumped through many rings of fire on the way to being classified as a full-fledged profession, and although progress may seem slow, we know that we are part of a huge continuum in the prevention of oral disease and the promotion of oral health.

Your RDH is a license to learn. Learn from your patients.

Dental hygienists and dentists are truly co-therapists—working together to provide comprehensive care to their patients.

To help people learn basic health behaviors for lifetime, oral disease control is a basic objective in dental hygiene practice.

Over the past 75 years, and especially the past 50 years, research advancements and practical application of prevention of preventive measures have brought a decline in the debilitating dental, periodontal and other oral conditions that were widespread in the past.

The image we create is especially characteristic within our health professions, because of the intimate nature of our work.

To the patient, you represent the entire profession.

✥ ADVICE FOR NEW DENTAL HYGIENISTS ✥

Fortune has favored you—you have selected a worthwhile, important profession. You are able to help others help themselves toward oral health. Your good fortune will be at least due in part to your stamina, good health, and integrity.

Congratulations on picking dental hygiene for your career.

You have changed. Not only has the scope of your knowledge about your chosen occupation widened, but you now have the opportunity to realize how WHAT you do, HOW you conduct yourself, and WHAT you say all have a marked impact in the professional word.

Everyone in this room has been looking forward eagerly to the milestone which this event [graduation] represents. Together we can think of the significance, it is a good time to take stock, think ahead, for it is not unlike a bride and groom saying "I do." When entering a health profession, there are responsibilities, loyalties, and ethical vows which must be pledged and promised, because health professionals are different, and we must realize that people look to us for a particular kind of leadership.

Your RDH is a license to learn. Learn from your patients.

To graduates: As you reshuffle your own personal goals and objectives, and start out on your new career, don't forget the idealism which we promulgate.

You have a right to be heard; it is your duty to be heard.

Of course, I can't come here tonight and pretend to give you all that wonderful advice about your date for tomorrow.

Show respect for all patients, especially senior citizens.

The next steps are yours to take. Best wishes on achieving your full potential and taking the path toward active participation in this dynamic profession.

Visit the exhibits at dental meetings to learn about new products. In addition to requesting a sample, ask questions and request copies of clinical research.

Aren't you proud to be joining a profession whose main purpose is HEALTH PROMOTION? The pride that I am talking about is the personal pride that implies dignified self-respect—a really modest, honest pride that comes from a special accomplishment.

In the years to come, you will look back on this day. You will realize that you have become a part of an industrious, health service group. You will have seen people's oral health change—and you can hum with satisfaction!

May your professional experiences be enjoyable and fulfilling.

You will hang up your diploma and your license where all can see!

Don't be afraid to be a perfectionist or an idealist.

You know that old expression: When one door closes another one opens to a new path for your life. Well reach out and turn that doorknob. It won't open unless you give it a push.

Recognize that you are a functioning, important, necessary member of this group.

Live a balanced life. Learn some, think some, work and play every day.

Fluoridation should be only one of your soapboxes.

A wholesome fear of failure is one of the best guarantees of success.

As much as the weather and your continued health permit—stay active and walk out into the world every day.

As you begin your career in this fine profession of dental hygiene, remember to keep a sense of wonder about what there is to learn and what you can accomplish. The chance for career growth and satisfaction is in your hands.

You have reason to be proud of your position—and you must never underestimate the power of your own influence.

Take good care of your hands. (Your work depends on them.)

Never call a new patient over 25 years of age by the first name unless suggested by the patient.

Develop partnerships with your patients; you do your part and they do their part.

The day of your capping brings you to another fork in your road. You can restate your objectives and approach your classwork with a new zest. You have been, and still are, quite dependent on your teachers; they guide your learning.

Join the fluoridation cause for yours or a neighboring community!

This is a highly significant time for all dental hygienists to join hands to strengthen the power of the ADHA, their professional organization. Membership and participation in the ADHA support efforts that are in the interest of the individual dental hygienist and, therefore, the entire united profession.

Continued membership and attending meetings can be very rewarding after years of being part of the dental hygiene network.

May those whose lives you touch be enriched!

❧ THE IMPORTANCE OF ORAL HEALTH ❧ AND OVERALL HEALTH

I am grateful to be here to share with you my belief that the purpose and indeed the very survival of dental hygiene as a profession and the dental profession as a whole is dependent on the increased, more effective functioning of procedure concerned with the prevention and control of oral problems and diseases.

MOUTH HEALTH contributes to TOTAL BODY health, and overall body health contributes to oral health.

Fluoride is definitely not only for children's teeth. Now we know all ages can benefit. When people live where there is fluoridation, there are much few cavities, especially at the root.

If people can live longer and contribute longer, they need their oral health.

I believe dental and oral diseases are preventable or at least controllable.

All my life I've been thinking how it *can* be done: People *can* save their teeth.

Our motivational interventions are the little sparks we light, or the big bonfires we torch off. If oral health is to improve, we need to utilize all of the preventive measures science has given us.

Health care is moving toward a more interdisciplinary focus in order to improve the quality of care while reducing costs. Effective collaboration between medical and dental professionals can lead to improved patient care.

The hope is that the overall health of the centenarians will permit a full quality of life so they can enjoy the bonus of time they have earned.

Developing social connections with colleagues, friends, and family members profoundly impacts personal happiness, health, and longevity.

There will be many more healthy older people with their natural teeth. They will need the loving care a dental hygienist can provide.

Dental hygienists can inform, inspire, and supervise their older patients by means of regularly scheduled motivational maintenance appointments.

We are fortunate as members of the dental hygiene profession to understand the significance of oral health in lifelong health.

Professional care by the dental hygienist has limited short-range benefits if not backed up by self-care by the patient.

We know that lifelong habits and practices greatly influence health throughout life and into the so-called "golden years."

Our profession of dental hygiene is growing. We are bonded together around the world by our mission to help people understand how the health of the oral tissues influences the health of the entire body and greatly changes the quality of life.

Advance the profession through practice in a collaborative relationship with the patient, other health care professions, and society in general to achieve and maintain optimal oral health as an integral part of well-being.

❧ THE IMPORTANCE OF LEARNING ❧ AND RESEARCH

I'll never forget my first lecture. I was scared, but once you get up there you have to forget yourself and think only of your audience.

The future of any profession depends on its faculty.

Those old paradigms—research has shoved them out!

Study hard, learn everything you can find, ask questions, and seek out the literature for new developments.

You have a tremendous amount of know-how that past students couldn't learn—because of the new scientific technology, research, new facts, techniques, and apparatus. There is just more to learn, and since, of course, we can't learn everything, we need to learn very well where to find it.

Taking a few continuing education courses as required for continued licensure can help to drive away the lonely feeling that goes with practice and the wonderful patients who have their teeth and healthy gingiva because of your devotion to complete dental care.

All dental hygienists benefit from research—and use the findings to provide their patients with the most up-to-date services possible.

What appears now as knowledge-carved-in-granite truth will be reshaped to something greater.

As professional people, we need to grab every opportunity to learn.

This is our professional life, and continued success in practice requires disciplined continuing education.

Advancing your education opens the door to professional opportunities.

The literature of the profession is extremely important to the future of our dental hygiene profession.

It is something of an addiction that I remain on the mailing lists for journals and bulletins for continued learning.

I have spent many years keeping in contact with new research, changing viewpoints and terminology for patient instruction, and new products as new scientific information replaces the old. Perhaps my generation of biologic and other scientific terminology has long since been replaced with words and theories I may not recognize, but the challenge to learn what's new is still there.

Teachers show and tell, coax, referee, invent, and especially provide role models.

Education is an essential consideration for the future of dental hygiene. At all levels, leaders with higher degrees will be required. Higher education opportunities for our dental hygiene educators, practicing dental hygienists, and the new ADHP specialists are clearly in the near future of dental hygiene.

A dental hygienist's education today is more complex. Instruction has gone from an emphasis on technique to an emphasis on understanding the science and theory behind what hygienists do.

Enjoy continuing education courses for their own sake—not only because they help renew your license.

❧ Esther's Humor ❧

After the course, let's you and I go for a beer!

Never let a patient suck the saliva ejector.

Get acquainted with the person behind the teeth!

I am uncovering my head swamped in emails.

I have never been in favor of complete retirement. When a friend said she could hardly wait to retire, move to Florida, and play golf every day, it sounded quite unappealing to me.

Back in the teal blue CPDH days, we had all the answers! Since then, the questions have been changed!

Some of your teaching influences the person for the rest of his or her life—we never know how far our little candle throws its beams.

Without a "care plan" or treatment plan, you cannot know where you are going. So you'll probably end up somewhere else, and not know where you are.

They used to say I could find calculus that wasn't there!

Open your mouth when you take a shower.

We know so much more now than we used to know when I first became a dental hygienist!

I've been like a kid in a candy shop . . . before they knew what caused cavities.

Everybody makes me feel good when they say I don't look 90. Or on the phone I don't *sound* 90.

I am working on book revisions still and seem to crawl inch by inch sometimes in the wrong direction.

I am passionate about people having the best knowledge—and the least expensive, too.

Most of you in this audience know me. And even if my topic is "Retirement," as you see I'm *still here*. Retirement would not be a good idea for me!

As Glickie used to say, You can't build bridges in swamps!

The old familiar "use it or lose it" has truth in it, and it needs attention.

My head is so swelled up and my shoes feel too tight—I am bursting . . . with wonder.

A man had two daughters: one was beautiful and the other went to Simmons!

❧ ESTHER'S REFLECTIONS ❧

On the way to 100, I am often asked how I have maintained my health into such an advanced age. The answer is eat right, drink lots of milk, no tobacco, exercise as much as possible, drink fluoridated water, avoid the major illnesses old people have, and, of course, maintain excellent oral health. Retirement is not on the list. The mind must keep busy and there is always more to be done in the promotion of oral health and prevention of oral diseases.

About the University of Washington: It was really a "Go West Young Woman" type of feeling, and the opportunity to be a dental hygiene director and teach dental hygienists appealed to me. I started the new program single-handed, nobody knew anything about how to do it, neither did I.

The contributions to my textbook, my students, university colleagues, and the many dental hygienists around the world, have all added greatly to my life.

There was an obvious need for a clinical dental hygiene text with more detail, more emphasis on total care, especially patient assessment.

It is wonderful to see the effects of fluoridation.

We all need to be accepting of change and contribute to it.

None of us can have a happy successful career by ourselves.

Thank you for the honor and compliment you pay me by collecting all the CPDHs and having me sign them. What a rare happening! You are an honorary member of the DHSC [Dental Hygiene Supporters Club]—Esther to Pam.

People have asked if I felt I was a pioneer. I didn't really feel it. I was just there to do it, get it done, and work hard.

I'm amazed at what's happened in my lifetime.

The connections I have made are some of my greatest treasures. The relationships I have developed with colleagues in dentistry and dental hygiene over the past 75 years are some of the most valued of all.